Anticancer

Anticancer

A NEW WAY OF LIFE

David Servan-Schreiber,
MD, PhD

VIKING

VIKING
Published by the Penguin Group
Penguin Group (USA) Inc., 375 Hudson Street, New York, New York 10014, U.S.A.
Penguin Group (Canada), 90 Eglinton Avenue East, Suite 700, Toronto,
Ontario, Canada M4P 2Y3 (a division of Pearson Penguin Canada Inc.)
Penguin Books Ltd, 80 Strand, London WC2R 0RL, England
Penguin Ireland, 25 St. Stephen's Green, Dublin 2, Ireland
(a division of Penguin Books Ltd)
Penguin Books Australia Ltd, 250 Camberwell Road, Camberwell,
Victoria 3124, Australia (a division of Pearson Australia Group Pty Ltd)
Penguin Books India Pvt Ltd, 11 Community Centre,
Panchsheel Park, New Delhi–110 017, India
Penguin Group (NZ), 67 Apollo Drive, Rosedale, North Shore 0632,
New Zealand (a division of Pearson New Zealand Ltd)
Penguin Books (South Africa) (Pty) Ltd, 24 Sturdee Avenue,
Rosebank, Johannesburg 2196, South Africa

Penguin Books Ltd, Registered Offices: 80 Strand, London WC2R 0RL, England

This edition published in 2009 by Viking Penguin,
a member of Penguin Group (USA) Inc.

10

Originally published in French by Éditions Robert Laffont, S.A. Paris, 2007.
First English-language edition published in Great Britain by Michael Joseph,
Penguin Books Ltd., 2008.

Illustration credits: Figure 2: Zheng Cui; 15: Dr. Richard Béliveau;
18: © Boehringer Ingelheim Pharma KG, Photo Lennart Nilsson; illustrations
(excluding figures 2, 10, 14, 15, 18) by Sylvie Dessert

Publisher's Note: Neither the publisher nor the author is engaged in rendering professional advice or services to the individual reader. The ideas, procedures, and suggestions contained in this book are not intended as a substitute for consulting with your physician. All matters regarding your health require medical supervision. Neither the author nor the publisher shall be liable or responsible for any loss or damage allegedly arising from any information or suggestion in this book.

LIBRARY OF CONGRESS CATALOGING IN PUBLICATION DATA
Servan-Schreiber, David.
Anticancer : a new way of life / David Servan-Schreiber.—1st American ed.
p. cm.
"Originally published in French by Éditions Robert Laffont, S.A. Paris."
Includes bibliographical references and index.
ISBN 978-0-670-02164-2
1. Cancer—Prevention. 2. Cancer—Adjuvant treatment.
3. Cancer—Alternative treatment. I. Title.
RC268.S475 2010
616.99'405—dc22   2009038748

Printed in the United States of America

While the author has made every effort to provide accurate telephone numbers and Internet addresses at the time of publication, neither the publisher nor the author assumes any responsibility for errors, or for changes that occur after publication. Further, publisher does not have any control over and does not assume any responsibility for author or third-party Web sites or their content.

This book is dedicated to:

MY FELLOW PHYSICIANS,
who tirelessly treat suffering and fear, sometimes with a courage as great as their patients'. Above all, I hope they will find this book useful and will want, as I did, to integrate these approaches into their practice.

AND MY SON SACHA,
born during this time of upheaval, whose enthusiasm for life is an inspiration to me every day.

Foreword

This book describes natural methods of health care that contribute to preventing the development of cancer or to bolstering its treatment. They are meant to serve as a complement to conventional approaches (such as surgery, radiotherapy, chemotherapy). The contents of this book cannot replace a physician's opinion. It is not intended to be used to make a diagnosis or to recommend a treatment.

All the clinical cases I refer to in the following pages are drawn from my own experience (except for a few cases described by fellow physicians in the medical literature, which are indicated as such). For obvious reasons, patients' names and other identifying features have been changed.

I have chosen to set forth our present understanding of cancer and of natural defenses in simple terms. In certain cases, this hasn't allowed me to describe the full complexity of biological phenomena or the details of controversies over existing clinical studies. Though I believe I have been faithful to the spirit of their research, I apologize to biologists and to oncologists for thus simplifying what for many of them represents their life's work.

Contents

I have always felt that the only trouble with scientific medicine is that it is not scientific enough. Modern medicine will become really scientific only when physicians and their patients have learned to manage the forces of the body and the mind that operate via vis medicatrix naturae [*the healing power of nature*].

—RENÉ DUBOS, professor of biology, Rockefeller University;
discoverer of the first antibiotic in clinical use (1939);
founder of the first earth summit (1972)
of the United Nations

Anticancer

Introduction to the Second Edition

Seventeen years ago, I discovered from my own brain-scanning experiment that *I* had brain cancer. From the waiting room on the tenth floor of the oncology building, I remember looking down at people in the street—distant and oblivious, going about their everyday life. I had been cast out of that life, separated from its goal-oriented busyness and from its promises of joy, by the prospect of a probable early death. No longer wrapped in the comfortable mantle of physician and scientist, I had become a cancer patient. This book is the story of what happened next—of the return to life and health—in fact, to a level of health I had never experienced before—while knowing I had cancer. It is the story of how I used my skills as a physician and a scientist to find out everything in the medical literature that would help me change the odds. Most important, it offers a new, scientifically based perspective on cancer that gives all of us a chance to better protect ourselves from this disease.

The publication of *Anticancer* two years ago launched a new chapter in my journey. After having kept my illness a secret for fourteen years, I was able to take what I had learned and bring it around the world to people who were frightened, depressed, or had lost hope. I was able to discuss these ideas with doctors, scientists, politicians, and activists and to compare my observations directly with their experiences. I also met a considerable number of patients who had changed the course of their illness with the advice that is given here. After publication in thirty-five languages in close to fifty countries, and after more than a million copies sold, my conviction that we can all powerfully strengthen our bodies' natural defenses against cancer has been reaffirmed. As has my belief that this approach should be a part of preventing or treating cancer for everyone. In the past two years, research has also yielded new proofs, explanations, and perspectives on how we can all learn to strengthen our health and improve our "terrain" by creating an anticancer biology within our body, and it has confirmed the importance of paying attention to how our emotions may affect the course of cancer.

So what exactly is new in this revised edition?

In my many discussions with my medical colleagues—doctors, oncologists, psychiatrists—and with the public, I realized that the book's message about nutrition has been much more easily grasped than the analysis of mind-body factors and the crucial role played by the feeling of helplessness in promoting cancer. If there is one single, clear, and emphatic message I'd like to send with this revised edition, it is that we must pay close attention to the mind-body connection, especially the negative impact of prolonged feelings of helplessness and despair. When left unattended, these feelings—not the stresses of life themselves—contribute to the inflammatory processes that can help cancer grow. There are truly effective and simple methods for taming those feelings, experiencing life on a more satisfying level, and reducing inflammation at the same time.

To address this, I've completely revised chapter 9, "The Anticancer Mind," and I've also updated it with new studies that confirm how important it is to treat feelings of helplessness and despair in order to fight the progression of cancer. I have taken this opportunity to share the story of Kelly, who, in her struggle against breast cancer, was able to rely on friends to give her the support and love she needed to get through her ordeal. Recent studies show, in fact, that it's not only the love of a husband, a wife, or children that can enable morale to remain strong and slow the progression of illness, but also the simple love and caring attention of friends old and new.

In terms of nutrition, promising recent studies have attested to a number of new anticancer foods. Large-stoned summer fruit, such as plums and peaches, can now be included in this category. New data about olive oil, which was already strongly recommended in the first edition, now make it a fully fledged anticancer food with activity against a variety of specific cancer types.

Also, two new studies have shown exactly how many cups of green tea need to be drunk per day to reduce the risk of breast or prostate cancer relapse by more than 50 percent. New natural sweeteners—acacia honey and coconut sugar, characterized by a low glycemic index—have appeared on the market alongside agave nectar. These are introduced in chapter 6.

New research has confirmed the importance of vitamin D3 in preventing cancer, particularly in countries where the lack of sunshine means that the skin cannot synthesize enough of this vitamin during the winter. I've therefore given more attention to this topic, and made new and more specific recommendations.

Finally, information has become available on how different cooking methods may preserve or, to the contrary, reduce the benefits of anticancer foods.

Almost every time I give a lecture, I'm asked whether cell phone use can cause cancer. In order to respond to these questions, in 2008 I brought together a group of cancer specialists, toxicologists, epidemiologists, and a physicist. We published an appeal recommending a number of precautions to take for better, safer use of cell phones, as they are now an unavoidable feature of everyday life. The appeal was quickly picked up around the world and even led to a House of Representatives hearing in the United States in September 2008 and a public roundtable organized by the Ministry of the Environment and the Ministry of Health in France in April 2009. This edition summarizes the scientific literature on this subject and reprises the precautions that can be taken toward safer cell phone use.

Animal studies have now clearly identified links between a number of chemical products present in our daily environment and the progression of existing tumors. They include bisphenol A, which is contained in polycarbonate plastics (present in reusable plastic bottles and baby bottles, plastic microwave-safe containers, and a wide range of containers with plastic inner linings, such as cans). This substance diffuses into liquids when they are heated in a lab. When human breast cancer cells are exposed to doses of bisphenol A (BPA) corresponding to levels often found in people's blood, the cells no longer respond to chemotherapy. Comparable data have been obtained in studies of food additives based on inorganic phosphates (found in sweetened sodas, processed baked goods, etc.), which promote the progression of non-small-cell lung cancers. I felt this new data was important to discuss for people who may be undergoing treatment for these cancers.

In early 2009, a statement by the French National Cancer Institute and a study at Oxford University in Britain concluded that alcohol can increase the risk of developing cancer *at any dose,* even one glass of red wine. Together with Professor Béliveau from Montreal and researcher Michel de Lorgeril—a cardiologist, nutritionist, and pioneer of the Mediterranean diet—I published my disagreement with these conclusions, and that position is detailed here as well.

Since the original publication of *Anticancer: A New Way of Life,* numerous studies have confirmed its core message about the importance of the "terrain" in preventing or controlling cancer. I have integrated the information from these studies into the various chapters of this new edition. For example, one study published in the journal *Nature* in 2007 concluded that cancer can be understood as a breakdown in the balance between cancer cells that have always been "dormant" in the body and the natural defenses that normally keep them at bay (see chapter 4). This type of study highlights how important it is to nourish and strengthen our "terrain," a topic revisited throughout *Anticancer.* To my mind, measures to reinforce the terrain should always accompany conventional treatments—which, of course, remain indispensable.

There was also a major, 517-page report published in 2007 by the World Cancer Research Fund that synthesized several thousand studies. This report concurred with *Anticancer* that at least 40 percent of cancers can be prevented by simple changes in nutrition and physical activity (not to mention environmental factors).[1] Another report, released in 2009 by the French National Cancer Institute, reached these same conclusions.[2]

Two major epidemiological studies, one conducted within eleven European countries and spanning twelve years (the HALE study)[3] and the other in a single region of the United Kingdom (twenty thousand subjects followed over the course of eleven years),[4] reported results that were even more dramatic: *a more than 60 percent reduction in cancer mortality over the course of the study among people who had adopted a healthier lifestyle.* Increased life expectancy wasn't the only benefit: the English researchers concluded that people who practiced healthier living were fourteen years younger in terms of their biological age throughout the duration of the study. That translates into more energy to devote to work and family, an increased ability to concentrate, improved memory, and a reduction in physical discomfort. In their conclusion, the Cambridge researchers explain, "The evidence that behavioral factors such as diet, smoking, and physical activity influence health is overwhelming."

The importance of limiting consumption of refined sugar and white flour has been confirmed by new analysis of the massive American Women's Health Initiative. This study demonstrated that the link between obesity and breast cancer is dependent on the level of insulin in the blood, and thus the level of sugar in the diet. The study also showed that sugar may be contributing more to cancer than hormone replacement therapy.

In November 2008 a research article in the journal *Cancer* made the perfect case for the legitimacy of the advice presented in *Anticancer*. Women whose breast cancer had spread to their lymph nodes were followed for eleven years after they had received conventional treatment. Over the years, those who followed, in addition to their medical treatment, a program of nutritional education, physical activity, and better stress management saw their risk of dying decrease 68 percent compared to those who received conventional treatment only (see chapter 9).

In another nicely executed study, in 2008 Professor Dean Ornish of the University of California at San Francisco demonstrated that lifestyle changes in diet and exercise and stress reduction actually modified gene expression deep within cancer cells (see chapter 2).

Since *Anticancer* was published, I've given over a hundred lectures in fifteen different countries. In talking with the people who have come to hear me speak, I've learned a great deal about how we experience fear of cancer, and I think I've come to understand what people have found worthwhile in this book. Simply put, we're used to receiving a message of despair. Cancer is perceived as a kind of unlucky draw in the grand genetic lottery, an illness that does not respond well to most treatments and for which all hopes are pinned on the advent of a miraculous new cure—one that only the largest research labs could possibly develop.

In this context, I realize that any approach that is not focused on conventional treatment risks being accused of arousing "false hope." But I know—having learned this when I faced my own cancer—that such thinking robs patients of their power to act; and I mean this in terms of real power, not some illusion. Promoting this mind-set of helplessness is psychologically demeaning, medically dangerous, and most important, it is not grounded in good science. In the past thirty years, science has made prodigious advances and has demonstrated that all of us have the ability to protect ourselves from cancer and to contribute by our own means to healing it. *Refusing* to explain that we have this ability contributes to a sense of false hopelessness, and it is because they reject that false hopelessness that so many people have found *Anticancer* appealing.

I have been heartened by the positive reaction of many institutional cancer specialists to the book's message. In Europe, Professor Jean-Marie Andrieu, who heads the department of Oncology at the Georges Pompidou European Hospital, told the daily newspaper *Le Monde,* "I learned an enormous amount from this book. And you know what? I've changed my diet. And I've already lost six kilos (13 pounds)."

In Italy, the national Anti-Cancer League* endorsed *Anticancer,* placed its logo on the book jacket, and organized the press launch in Rome in October 2008. The League emphasized the importance of the book's message in terms of how best to prevent cancer, bolster the benefits of conventional treatment, and minimize relapses.

And in the United States, Professor John Mendelsohn, the president of the M. D. Anderson Cancer Center—the largest cancer treatment and research center in the country—wrote, "I found *Anticancer* to be a highly readable and well-researched book. It provides the understanding needed for the practice of evidence-based cancer prevention and risk reduction. It also fills an important gap in our knowledge of how patients can contribute to their own care by supplementing conventional medical treatment."

I've lost some friends since this book was first published. Some of them

---

* Lega Italiana per la Lotta contro i Tumori

were people who applied its principles in their own lives. Unfortunately, the methods and principles outlined here do not guarantee success against cancer. Yet I was deeply moved when I heard from them, or from their families, that they never regretted having tried all the suggestions in the book. One family member wrote to me: "Right up until the end, it's given her the feeling that she still held her life in her own hands." It's been a relief for me to learn that I had not encouraged false hopes, and it has confirmed my conviction that even if the *Anticancer* program cannot (and does not) claim to hold cancer at bay for everyone, it does help sustain life, whatever the outcome.

An amazing number of patients and their families have sent me messages—in person, by e-mail, or through my blog—bearing witness to the benefits they've gained from reading *Anticancer* and applying its advice. A fifty-year-old salesman who does not have cancer told me how much his life has changed since he started drinking green tea, adding turmeric to his food every day (with black pepper!), and managing his stress with cardiac coherence. A woman suffering from lymphoma wrote that she has read and reread *Anticancer,* in snippets, before going to sleep, like a book you might read to soothe a child. An engineer with prostate cancer sent me a graph of his blood tests from the past three years: His blood marker of cancer activity (PSA) has been dropping regularly since he began applying *Anticancer* principles, and his oncologist has been repeatedly persuaded to delay the surgery that was initially scheduled two years ago. A thirty-two-year-old woman, undergoing chemotherapy for a relapse of her breast cancer—so young!—wrote to tell me about the positive effects of the aerobic exercises she's been doing since she read the story of Jacqueline, who started practicing karate during her own treatment (see chapter 11).

Last, and a very particular source of satisfaction for me, is that two of the oncologists I consulted over the years for my own treatment contacted me after having read *Anticancer*. They asked me how best to slow down the progression of their own cancer by improving their "terrain." It was a great pleasure to be able to draw upon my research and return a measure of the compassion these doctors once showed me when I needed it most.

I'm happy and proud to present this second edition. The task of rereading the manuscript and improving it was a light one. Several times I noted with surprise that I had forgotten the details of a particular study, or of a story, since writing it. Reading all of them again has encouraged me to hold the course toward what I hope will continue to be full health. And I wish the same for you.

Introduction

Cancer lies dormant in all of us. Like all living organisms, our bodies are making defective cells all the time. That's how tumors are born. But our bodies are also equipped with a number of mechanisms that detect and keep such cells in check. In the West, one person in four will die of cancer, but three in four will not. Their defense mechanisms will hold out, and they will die of other causes.[1, 2]

I have cancer. I was diagnosed for the first time fifteen years ago. I received conventional treatment and the cancer went into remission, but I relapsed after that. Then I decided to learn everything I could to help my body defend itself against the illness. As a physician, established researcher, and former director of the Center for Integrative Medicine at the University of Pittsburgh, I had access to invaluable information about natural approaches to prevent or help treat cancer. I've kept cancer at bay for seven years now. In this book, I'd like to tell you the stories—scientific and personal—behind what I learned.

After surgery and chemotherapy for cancer, I asked my oncologist for advice. What should I do to lead a healthy life and what precautions could I take to avoid a relapse? "There is nothing special to do. Lead your life normally. We'll do MRI scans at regular intervals and if your tumor comes back, we'll detect it early," replied this leading light of modern medicine.

"But aren't there exercises I could do, a diet to follow or to avoid? Shouldn't I be working on my mental outlook?" I asked. My colleague's answer bewildered me: "In this domain, do what you like. It can't do you any harm. But we don't have any scientific evidence that any of these approaches can prevent a relapse."

In reality, what my doctor meant was that oncology is an extraordinarily complex field that is changing at breakneck speed. He was already hard pressed to keep up with the most recent diagnostic and therapeutic procedures. We had used all the drugs and all recognized medical practices relevant to my case. In our present state of knowledge, we had reached the limits. As for more theoretical mind-body or nutritional approaches, he clearly lacked the time or interest to explore these avenues.

I know this problem as an academic physician myself. Each in our own specialty, we are rarely aware of fundamental discoveries recently published in prestigious journals such as *Science* or *Nature*. Not until they have been the subject of large-scale human studies do we take note. Still, these major breakthroughs may sometimes enable us to protect ourselves long before they have led to new drugs or protocols that will become the mainstream treatments of tomorrow.

It took me months of research to begin to understand how I could help my body protect itself from cancer. I participated in conferences in the United States and in Europe that brought together researchers who were exploring this type of medicine, which works with the "terrain" at the same time that it addresses the disease. I scoured medical databases and combed scientific publications. I soon perceived that the available information was often incomplete and widely dispersed. It only took on its full meaning when it was brought together and combined.

Taken as a whole, the mass of scientific data reveals an essential role for our natural defenses in the battle against cancer. Thanks to key encounters with other physicians or practitioners who were already working in this field, I managed to put all this information into practice along with my treatment.

This is what I learned: If we all have a potential cancer lying dormant in us, each of us also has a body designed to fight the process of tumor development. It is up to each of us to use our body's natural defenses. Other cultures do this much better than ours.

The cancers that afflict the West—for example, breast, colon and prostate cancer—are seven to sixty times more frequent here than in Asia.[3] Nevertheless, statistics reveal that relative to men in the West, just as many precancerous microtumors are found in the prostates of Asian men who die before fifty from causes other than cancer.[4] Something in *their* way of life prevents these microtumors from developing. On the other hand, the cancer rate among Japanese people who have settled in the West catches up with ours in one or two generations.[5] Something about our way of life weakens our defenses against this disease.

We all live with myths that undermine our capacity to fight cancer. For example, many of us are convinced that cancer is primarily linked to our genetic makeup, rather than our lifestyle. When we look at the research, however, we can see that the contrary is true.

If cancer was transmitted essentially through genes, the cancer rate among adopted children would be the same as that among their biological—not their adoptive—parents. In Denmark, where a detailed genetic register traces each individual's origins, researchers have found the biological parents of more than a thousand children adopted at birth. The researchers' conclusion, published in the prestigious *New England Journal of Medicine,* forces us to change all our assumptions about cancer. They found that the genes of biological parents who died of cancer before fifty had *no influence* on an adoptee's risk of developing cancer. On the other hand, death from cancer before the age of fifty of an adoptive parent (who passes on habits but not genes) increased the rate of mortality from cancer fivefold among the adoptees.[6] This study shows that lifestyle is fundamentally involved in vulnerability to cancer. All research on cancer concurs: Genetic factors contribute to at most 15 percent of mortalities from cancer. In short, there is no genetic fatality. We can all learn to protect ourselves.*

It must be stated at the outset that to date, there is no alternative approach to cancer that can cure the illness. It is completely unreasonable to try to cure cancer without the best of conventional Western medicine: surgery, chemotherapy, radiotherapy, immunotherapy, and soon, molecular genetics.

At the same time, it is completely unreasonable to rely *only* on this purely technical approach and neglect the natural capacity of our bodies to protect against tumors. We can take advantage of this natural protection to either prevent the disease or enhance the benefits of treatments.

In these pages I will tell you the story of how I changed from a scientist-researcher, completely ignorant of the body's natural defenses, to a physician who relies above all on these natural mechanisms. My cancer helped me make that change. For fifteen years I protected the secret of my disease ferociously. I love my work as a neuropsychiatrist, and I never wanted my patients to feel they had to look after me instead of letting me help them. Nor, as a researcher and teacher, did I want my ideas and my opinions to be seen as the fruit of my personal experience instead of the scientific approach that has always guided me. From a personal point of view, as everybody who has had cancer knows, I wanted to be able to go on living, fully alive, among the living. Today it is not without apprehension that I've decided to talk about it. But I am convinced that it is important to make the information that I've benefited from available to those who may wish to use it.

The first part of this book presents a new view of the mechanisms of cancer. This view is based on the fundamental but still little-known workings of the immune system, on the discovery of the inflammatory mechanisms

---

* Another Scandinavian study was conducted at the Karolinska Institute in Sweden, where Nobel Prize candidates are selected. It shows that genetically identical twins, who share every single gene in their bodies, usually do not share the risk of developing cancer. Researchers conclude, again in the *New England Journal of Medicine:* "Inherited genetic factors make a minor contribution to susceptibility to most types of neoplasms." (NB: "neoplasm" means "cancer.") This finding indicates that environment plays the principal role among the causes of common cancers.[7]

underlying the growth of tumors, and on the possibility of blocking their spread by preventing new blood vessels from nourishing them.

From this new perspective on the illness follow four new approaches. Anyone can put them into practice and engage both body and mind to create their own anticancer biology. These four approaches consist of: (1) guarding ourselves against the imbalances of our environment that have developed since 1940 and promote the current epidemic of cancer, (2) adjusting our diet so as to cut back on cancer promoters and include the greatest number of phytochemical components that actively fight tumors, (3) understanding and healing the psychological wounds that feed the biological mechanisms at work in cancer, and (4) creating a relationship with our bodies that stimulates the immune system and reduces the inflammation that makes tumors grow.

But this is not a biology textbook. Confrontation with illness is a searing inner experience. I wouldn't have been able to write this book without going back over the joys and sorrows, the discoveries and failures that have made me a lot more alive today than I was fifteen years ago. I hope that by sharing them with you, I will help you find pathways of healing for your own adventure, and that it will be filled with beauty.

CHAPTER 1

One Story

I had been in Pittsburgh for seven years, and away from my native country for more than ten. I was doing my internship in psychiatry while continuing research I had begun for my PhD in neuroscience. With my friend Jonathan Cohen, I ran a laboratory of functional brain imaging funded by the National Institutes of Health. Our goal was to understand the mechanisms of thought by linking them to the workings of the brain. I could never have imagined what this research would reveal—my own disease.

Jonathan and I were very close. We were both physicians specializing in psychiatry. We had enrolled together in the PhD program in Pittsburgh. He came from the cosmopolitan world of New York via San Francisco, and I from Paris via Montreal. We had suddenly found ourselves in Pittsburgh, in the remote heartland of America, which was foreign to both of us. We had recently published a paper in the prestigious *Psychological Review* on the role of the prefrontal cortex, a rather unexplored area of the brain, which helps to bridge consciousness of the past and the future. Thanks to our computer simulations of brain function, we proposed a new theory in psychology. The article had caused something of a stir, which had enabled us, though still mere students, to get government grants and set up the research lab.

To Jonathan, computer simulations were no longer enough if we wanted to move ahead in this field. We had to test our theories by observing brain function directly, using state-of-the-art technology—functional magnetic resonance imaging (MRI). At the time, that technique was only just beginning to be used. Only research centers at the cutting edge had high-precision scanners. Hospital scanners were much more common but also significantly less accurate. In particular, no one had been able to measure prefrontal cortex activity—the object of our research—on a hospital scanner. In contrast to the visual cortex, whose variations are very easy to measure, the prefrontal cortex is very difficult to observe in action. In order for it to display its activity on MRI images, complex tasks have to be invented to "goad" it into revealing itself. At the same time, Doug, a young physicist specializing in MRI techniques, had an idea for a new method of recording images that might make it possible to get around this difficulty. Our hospital agreed to lend us its scanner between eight and eleven in the evening, after consulting hours, so we could test our ideas.

Doug worked out the mechanics while Jonathan and I invented mental tasks to stimulate this area of the brain to the maximum. After several failures, we were able to catch sight of the famous prefrontal cortex at work on our screens. It was a rare moment, the culmination of a phase of intense research, all the more exciting because it was part of our friendship.

We were a little arrogant, I have to admit. All three of us were in our early thirties, we had just gotten our PhDs, and we already had a laboratory. With our new theory that interested everyone, Jonathan and I were rising stars of American psychiatry. We had mastered the latest technology that no one was using yet. Computer simulations of neural networks and functional brain imaging by MRI were still little known to university psychiatrists. That year, Jonathan and I had even been invited by Professor Widlöcher, the leading light of French psychiatry at the time, to come to Paris and conduct a seminar at the Hospital La Pitié-Salpêtrière, where Freud had studied with Charcot. For two days, in front of an audience of French psychiatrists and neuroscientists, we had explained how computer simulations of neural networks could help us understand psychological and pathological mechanisms. At thirty, there was cause enough to be proud.

I was living life to the fullest—a certain life that now seems a little strange to me. Quite sure of success, confident in hard science, I was not really interested in having contact with patients. As I was busy with both my internship in psychiatry and the research laboratory, I was trying to do as little clinical work as possible. I recall a certain rotation in the training program that I had been asked to do. Like most residents, I wasn't enthusiastic. The workload was too heavy, and anyway, it wasn't real psychiatry. The program consisted of spending six months at the general hospital looking after the psychological problems of patients hospitalized for physical problems—they had undergone a coronary bypass, received a liver transplant, or had cancer, lupus, multiple sclerosis . . . I had no desire to do a rotation that was going to prevent me from running my laboratory. Besides, all those people with medical problems didn't really interest me. I wanted to do research on the brain, write papers, speak at conferences, and contribute to the advancement of knowledge.

A year earlier, I had gone to Iraq as a volunteer with Doctors Without Borders. I had witnessed the horror there, and I had thrown myself into trying to alleviate the suffering of so many people day after day. But the experience hadn't really woken me up to what I could do once back at my hospital in

Pittsburgh. It was as if they were two completely different worlds. Above all, I was young and ambitious.

The dominant importance of work in my life surely played a role in the painful divorce that I was just emerging from at that time. Among other reasons for our breakup, my wife couldn't bear the fact that I wanted to go on living in Pittsburgh for the sake of my career. She wanted to return to France, or at least move to a city like New York, which would be more exciting. But to me, Pittsburgh meant the fast track, and I didn't want to leave my laboratory and my colleagues. We wound up in front of a judge, and I lived alone for a year in my tiny house between a bedroom and a study.

And then one day, when the hospital was practically deserted—between Christmas and New Year's, the quietest week of the year—I saw a young woman in the cafeteria reading Baudelaire. Someone reading a nineteenth-century French poet at lunchtime is a rare sight in the United States. I sat down at her table. She was Russian, with high cheekbones and large black eyes, and an air both reserved and extremely sharp. At times she would stop talking altogether and leave me disconcerted. I'd ask her what she was doing and she'd reply, "I'm running a sincerity check on what you just said." That made me laugh, and I liked being kept in check. That was the beginning of our relationship. It took time to develop. I wasn't in a hurry, and neither was she.

Six months later, I left for the University of California at San Francisco to work for the summer in a psychopharmacology laboratory. The head of the laboratory was getting ready to retire, and he would have liked me to take over from him. I remember telling Anna that if I met someone in San Francisco, it might mean the end of our relationship, that I would understand if she did the same thing. I think that this saddened her, but I wanted to be perfectly frank.

When I returned to Pittsburgh in September, Anna moved in with me and shared my doll's house. I felt something developing between us, and I was happy. I wasn't sure where this relationship was heading. I still remained somewhat on my guard—I hadn't forgotten my divorce. But my life was looking up. In October we had two magical weeks. It was Indian summer. I was working on a movie script that I'd been asked to write about my experience with Doctors Without Borders. Anna was writing poetry. I was falling in love. Then my life took a sudden turn.

I remember that glorious October evening in Pittsburgh, gliding on my motorcycle down avenues lined with flaming autumn leaves toward the MRI center. Jonathan and Doug were meeting me there for one of our sessions of experiments with student "guinea pigs." For a minimum fee, our subjects slid into the scanner and we asked them to carry out mental tasks. Our research excited them, and so did the expectation of receiving a digital image of their brain at the end of the session that they could dash home and put up on their computer. The first student arrived around eight o'clock. The second, scheduled for nine to ten, didn't show up. Jonathan and Doug asked me if I would be willing to step in. Naturally, I accepted. Of the three of us, I was the least "technical." I lay down in the scanner, a narrow tube where my arms were held tight against my body, a little like a coffin. Many people can't bear the confinement of a scanner: 10 percent to 15 percent of patients are so claustrophobic that an MRI is out of the question.

There I am, in the scanner. We begin as we always do, with a series of images that aim to identify the subject's brain structure. Brains, like faces, are all different. Before taking any measurements, a sort of map of the brain at rest (called the anatomic image) must first be recorded. This is then compared to pictures (known as functional images) taken while the subject is executing the mental tasks. Throughout the process, the scanner emits a loud clanging sound, like that of a metal staff striking the floor repeatedly. It corresponds to the movements of the electronic magnet that quickly turns on and off to induce variations in the magnetic field in the brain. Depending on whether anatomic or functional images are involved, the pace of the clanging varies. From what I can hear, Jonathan and Doug are doing anatomic images of my brain.

After ten minutes, the anatomic phase is complete. In the small screen just above my eyes, I expect to see the mental task we have programmed to stimulate activity in the prefrontal cortex—which is the object of the experiment. It consists of pushing a button each time consecutive letters that appear in a rapid sequence on the screen are identical (the prefrontal cortex is activated to remember for a few seconds the letters that have disappeared from the screen so they can be compared to those coming after them). I'm waiting for Jonathan to send me the task and for the particular pulsing sound of the scanner registering the functional activity of the brain. But the pause goes on. I don't understand what is happening. Jonathan and Doug are behind a shielded glass in the control room; we can communicate only by intercom. Then I hear in the headphone: "David, we have a problem. There's something wrong with the images. We have to do them over." Fine. I wait.

We begin over again. We do ten more minutes of anatomic images, and then comes the time for the mental task to begin. I wait. Jonathan's voice says: "Listen, there's something wrong. We're coming in." They come into the scanner room and slide out the table I am lying on. Emerging from the tube, I see that they have strange expressions on their faces. Jonathan puts his hand on my arm and says, "We can't do the experiment. There's something in your brain." I ask them to show me on the screen the images they had just recorded twice by computer.

I was neither a radiologist nor a neurologist, but I'd seen a lot of brain images; it was our daily work. In the right-hand region of my prefrontal cortex there was a sort of ball the size of a walnut. Placed in that position, it was not one of those benign brain tumors that one sometimes sees that are operable or not among the most virulent—such as meningiomas or adenomas of the pituitary gland. In that location it could be a cyst or an infectious abscess, provoked by certain diseases such as AIDS. But my health was excellent. I got a lot of exercise, and I was even captain of my squash team. So it couldn't be that.

It was impossible to deny the gravity of what we had just discovered. At an advanced stage, a brain tumor can kill in six weeks without treatment, in six months to a year with treatment. I didn't know what stage I was at, but I knew the statistics. Not knowing what to say, all three of us remained silent. Jonathan sent the films to the radiology department so that they could be evaluated the next day by a specialist, and we said good night.

I set out on my motorcycle toward my little house at the other end of town. It was eleven o'clock; the moon was very beautiful in a bright sky. In the bedroom, Anna was asleep. I lay down and looked at the ceiling. It was really very strange that my life might end like this. It was inconceivable. There was such an abyss between what I had just found out and what I had been building up over so many years—the momentum I had accumulated for what promised to be a long race and should have led on to meaningful achievements. I felt like I was only just beginning to make a useful contribution. In pursuing my education and my career, I had made many sacrifices, invested a lot in the future. And suddenly I was facing the possibility that there would be no future at all.

And besides, I was alone. My brothers had been students in Pittsburgh for a time but had since graduated and moved away. I no longer had a wife. My relationship with Anna was very new, and she was surely going to leave me, for who would want a partner who is condemned at thirty-one? I saw myself like a piece of wood floating down a river, suddenly tossed against the shore, caught in a stagnant pool. It would never go all the way to the ocean. By a twist of fate, I was a captive in a place where I didn't have any real ties. I was going to die. Alone. In Pittsburgh.

I remember something extraordinary happening as I lay there, contemplating the smoke from my little Indian cigarette. I didn't really want to sleep. I was caught up in my thoughts when suddenly I heard my own voice speaking in my head, gently, with self-assurance, conviction, clarity, a certitude that I didn't recognize. It wasn't me, and yet it was definitely my voice. Just as I was repeating, "It can't be happening to me; it's impossible," the other voice said, "You know what, David? It's perfectly possible, and it's all okay." Something happened then that was both astonishing and incomprehensible. From that second onward, I was no longer paralyzed. It was obvious; yes, it was possible. It was part of the human experience. Many others had experienced it before me, and I wasn't special. There was nothing wrong with being simply, completely human. All by itself, my mind had found the path to some relief. Later on, when I was frightened again, I had to learn to tame my emotions. But that night I went to sleep, and the next day I was able to go to work and take the necessary steps to begin to face the disease, and to face my life.

CHAPTER 2

Escaping Statistics

Stephen Jay Gould was a professor of zoology at Harvard University and a specialist in the theory of evolution. He was also one of the most influential scientists of his generation, considered by many to be the "second Darwin" for his more complete rendition of the evolution of species.

In July 1982, at the age of forty, he found out that he was suffering from a mesothelioma of the abdomen—a rare and serious cancer attributed to exposure to asbestos. After his operation he asked his doctor, "What are the best technical articles on mesothelioma?" Whereas until then she had always been very frank, the oncologist answered that "the medical literature on the subject contains nothing really worth reading." But trying to prevent an academic of his caliber from going over the literature on a subject that concerns him or her is, as Gould would later write, a little like "recommending chastity to *Homo sapiens,* the sexiest primate of all."

When he left the hospital, he went straight to the campus medical library and sat down at a table with a pile of recent medical journals. An hour later, horrified, he understood the reason for his doctor's vague response. The scientific studies left no room for doubt: Mesothelioma was "incurable," with a median survival time of eight months after diagnosis. Like an animal suddenly caught in the claws of a predator, Gould could feel a panic taking over. He was physically and mentally stunned, and it took him a good fifteen minutes to recover.

Eventually, his training as a scholar asserted itself and saved him from despair. After all, he had spent his life studying and quantifying natural phenomena. If there was one lesson to be learned from that, it was that there is no fixed rule in nature that applies in like manner to everything. Variation is the very essence of nature. In nature, the *median* is an abstraction, a "law" that the human mind tries to impose on the diverse profusion of individual cases. To the individual Gould, distinct from all other individuals, the question was where he was located in the range of variations surrounding the median.

The fact that the median survival was eight months, Gould reflected, meant that half of individuals with mesothelioma survived less than eight months. Thus, the other half survived more than eight months. Now, in which half did he belong? He was young, he didn't smoke, he was in good health (except for this cancer), his tumor had been diagnosed at an early stage, and he could count on the best available treatment. So Gould concluded with relief that he had every reason to believe that he was in the promising half. So far, so good.

Then he became aware of a more fundamental issue. All curves plotting the survival time of each individual—so-called survival curves—have the same asymmetrical shape: By definition, half the cases are concentrated on the left-hand side of the curve, between zero and eight months.

But the other half, on the right, naturally spreads out beyond eight months, and the curve—the distribution, as it is called in statistics—always has a long tail that can extend to a considerable length of time. Nervously, Gould set about looking in the journals for a complete survival curve for mesothelioma. When he finally found one, he observed that the tail of the distribution actually spread out over several years. Thus, even if the median was only eight months, at the end of the tail a small number of people survived for *years* with this disease. Gould didn't see any reason why he too could not be found at the end of that long tail, and he breathed a sigh of relief.

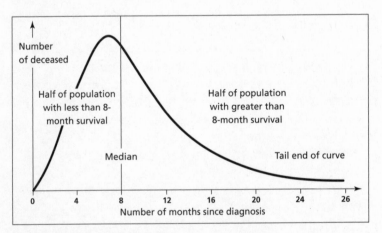

Figure 1. Survival curve for mesothelioma as seen by Gould.

Reinvigorated by these discoveries, the biologist in him came to a third realization that was as important as the other two: The survival curve he was looking at concerned people who had been treated ten to twenty years earlier. They had benefited from the treatments available then, under the conditions of that earlier time. In a domain like oncology, two things are continually changing: conventional treatments and our knowledge of what each of us can do individually to reinforce the effect of these treatments. If the circumstances change, the survival curve changes too. Perhaps with the new treatment he would receive, and with a little luck, he would be part of a new curve with a higher median and a longer tail, which would go far, very far, as far as natural death in old age.

Stephen Jay Gould died twenty years later of another disease. He had had time to pursue one of the most admirable scientific careers of his era. Two months before his death, he was able to witness the publication of his magnum opus, *The Structure of Evolutionary Theory*. He had lived thirty times longer than the oncologists had predicted.*

The lesson that this great biologist teaches us is simple: Statistics are information, not condemnation. The objective, when you have cancer and want to combat fatality, is to make sure you find yourself in the long tail of the curve.

No one can predict precisely the course a cancer will follow. Professor David Spiegel of Stanford University has been organizing psychological support groups for women with metastatic breast cancer for thirty years. In a lecture at Harvard in front of an audience of oncologists (published in the *Journal of the American Medical Association*), he explains his uneasiness: "Cancer is a very puzzling illness. We have some patients who had brain metastases [a frequently ominous development in breast cancer] eight years ago and are fine now. Why is that? Nobody knows. One of the great mysteries of chemotherapy is that sometimes you can make tumors melt away and have very little effect on survival time. The link between somatic resistance and disease progression, even from a purely oncological point of view, is still very hard to tease apart."[1]

We have all heard of miracle cures, of people who had no more than a few months to live and who nevertheless survived for years, even decades. "Don't forget," we are warned, "that these are very rare cases." Or else we are told that these cases may not really be cancer but are more likely mistaken diagnoses. In the eighties, to clarify the matter, two researchers from Erasmus University in Rotterdam systematically researched cases of spontaneous remission from cancer whose diagnosis could not be called into question. To their great surprise, in eighteen months of research in their small region of

---

* Stephen Jay Gould talks about his reaction to the statistics on his cancer in a fine essay entitled "The Median Isn't the Message," which can be found on the Web site www.cancerguide.org. I am grateful to Steve Dunn and his Web site for making this information available to the general public.

the Netherlands, they counted seven cases, as indisputable as they were unaccountable.[2] It is clear that such cases are much more common than is generally admitted.

By participating in certain programs, such as that of the Commonweal Center in California (which we'll discuss later), patients try to take charge of their cancer, to learn to live in greater harmony with their bodies and their past, to seek peace of mind through yoga and meditation, and to choose foods that fight cancer while avoiding those that promote its development. Their case histories show that they live two or three times longer than the average person with the same cancer at the same stage of development.*

An oncologist friend at the University of Pittsburgh, whom I told about these figures, objected: "These aren't ordinary patients. They're better educated, more motivated, and in better health. The fact that they live longer doesn't prove anything." But that is precisely the point: If patients are better informed about their disease, if they look after body and mind, and if they are given what they need to improve their health, then they can mobilize the body's vital functions to fight cancer. They live better, and for longer.

Since then, more formal proof has been provided by Dr. Dean Ornish, a major forerunner of integrative medicine and a clinical professor of medicine at the University of California at San Francisco. In 2005 he published the results of an unprecedented study in oncology.[4] Ninety-three men with early-stage prostate cancer—confirmed by biopsy—had chosen, under the supervision of their oncologists, *not* to undergo surgery but simply to keep the tumor under surveillance. This meant measuring the blood level of PSA (prostate-specific antigen), an antigen secreted by the tumor, at regular intervals. An increase in PSA would suggest that the cancer cells were multiplying and the tumor growing.

As these men had refused all conventional medical treatment during this observation period, they made it possible to evaluate the benefits of natural approaches. The patients were split into two groups by drawing lots, so as to establish that they were, at the outset, strictly comparable. The control group simply continued under surveillance with regular measurements of PSA. For the other group, Dr. Ornish set up a complete program of physical and mental health. Over the course of one year, these men followed a vegetarian diet with supplements (the antioxidants vitamins E and C and selenium, and a gram of omega-3 fatty acids a day), physical exercise (thirty minutes of walking, six days a week), practice in stress management (yoga movements, breathing

---

* These observations are not from a scientific study but are drawn from follow-up with patients participating in the program.[3]

exercises, mental imagery, or progressive relaxation), and one hour of weekly participation in a support group with other patients in the same program.

This amounted to a radical change in lifestyle, especially for stressed executives or heads of families with many responsibilities. These were methods long considered outlandish, irrational, or based on superstition. Twelve months later, the results left no room for doubt.

Of the forty-nine patients who hadn't changed anything in their lifestyles and who had relied simply on regular surveillance of the disease, six saw their cancer worsen and had to undergo the ablation of their prostate, followed by chemotherapy and radiotherapy. Conversely, *none* of the forty-one patients who had followed the program of physical and mental health required recourse to such treatments. In the first group, the PSA level (which reflects the tumor's growth) had increased by 6 percent on average, not including the men who had had to withdraw from the study because of the increase in their disease (their level of PSA was still more worrisome and would have greatly increased that number). This first group's progression suggested that the tumors were growing, slowly but surely. As for the second group, whose lifestyle had changed, the PSA had *decreased* by an average of 4 percent, indicating a regression in the tumors of most patients.

But what was more impressive still was what happened in the bodies of the men who had changed their lifestyles. Their blood, presented with typical cancerous prostate cells (cells from the LNCaP line used to test various chemotherapy agents) was *seven times* more capable of inhibiting the growth of cancer cells than the blood of men who hadn't changed anything in their lifestyles.

The best proof of a link between changes in lifestyle and the arrested development of cancer cells is that the more diligently these men had absorbed Dr. Ornish's advice and applied it to their daily lives, the *more active* their blood was against the cancer cells!

In scientific terms, this is what we call a "dose-response effect" and is a major argument in favor of a causal link between lifestyle and cancer.

To understand the molecular mechanisms behind these data, Dr. Ornish decided to investigate how changes in behavior influence the expression of genes within the prostate cells themselves. He took RNA samples from the prostates of test subjects before the start of his lifestyle modification program and again three months later. The results of this study, published in 2008, lived up to expectations: They indicated that Ornish's lifestyle program modified the functioning of *more than five hundred genes* in the prostate.[5] It stimulated genes that had a preventive effect against cancer and inhibited those that favored the development of the disease. One of the subjects, Jack McClure, had been diagnosed with prostate cancer six years earlier. After three months on the program, he no longer showed any symptoms of the disease: "My latest biopsy, they couldn't find any cancer cells at all. I'm not ready to say I'm cured of cancer. They just can't find it anymore." Dean Ornish feels this study should give hope to those afraid that their genetic predisposition condemns them to develop the disease: "So often people say, I have bad genes, what can I do? Turns out you can do a lot more than you thought."

Cancer genes may not, in fact, be defective parts of our biological machinery that condemn us to become ill. In 2009, two independent research groups, one in Quebec and the other in California, completely shook up our understanding of the genetic causes of breast and prostate cancer and the very idea that our genes condition our risk of dying of cancer. Reading these studies, we're reminded of the traditional notion of the "ancestors," as seen in Asian cultures or in ancient Rome. In these cultures, ghosts of ancestors were believed to inhabit the places where they had lived. If they weren't continually honored with offerings of food, they could inflict all kinds of evil on the household. Cancer genes may act a little like these "hungry ghosts," showing up and wreaking havoc only when we forget to tend to them properly.

At the University of Montreal, a team headed by Dr. Parviz Ghadirian studied women who carried the BRCA-1 and BRCA-2 genes—genes that terrify so many women because almost 80 percent of carriers risk developing breast cancer during their lifetimes. Many women who learn they are carriers choose to have both breasts amputated rather than live with the near certainty that they will fall sick at some point. However, Ghadirian and his team observed that the risk of cancer development diminished sharply for some women who carried the BRCA gene. Their main discovery? The more fruits and vegetables these genetically at-risk women ate, the lower their risk of developing cancer. Women who consumed up to twenty-seven different fruits and vegetables a week (and variety does seem to be important here) saw their risk diminished by fully 73 percent.[6]

At the University of San Francisco, Professor John Witte's team made a similar discovery about prostate cancer.[7] Certain genes trigger an extreme sensitivity to inflammation and stimulate the transformation of slow-growing micro-tumors of the prostate into aggressive and metastatic cancers.* However, when men who carried such genes consumed oily, omega-3-rich fish at least twice a week, their dangerous genes remained in check. Their cancers were five times less likely to become aggressive than those of men who ate no oily fish at all.

---

* These are genes that control the activity of the enzyme responsible for transforming omega-6 fatty acids, found in food, into factors of inflammation.

These recent findings support the notion that "cancer genes" may not be so harmful if not triggered by our unhealthy lifestyle. They behave a little like the irascible ghosts of ancestors, who required regular offerings in order to stay calm. In fact, they may simply be genes who have responded poorly to the transition from our ancestral forms of nutrition, which were perfectly adapted to our organism, to our modern-day industrial, processed diet (see chapter 6). This would explain, for example, why BRCA-carrying women born prior to World War II have two to three times less risk of developing breast cancer than their daughters and granddaughters, born in the fast-food era.[8] Perhaps these much-feared genes are not, in the end, "cancer genes" at all, but rather "fast-food intolerant genes." . . . And the same may be true of other lifestyle choices beyond diet, such as exercise and stress management.

In short, the statistics we are shown on cancer survival don't distinguish between people who are satisfied with passively accepting the medical verdict and those who mobilize their own natural defenses. In the same median are found those who go on smoking, who continue to expose themselves to other carcinogenic substances, whose diet is typically Western—a fertilizer for cancer, as we will see—who continue to sabotage their immune defenses with too much stress and poor management of their emotions, or who abandon their bodies by depriving them of physical activity. And within this median are those who live much longer. This is most likely because, along with the benefits of the conventional treatments they receive, they have somehow galvanized their natural defenses. They have found harmony in this simple quartet: detoxification of carcinogenic substances, an anticancer diet, adequate physical activity, and a search for emotional peace.

There is no natural approach capable of curing cancer by itself. But there is no inherent fatality either. Like Stephen Jay Gould, we can put statistics in perspective and aim for the long tail on the right-hand side of the curve. There is no better path to this objective than to learn to use our bodies' resources to live a richer, longer life.

Not everyone follows this route through conscious decision. Sometimes the disease itself leads us there. In Chinese, the notion of "crisis" is written as a combination of the two characters "danger" and "opportunity." Cancer is so threatening that its effect is blinding; it is hard for us to grasp its creative potential. In many ways, my illness has changed my life for the better, and in a way that I could never have imagined when I thought that I was condemned. It started shortly after the diagnosis. . . .

CHAPTER 3

Danger and Opportunity

Turning into a "Patient"

When I found out I had a brain tumor, I discovered overnight a world that looked familiar but in fact I knew little about—the world of the patient. I had known casually the neurosurgeon I was immediately referred to. We'd had patients in common, and he was interested in my research. After my tumor was discovered, our conversations changed completely. No more allusions to my scientific experiments. I was asked to lay bare the intimate details of my life, describe my symptoms in full. We discussed my headaches, nausea, the chances I might have seizures. Stripped of my professional attributes, I joined the ranks of ordinary patients. I felt the ground giving way beneath me.

I clung as best as I could to my status as a physician. Rather pitifully, I wore my white coat with my name and degrees embroidered in blue lettering to my appointments. In my hospital, where hierarchy was often quite pronounced, the nurses and orderlies who knew your status called you "Doctor" respectfully. But when you were on a stretcher and no longer wearing your white coat, you became "Mr. So-and-so" or, more often, "honey." Like everyone else, you waited in the waiting room that as a doctor you had breezed through, head high, avoiding eye contact with patients so as not to be waylaid. Like everyone else, you were taken to the examination room in a wheelchair. What did it matter if the rest of the time you moved around these same corridors on the run? "It's hospital policy," the orderly would say. You resigned yourself to being treated as someone who could not be trusted to walk.

I entered a colorless world. It was a world where people were afforded no recognized qualifications, no profession. A world in which nobody was interested in what you did in life or what might be going through your mind. Often the only interesting thing about you was your latest scan. I discovered that most of my doctors didn't know how to treat me as a patient and a colleague at the same time. At a dinner party one evening, my oncologist at the time, a brilliant specialist I very much liked, also turned out to be a guest. When I arrived I saw him turn pale, then get up and leave after some vague excuse. Suddenly I had the feeling that there was a club of the living and I was getting the message that I wasn't a member. I began to feel frightened that I was in a category apart, a category of people defined primarily by their disease. I was afraid of becoming invisible. Afraid of no longer existing, even before dying. Perhaps I was going to die soon, but I still wanted to live fully up to the end.

A few days after the scan session with Jonathan and Doug, my brother Edward was passing through Pittsburgh for his work. I hadn't broken the news to anyone except Anna. With a lump in my throat, I struggled to talk to Edward as best I could. I was afraid of causing him pain and, strangely, of jinxing myself. His beautiful blue eyes filled with tears, but he didn't panic. He simply took me in his arms. We cried for a while, then discussed treatment options, statistics, everything I would have to face from this point onward. And then he got me to laugh, as he could do so well. He reminded me that with my head shaved I would finally have that punk look I had toyed with when I was eighteen but hadn't dared to take on. With him, at least, I was still alive.

The next day Anna, Edward, and I went to lunch near the hospital. We were in high spirits leaving the restaurant. The old memories we recalled made us laugh so hard that I had to hang on to a lamppost. At that very moment, Doug crossed the street in our direction. He looked both gloomy and taken aback. There was even a touch of disapproval in his eyes. They seemed to be asking, "How can you be laughing like this when you've just gotten such bad news?"

I was dismayed. Most people seemed to think it was wrong to have a good laugh when you had a serious illness. From this day forward, for the rest of my life, I would be marked as a person condemned to die.

Dying? Impossible . . .

And then there was the nagging question of death itself. The first reaction to the diagnosis of cancer is often disbelief. When we try to imagine our own death, our mind rebels. As if death could only come to others. Tolstoy describes this reaction perfectly in *The Death of Ivan Ilych*. Like many before me, I recognized myself in this story. Ivan Ilych is a judge in Saint Petersburg. He leads a well-ordered life up until the day he falls ill. No one tells him how sick he is. When, in the end, he realizes he is dying, his whole being revolts against this idea. Impossible!

In the depth of his heart he knew he was dying, but not only was he not accustomed to the thought, he simply did not and could not grasp it. The syllogism he had learnt from Kiezewetter's Logic: "Caius is a man, men are mortal, therefore Caius is mortal," had always seemed to him correct as applied to Caius, but certainly not as applied to himself. That Caius—man in the abstract—was mortal, was perfectly correct, but he was not Caius, not an abstract man, but a creature quite, quite separate from all others. He had been little Vanya, with a mamma and a papa, with Mitya and Volodya, with the toys, a coachman and a nurse, afterwards with Katenka and with all the joys, griefs, and delights of childhood, boyhood, and youth. What did Caius know of the smell of that striped leather ball Vanya had been so fond of? Had Caius kissed his mother's hand like that, and did the silk of her dress rustle so for Caius? Had he rioted like that at school when the pastry was bad? Had Caius been in love like that? Could Caius preside at a session as he did? Caius really was mortal, and it was right for him to die; but for me, little Vanya, Ivan Ilych, with all my thoughts and emotions, it's altogether a different matter. It cannot be that I ought to die. That would be too terrible.

Eyes Opened

Until we have brushed up against mortality, life seems boundless and we'd prefer to keep it that way. It seems that there will always be time to set out in search of happiness. First I have to get my degree, pay off my loans, let the children grow up, retire. . . . I'll worry about happiness later. When we put off till tomorrow the quest for the essential, we may find life slipping through our fingers without ever having savored it.

Cancer sometimes cures this strange nearsightedness, this dance of hesitations. By exposing life's brevity, a diagnosis of cancer can restore life's true flavor. A few weeks after my diagnosis, I had the odd feeling a veil had been lifted that until then had dimmed my sight. One Sunday afternoon, in the small, sunny room of our tiny house, I was looking at Anna. Focused and peaceful, she was sitting on the floor near the coffee table, trying her hand at translating French poems into English. For the first time, I saw her as she was, without wondering whether I should prefer someone else. I simply saw the lock of hair that slipped gracefully forward when she leaned her head on her book, the delicacy of her fingers gently grasping the pen. I was surprised that I had never noticed how touching the slightest contractions of her jaw could be when she had trouble finding the word she was looking for. I suddenly saw her as herself, apart from my questions and doubts. Her presence became incredibly moving. Simply being allowed to witness that moment came to me as an immense privilege. Why hadn't I seen her that way before?

In *Existential Psychotherapy*, his book on the transforming power of approaching death, Irvin Yalom, an eminent psychiatrist at Stanford University, quotes a letter written by a senator in the early sixties shortly after he had been told he had a very serious cancer.

> A change came over me which I believe is irreversible. Questions of prestige, of political success, of financial status, became all at once unimportant. In those first hours when I realized I had cancer, I never thought of my seat in the Senate, of my bank account, or of the destiny of the free world. . . . My wife and I have not had a quarrel since my illness was diagnosed. I used to scold her about squeezing the toothpaste from the top instead of the bottom, about not catering sufficiently to my fussy appetite, about making up guest lists without consulting me, about spending too much on clothes. Now I am either unaware of such matters, or they seem irrelevant. . . .
>
> In their stead has come a new appreciation of things I once took for granted—eating lunch with a friend, scratching Muffet's ears and listening for his purrs, the company of my wife, reading a book or magazine in the quiet cone of my bed lamp at night, raiding the refrigerator for a glass of orange juice or a slice of coffee cake. For the first time I think I actually am savoring life. I realize, finally, that I am not immortal. I shudder when I remember all the occasions that I spoiled for myself—even when I was in the best of health—by false pride, synthetic values, and fancied slights.[1]

Thus the approach of death can sometimes lead to a kind of liberation. In its shadow, life suddenly takes on an intensity, resonance, and savor we may never have known before. Of course, when the time comes, we feel the despair of taking leave, much as we would in saying farewell to someone we loved, knowing we would never see them again. Most of us dread that sadness. But, in the end, wouldn't it be worse to leave without having tasted of life's full flavor? Wouldn't it be far worse to have no reason to be sad at that moment of parting?

I confess that at the start I had a long way to go. As I was helping Anna put away her books when she moved in, I came across *What the Buddha Taught*. Dumbfounded, I asked, "Why do you waste your time on stuff like this?" At a distance, it's hard for me to believe. But the incident comes back to me clearly: My rationalism verged on the obtuse. In my culture, Buddha and Christ were, at best, outdated moralists and preachers and, at worst, agents of moral repression in the service of the bourgeoisie. I was almost shocked to see that the companion I was going to live with was drugged on such nonsense—concepts I'd learned to think of as "the opium of the masses." Anna cast a sidelong glance at me. She put the book back on the shelf and said, "I think that one day you'll understand."

Changing Paths

All this while, I went on seeing doctors and weighing the pros and cons of different treatments. I finally decided on surgery. I looked for the surgeon who inspired the most confidence in me. The one I was willing to entrust my brain to in the end was not the one most highly recommended for his surgical technique. But it seemed to me that he was the one who understood best who I was and where I was coming from. I sensed that he wouldn't drop me if things went badly. He couldn't operate right away. Luckily, at that point the tumor was not growing rapidly. I waited a few weeks for an opening in his schedule. I spent this time exploring writers who had thought about what we can learn from confronting death. I threw myself into a reading list of books that weeks earlier I would have put back unopened on the shelf. I read Tolstoy, thanks to Anna, who loved authors from her homeland, and also Yalom, who'd cited him frequently in his masterful book on existential psychotherapy.[2] I first read *The Death of Ivan Ilyich,* then *Master and Man,* which made a profound impression on me.

In this work, the master is a landowner obsessed with his own interests. Tolstoy tells the story of his transformation. Determined to finalize a deal he has negotiated for a pittance, the master sets out in his sled at nightfall, despite threatening weather. With his servant, Nikita, he gets lost in a blizzard. When he realizes this may be his last night, his vision changes radically. He lies on the freezing body of his valet in a final, life-giving gesture, to protect him with his own warmth. He dies, but he succeeds in saving Nikita. Tolstoy describes how, with this gift of himself, the shrewd businessman attains a feeling of grace he had never before experienced in his whole life. For the first time, the master lives in the present. As the cold creeps up on him, he feels at one with Nikita. His own death no longer matters because Nikita lives. Beyond his egoism, he discovers a truth touching the essence of life. And at the moment of death he sees the light—a great white light at the end of a dark tunnel.

During this time, my work changed direction. Until then most of my activities had been devoted to science, almost mostly for its own sake. Little by little I gave it up. Like most medical research, the work in my lab was only distantly related to the relief of suffering. Many researchers like me, in the beginning of their careers, get caught up enthusiastically and naively in work that they believe will lead to a cure for Alzheimer's, diabetes, or cancer. But then, without quite knowing how, they wake up one day working arduously on better measuring techniques for cellular receptors targeted by medications. In the process, they gather enough material to publish articles in scientific journals, get subsidies, and keep their labs humming. But they have drifted miles away from human suffering.

The hypothesis that Jonathan and I were exploring—the role of the prefrontal cortex in schizophrenia—is now a generally accepted theory in neuroscience. It continues to generate research programs in a variety of labs around the world. It was certainly solid scientific work. But it didn't help cure anyone. It didn't even help improve anyone's condition. And now that I was living day to day with the fear of disease, of suffering, and of dying, this was what I wanted to be working on.

After my surgery, I went back to my research and my hospital consulting. I discovered that, contrary to what I had thought, it was my work as a clinician that now interested me most. As if my own distress was relieved in some measure every time I helped a patient who couldn't sleep or whose incessant pain was driving him to think of suicide. As if I'd become one with him. From that angle, a doctor's work no longer seemed like an obligation but became a marvelous privilege. A feeling of grace came into my life.

Vulnerability

I remember having one of those fleeting incidents, the kind that lead us to sense the frailty of life and the miracle of our connection to our fellow mortals. It was a tiny thing—a brief encounter in a parking lot on the eve of my first operation. From the outside it would seem trifling, but to me it took on a particular significance.

Anna and I had driven to New York, and I'd parked in the hospital lot. I was standing there, breathing the fresh air during those final few minutes of freedom before admission, tests, and the operating room. I noticed an elderly woman who was obviously on her way home after a hospital stay. She was alone, carrying a bag and walking with crutches. Unaided, she couldn't manage to get into her car. I stared at her, surprised that they had let her leave in that state. She noticed me, and I saw in her look that she wasn't expecting anything of me. Nothing. We were in New York, after all, where it's everyone for himself. I felt drawn toward her by a surprising momentum that sprang from my situation as a fellow patient. This wasn't compassion, it was a gut feeling of fraternity. I felt close to this woman, made of the same fabric as this person who needed help and wasn't asking for any. I put her bag in the trunk, backed her car out of its space, then helped her while she settled into the driver's seat. I shut her door with a smile. For those few minutes, she hadn't been alone. I was happy to perform this tiny service. In fact, she was the one who did me a favor by needing me exactly at that instant. It gave me a chance to feel that we were part of the same human condition. We made that gift to each other. I can still see her eyes, in which I had awakened a sort of confidence in others, a sense that life could be trusted if it put in her path—as it just had—the help she needed when she needed it. We hardly spoke to each other, but I am sure she shared with me the sense of a precious connection. That encounter warmed my heart. We, the vulnerable, could help each other and smile. I went into surgery in peace.

Saving One's Life, Right Up to the End

We all need to feel useful to others. It's an indispensable nourishment for the soul. When this need isn't satisfied, it leads to pain that is all the more searing if death is near. A large part of what is called the fear of death comes from a fear that our life hasn't had any meaning, that we have lived in vain, that our existence hasn't made any difference to anyone or anything.

One day I was called in to see Joe, a young man covered with tattoos who had a long history of alcoholism, drugs, and violence. He'd become unhinged when he was told he had brain cancer, and he had started to trash everything in his room. The terrified nurses wouldn't go near him. Joe seemed like a caged lion when I introduced myself to him as a psychiatrist. But he agreed to talk to me. I sat down next to him and said, "I've heard the news that you've just been given. I know you are very upset. I imagine that it can be quite frightening." He launched into a long diatribe, but after twenty minutes he started to cry. His father was an alcoholic, his mother withdrawn and emotionally absent. He had no friends and his fellow barflies were surely going to turn their backs on him. He was lost. I said, "I don't know what I'm going to be able to do for you. But I can promise to see you every week as long as that helps." He calmed down and came to see me every week for six months until he died.

During those meetings, I didn't have much to say, but I listened. He had worked a bit as an electrician. For years he hadn't held down a job and had lived on welfare. He wasn't speaking to his parents. He spent his days watching TV. He was terribly alone. It soon became clear that what made his death intolerable was the fact that he hadn't done anything with his life. I asked if, in the time remaining to him, he could do something that would be useful to someone. He had never thought about it. He considered it for a while.

Then he answered, "There's a church in my neighborhood. I think I could do something for them. They need an air-conditioning system. I know how to do that." I encouraged him to go and see the minister, who was delighted with the offer.

Joe got up every morning to go to his rooftop job, installing air-conditioning for the church. His work moved ahead slowly. Because of his large brain tumor, he had trouble concentrating. But there wasn't any hurry. The parishioners got used to seeing him up there on their roof. They spoke to him, brought him a sandwich and coffee at lunchtime. He was teary when he talked about it. For the first time in his life, he was doing something that really mattered to others. He turned into a different person and never again exploded in anger. In reality, underneath his rough appearance he had a big heart.

One day, Joe couldn't go to work. His oncologist called me to say that he was in the hospital, the end was near, and he was going into hospice care. I went up to his room in the hospital and found it flooded with sunshine. He lay there very calmly, almost asleep. They had removed all his IVs. I sat down on his bed to say goodbye, and he opened his eyes. He tried to speak to me, but he didn't have the strength. Lifting a weak hand, he signaled for me to come closer. I brought my ear right next to his lips and heard him murmur, "God bless you for saving my life."

I still carry with me the lesson he taught me: On the threshold of death, one can still save one's life. That gave me enough confidence to take on the task I had to carry out for myself, to be ready when the time came. In a certain way, Joe saved my life, too.

I've now been celebrating the anniversary of my cancer diagnosis for fourteen years. I can't remember the exact date of the scanner session with Jonathan and Doug. I only recall that it was around October 15. So the period between the fifteenth and the twentieth is a special time for me, a little like Yom Kippur or Holy Week or fasting for Ramadan. It's a private ritual. I take the time to be alone. I sometimes go on a sort of private "pilgrimage" to a church, a synagogue, a holy place. I think about what happened to me, the pain, the fear, the crisis. I give thanks because I was transformed, because I am a much happier man since that second birth.

CHAPTER 4

Cancer's Weaknesses

I n cancer's grip, the whole body is at war. Cancer cells really do act like armed bandits, roving outside the law. They are unhindered by any of the restraints a healthy body respects. With their abnormal genes, they escape the mechanisms controlling normal, healthy tissues. For example, they lose the obligation to die after a certain number of divisions. They become "immortal." They ignore signals from surrounding tissues—alarmed by the overcrowding—that tell them to stop multiplying. Still worse, they poison these tissues with the particular substances they secrete. These poisons create a local inflammation that stimulates the cancerous expansion even more, at the expense of neighboring territories. Finally, like an army on the march seeking fresh supplies, they requisition nearby blood vessels. They force them to proliferate and furnish the oxygen and nutrients needed for the growth of what will soon become a tumor.

There are certain circumstances under which these savage bands are disrupted and lose their virulence: (1) when the immune system mobilizes against them, (2) when the body refuses to create the inflammation without which they can neither grow nor invade new territories, or (3) when blood vessels refuse to reproduce and provide the supplies the cells need to grow. These are the mechanisms that can be reinforced to prevent the disease from taking hold. Once a tumor is installed, none of these natural defenses can replace chemotherapy—or radiotherapy. But they can be exploited, accompanying conventional treatments, to fully mobilize the body's resistance to cancer.

PART ONE: THE BODY'S SENTRIES: POWERFUL IMMUNE CELLS
The Ravages of S180 Cells
Of all the strains of cancer cells researchers use, the most virulent are the S180—for "sarcoma 180"—cells. Stemming from one particular mouse in a Swiss laboratory, they are bred on a large scale. Throughout the world, they are used to study cancer under identical conditions. They are particularly abnormal, containing an unusual number of chromosomes. They secrete great

quantities of cytokines, toxic substances that destroy the envelopes of cells they come into contact with. Once S180 cells are injected into a mouse, they reproduce so fast that the tumor mass doubles every ten hours. They invade the surrounding tissues and destroy everything they find along the way. Inside the abdominal cavity their growth rapidly overwhelms the drainage capacity of the lymphatic system. Fluids, called ascites, build up in the abdomen, as in a clogged bathtub. These light-colored fluids provide an ideal environment for S180 cells to grow. They go on reproducing dangerously until a vital organ breaks down or a major blood vessel bursts, leading to death.

ANIMAL RIGHTS

This book, and this chapter in particular, refer to a number of studies conducted on laboratory mice and rats. I love animals, and I don't like to think about all the suffering they endure in the course of these experiments. But up to now, neither animal rights defense groups nor the scientists concerned by the animals' plight have found satisfactory alternatives to these experiments. As you will see, because of them, an extraordinary number of children, men, and women will one day be treated more effectively and humanely. A great many animals will benefit too, since, like us, they often suffer from cancer.

The Mouse That Resists Cancer

In his laboratory at Wake Forest University in North Carolina, Zheng Cui, PhD, professor of biology, did not study cancer, but the metabolism of fats. Antibodies were needed for his experiments, and in order to obtain them, the famous S180 cells were injected into mice. The injected cells provoked the production of ascites, where the antibodies could easily be extracted. None of the mice injected with several thousand S180 cells would survive more than a month, so this standard procedure required a continual renewal of "livestock." Until the day when a strange event took place.

A young researcher, Liya Qin, PhD, had injected two hundred thousand S180 cells into a group of mice. It was the usual dose for this common procedure. But one of them, mouse number 6, had resisted the effects of the injection. He kept a resolutely flat abdomen. Liya Qin repeated the injection, unsuccessfully. On the advice of Zheng Cui, who was supervising her research, she doubled the dose, still to no effect. She then injected ten times the dose, amounting to two million cells. To her amazement, there was still neither cancer nor ascites in the recalcitrant mouse. Zheng Cui began to doubt his assistant's competence. He decided to give the injection himself. For good measure, he injected twenty million cells and made sure the liquid had really penetrated the abdomen. Two weeks later, still nothing! He then tried two hundred million cells—a thousand times the usual dose—to no avail.

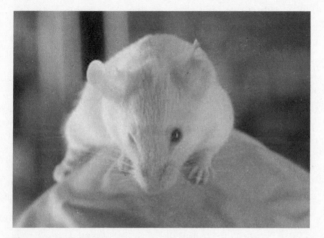

Figure 2. "Mighty Mouse," mouse number 6, which resists cancer. Courtesy of Zheng Cui, PhD, Wake Forest University.

No mouse had lived more than two months in this lab after being injected with the S180 cells. Mouse number 6 was now in his eighth month, despite the astronomic doses of cancer cells injected directly into his abdomen, where they typically reproduce the fastest. Zheng Cui began to suspect that they might have encountered the impossible—a mouse that was naturally resistant to cancer.

Over the past century, medical and scientific literature has reported cases of patients whose cancer, considered "terminal," suddenly retreated and ultimately disappeared completely.[1-7] But these cases are extremely rare. Obviously, it's hard to investigate them because they are unpredictable and they can't be reproduced on demand. Ordinarily, they are attributed to errors in diagnosis ("it probably wasn't cancer") or to a delayed response to earlier conventional treatments ("it was probably last year's chemotherapy that finally worked").

Still, in these unexplained remissions, anyone in good faith has to admit that there are poorly understood mechanisms at work countering the cancer's growth. Over the last ten years, some of these mechanisms have been brought to light and examined in the laboratory. Professor Zheng Cui's mouse number 6 shed light on the first one: the power of the immune system when it is totally mobilized.

Once convinced that the famous mouse—now known as Mighty Mouse (see Figure 2)—was resistant to cancer, Zheng Cui turned to a new concern. There was only one Mighty Mouse, and a mouse lives two years at most. Once he was dead, how could his extraordinary resistance be examined? And what if he caught a virus or pneumonia? Zheng Cui was thinking about preserving his DNA or cloning him. The first successful mouse clones had just been announced. Then one of his colleagues asked, "Have you thought about breeding him?"

Not only did Mighty Mouse go on to have a family—with a normal, nonresistant female—but half of his grandchildren inherited his resistance to S180 cells.* Like their grandfather, these mice could take in and perfectly resist two million S180 cells, a dose that had become fairly ordinary in the laboratory. They even tolerated two *billion* S180 cells, amounting to 10 percent of their total weight. This is the equivalent, in a human being, of injecting a twelve- to seventeen-pound mass of an ultravirulent tumor.

The Mysterious Mechanism

At one point, Zheng Cui had to be away from the lab on a sabbatical for several months. When he returned and picked up his experiments with the resistant mice, a serious disappointment was awaiting him. Two weeks after the usual injection, he observed that the mice had all developed cancerous ascites. All, without exception. What had happened? How had they managed to lose their resistance during his absence? For days he thought constantly about this setback and wondered what mistake he might have made. As most of his colleagues had predicted, perhaps the "discovery" really was too good to be true. He was so disappointed that he stopped going to see the mice. They were probably all dying, four weeks after the injections. Heavy-hearted, when he eventually returned to the laboratory, he raised the cover and froze: The mice were unquestionably alive, and their ascites had disappeared.

After several days of feverish experiments, the explanation emerged. At a certain age—six months for a mouse, the equivalent of fifty years for a human—the mechanism of resistance is weakened. At first, the cancer started to develop, which explained the abdomen swollen with ascites. But about two weeks later (one or two years on a human scale), the tumor's mere presence eventually activated the body's resistance. The tumor melted away by

---

* Zheng Cui did not test the mouse's children with the cancer cells, for fear that they might all die if the gene carrying the resistance was recessive.

the minute and vanished in less than twenty-four hours (one or two months on a human scale). The mice returned to their customary activities, including a highly active sex life. For the first time, science had an experimental model, reproducible on demand, of the spontaneous regression of cancer.[8] However, the mechanisms underlying this mysterious resorption still needed to be explained. It was Zheng Cui's colleague Mark S. Miller, PhD, a specialist in the development of cancer cells, who penetrated the mystery.

By examining under the microscope samples of S180 cells taken from the abdomens of the miraculous mice, Miller discovered a real battlefield. Instead of the usual cancer cells—rounded, hairy, and aggressive—he saw cells that were smooth, dented, and full of holes. They were locked in combat with white blood cells of the immune system, including the famous "natural killer," or "NK," cells. Miller was even able to film the white blood cells' attack on the S180 cells by video microscopy. He had found the explanation for the enigma. The resistant mice were able to mount a powerful defense, thanks to their immune system, even after cancer had taken hold.[9]

Very Special Agents Against Cancer

Natural killer (NK) cells are very special agents of the immune system. Like all white blood cells, they patrol the organism continually in search of bacteria, viruses, or new cancer cells. But while other cells of the immune system need previous exposure to disease agents in order to recognize and combat them, NK cells don't need prior introduction to an antigen in order to mobilize. As soon as they detect an enemy, they gather around the intruders, seeking membrane-to-membrane contact. Once they make contact, NK cells aim their internal equipment at their target, like a tank turret. This equipment carries vesicles filled with poisons.

On contact with the cancer cell's surface, the vesicles are released and the chemical weapons of the NK cells—perforin and granzymes—penetrate the membrane. The molecules of perforin take the shape of tiny circles, or microrings.

They are assembled in the shape of a tube, forming a passage for the granzymes through the cancer cell's membrane. At the core of the cancer cell, the granzymes then activate the mechanisms of programmed self-destruction. It's as if they give the cancer cell an order to commit suicide, an order it has no choice but to obey. In response to this message, its nucleus crumbles, leading to the cancer cell's collapse. The deflated remains of the cell are then ready to be digested by macrophages, which are the garbage collectors of the immune system and are always found in the wake of NK cells.[10, 11]

Like the immune cells of Zheng Cui's resistant mice, human NK cells are capable of killing different types of cancer cells, in particular sarcoma cells as well as those of breast, prostate, lung, or colon cancer.[12]

An investigation of seventy-seven women with breast cancer who were studied over a twelve-year period suggests how important these cells may be for recovery. First, samples of each woman's tumor taken at the time of diagnosis were cultivated with her own NK cells. Certain patients' NK cells did not react, as if their natural vitality had been mysteriously sapped. The NK cells of other patients, in contrast, went about a serious cleanup, indicating an active immune system. Twelve years later, at the end of the study, almost half (47 percent) of the patients whose NK cells had not reacted in the laboratory had died. On the other hand, 95 percent of those whose immune systems had been active under the microscope were still alive.[13]

Other studies reached similar conclusions: The less active the NK and other white blood cells were under the microscope, the more rapid the cancer's progress and the more it spread throughout the body in the form of metastases,[14] and the lower the chances of survival eleven years later.[15] Lively immune cells thus seem essential to countering the growth of tumors and the spread of metastases.[16, 17]

Cancer Kept at Bay

In a cruel way, Mary-Ann, a Scottish woman who wasn't suffering from cancer, learned how crucial the immune system is in preventing tumors from taking hold. She suffered from renal failure, a serious disease of the kidneys that makes them incapable of filtering blood. This leads to the accumulation of toxins in the body. To avoid the dialysis that she had to undergo at the hospital several times a week, she had a kidney transplant. For a year, Mary-Ann was able to live almost normally. The only constraint was a daily intake of immune-suppressing drugs. Their purpose, as their name suggests, was to weaken her immune system in order to prevent it from rejecting the transplant that was keeping her alive. After another six months, a gnawing pain developed around the transplanted kidney and an abnormal nodule was identified on her left breast in a routine mammogram. A biopsy revealed the appearance of a double metastasis of melanoma—a serious cancer of the skin. However, there was no primary melanoma that might have been the source of these metastases. Called in by the surgeons, dermatologist Rona MacKie was no better* able to explain this mysterious case of phantom melanoma.

---

* Dr. Miller's video showing how white blood cells in the human immune system detect and attack cancer cells can be viewed on my blog at www.anticancerbook.com (go to the Web site and search for "immune system video").

Everything was done to save Mary-Ann. The immunosuppressants were stopped, the diseased kidney removed. But it was too late. Six months later, she died of the general invasion of a melanoma whose original site could never be found.

Shortly afterward, George, a second patient who had had a kidney transplant in the same hospital, developed a metastatic melanoma with no original tumor. This time Dr. MacKie could no longer believe in simple coincidence or blame the impenetrable mysteries of medicine. Thanks to a register of transplanted organs, she traced the two kidneys back to their original donor. The donor's general health had indeed met all the usual requirements: no hepatitis, no HIV, and, of course, no cancer. But Dr. MacKie persevered, and she finally discovered the donor's name in a Scottish database of patients with melanoma. Eighteen years earlier, the donor had been operated on for a tiny 0.26 cm (1/10 of an inch) skin tumor. The woman had then received care for fifteen years at a melanoma clinic. Finally, she had been declared "completely cured" a year before her accidental death, unrelated to this old, extinct cancer. In this patient, who was for all intents and purposes "cured" of cancer, organs healthy in appearance still carried microtumors that her immune system kept in check. These microtumors were transplanted to new bodies—George's and Mary-Ann's—whose immune systems had been weakened on purpose to prevent rejection of the transplanted kidneys. In the absence of a normally functioning immune system, the microtumors rapidly went back to their chaotic, invasive ways.

Thanks to her detective work, Dr. MacKie convinced her colleagues in the department of renal transplants to stop the second patient's daily immunosuppressants. They gave him instead an aggressive immunostimulant, so that he would reject the melanoma-bearing transplant as fast as possible. A few weeks later, they were able to remove the kidney. Even though he had to go back to dialysis, two years later George was still alive and showed no sign of melanoma. Once it had recovered its natural power, his immune system fulfilled its mission and expelled the tumors.*

Nature Hasn't Read Our Textbooks

With Professor Zheng Cui's mice, researchers were able to show that their white blood cells could eliminate as many as two billion cancer cells in a few weeks.

---

* The case histories of Mary-Ann and George (not their real names) are described in an article in the *New England Journal of Medicine*, from which these elements were drawn.[18]

Barely six hours after the injection of cancer cells, the abdomens of these special mice are invaded by 160 million white blood cells. In the face of this onslaught, twenty million cancer cells vanish in half a day! Prior to these experiments on Mighty Mouse and his descendants, no one would have dared hope that the immune system was capable of mobilizing to such an extent. Not to the point of coming to terms with a cancer weighing 10 percent of the body's total weight. No one would have even imagined this was possible, the immunologists least of all. The reigning consensus on the limits of the immune system would probably have prevented a conventional immunologist from paying any attention to the phenomenal health of mouse number 6. That's what Lloyd Old, MD, professor of cancer immunology at Memorial Sloan-Kettering Cancer Center in New York, thought. To Zheng Cui—who didn't know anything about immunology before coming across mouse number 6—he wrote, "We can be thankful that you are not an immunologist. Otherwise, you would have definitely thrown away this mouse without hesitation." To which Professor Cui replied: "We should just be grateful that Nature never read our textbooks!"[19]

The body's resources and its potential for dealing with disease are still too often underestimated by modern science. Of course, in the case of Mighty Mouse, his extraordinary resistance is related to his genes. What about all those who, perhaps like you and me, are not endowed with these exceptional genes? To what extent can we count on an "ordinary" immune system to perform extraordinary tasks?

A study published in 2007 in the journal *Nature* investigated the immune potential of completely ordinary mice deprived of Mighty Mouse's extraordinary defenses. Catherine Koebel and her team at Washington University in Saint Louis injected a number of normal mice with a tar that's even more carcinogenic than that found in cigarette smoke.* As was expected, one group of mice quickly developed fatal tumors. But surprisingly, a group of surviving mice had *no tumors at all*. The researchers discovered that these healthy mice were, in reality, carriers of cancer cells but that these cells remained "dormant"—held in check by the immune system. Dr. Koebel's data indicate that when the immune system is weakened, microtumors are more likely to break free and begin to proliferate.[20] The cases of Mary-Ann and George, discussed earlier, illustrate this "dormant tumor" concept.

Catherine Koebel's team demonstrated for the first time in a laboratory environment a radical new concept in the field of oncology. The results of their

* The exact name is methylcholanthrene (MCA).

research suggest that cancer arises only from those cancer cells that find fertile "terrain" in which to grow. That is, cancer cells will flourish only within an individual whose immune defenses have been weakened. It may be primarily the lack of healthy defenses that allows otherwise dormant cancer cells to become aggressive tumors.

This opens up entirely new approaches to treatment. The aim of such new approaches would be not to eradicate tumors by targeting cancer cells themselves, but to "stabilize" these tumors over very long periods by strengthening and mobilizing our natural defenses.

We cannot overestimate how important it is that our white blood cells stay battle ready. They are the key elements in our body's ability to withstand and defeat cancer. We can arouse their vitality or, at the very least, stop slowing them down. The supermice succeed at this better than anyone else, but each of us can "urge on" our white blood cells so that they give their all in their confrontation with cancer. Several studies show that, like soldiers, human immune cells fight all the harder when (1) they are treated with respect (they are well fed and protected from toxins) and (2) their commanding officer keeps a cool head (he deals with his emotions and acts with poise).

As we'll see further on, studies on the activity of immune cells (including NK cells and white blood cells targeted against cancer) show that they are at their best when our diets are healthy, our environment is "clean," and our physical activity involves the entire body (not just our brains and our hands). Immune cells are also sensitive to our emotions. They react positively to emotional states characterized by a sense of well-being and a feeling that we are connected to those around us. It's as if our immune cells mobilize all the better when they are in the service of a life that is objectively worth living. We will encounter these faithful sentries throughout the following chapters when we examine the natural approaches to care that should accompany all cancer prevention and treatments.*

---

* The connection between the activity of the immune system and the progression of cancer is better established in mice than it is in people. Some cancers (such as liver or cervical cancer) are clearly linked to viruses and are thus highly dependent on the state of the immune system, but the link is not as clear for others. When the immune system is weakened—as in AIDS or in patients receiving high doses of immunosuppressant drugs—some cancers develop (lymphomas, leukemias, or melanomas in particular) but not most others. At the same time, a number of studies continue to show that people whose immune systems are particularly active against cancer cells seem to be protected against a wide variety of cancers (breast, ovary, lung, colon, and stomach, for example), unlike those whose immune cells are more passive. And when they do develop a tumor, it is less likely to spread in the form of metastases.[21-25]

TABLE 1. WHAT INHIBITS AND WHAT ACTIVATES IMMUNE CELLS	
Inhibits	Activates
Traditional Western diet (proinflammatory)	Mediterranean diet, Indian cuisine, Asian cuisine (antiinflammatory)
Persistent anger or despair	Serenity, joy
Social isolation	Support from family and friends
Denial of one's true identity (for example, one's homosexuality)	Acceptance of self with one's values and past history
Sedentary lifestyle	Regular physical activity

PART TWO: CANCER: A WOUND THAT DOESN'T HEAL

The Two Faces of Inflammation

All living organisms are naturally capable of repairing their tissues after a wound. In animals and humans, the basic mechanism of this process is inflammation. Dioscoride, a Greek surgeon in the first century A.D., described inflammation in terms so simple that they are still taught in all medical schools: *rubor, tumor, calor, dolor*. It's red, it's swollen, it's warm, and it's painful. Beneath these simple outward signs, complex and powerful operations go on.

As soon as a lesion—from shock, cutting, burning, poison, infection—affects a tissue, it is detected by blood platelets. As they gather around the damaged segment, they release a chemical substance—PDGF, or platelet-derived growth factor. PDGF alerts the white cells of the immune system. The white cells in turn produce a series of other transmitter substances. They have odd names and many effects. These cytokines, chemokines, prostaglandins, leukotrienes, and thromboxanes coordinate the repair operations. First, they dilate the vessels surrounding the damaged site to facilitate the influx of other immune cells called in as reinforcements. Next, they seal off the opening by provoking the coagulation of blood around the built-up pile of platelets. Then they render the neighboring tissue permeable so that the immune cells can enter and pursue the intruders wherever they may be. Finally, they trigger growth of the damaged tissue's cells. The tissue can then regenerate the missing piece and grow small blood vessels locally to deliver oxygen and food to the construction site.

These mechanisms are absolutely essential to the body's integrity. The body undergoes this rebuilding process all the time in dealing with insult and aggression, which is unavoidable. When these processes are well regulated and adjusted to the cells' other functions, they are beautifully harmonious and self-limiting. This means that the growth of new tissue stops as soon as the essential replacements have been carried out. The immune cells activated to deal with intruders return to their watchful, standby mode. This is an essential step to prevent the immune cells from continuing on and attacking healthy tissue (see figure 3).

In recent years, we have learned that cancer, like a Trojan horse, exploits this repair process to invade the body and drive it to destruction. That's the double face of inflammation: Whereas it is meant to heal by helping create new tissue, it can also be diverted to promote cancerous growth.

Wounds That Don't Heal

Rudolf Virchow, MD, was a great German physician and founder of modern pathology—the science that studies the relationship between disease and the processes that affect tissues. In 1863 he observed that several patients seemed to have developed cancer at the exact spot where they had received a blow or where a shoe or a tool had rubbed repeatedly. Under the microscope, he noticed the presence of a number of white cells in the cancerous growths. He advanced the hypothesis that cancer was a wound-repairing attempt that had gone wrong. His description seemed too anecdotal, almost too poetic, and was never really taken seriously. Some 130 years later, Harold Dvorak, MD, professor of pathology at Harvard Medical School, returned to this hypothesis. In "Tumors: Wounds That Do Not Heal,"[26] he presented forceful arguments in support of Virchow's original theory. In the article, he demonstrated the surprising similarity between mechanisms sparked by naturally occurring inflammation and the manufacture of cancerous growths.

Dvorak also noted that more than one cancer in six is *directly* linked to a chronic inflammatory state (see table 2). This is true for cervical cancer, which most commonly follows a chronic infection of papillomavirus. It is true too for colon cancer, which is very often found in subjects suffering from a chronic inflammatory disease of the intestine. Cancer of the stomach is linked to infection by the bacterium *Helicobacter pylori* (also a cause of ulcers). Cancer of the liver is related to infection by hepatitis B or C; mesothelioma to inflammation caused by asbestos; lung cancer to bronchial inflammation caused by the many toxic additives in cigarette smoke.

Nearly twenty years after Harold Dvorak's pioneering article, the National Cancer Institute brought out a report highlighting inflammation research too

TABLE 2. SOME CANCERS DIRECTLY RELATED TO
INFLAMMATORY CONDITIONS

Cancer Type	Cause of Inflammation
MALT lymphoma	*Helicobacter pylori*
Bronchial	Silica, asbestos, cigarette smoke
Mesothelioma	Asbestos
Esophageal	Barrett's metaplasia
Liver (hepatocellular)	Hepatitis virus (B and C)
Gastric	*Helicobacter pylori*–induced gastritis
Kaposi's sarcoma	Human herpesvirus type 8
Bladder	Schistosomiasis
Colon and rectum	Inflammatory bowel disease
Ovarian	Pelvic inflammatory disease, talc, tissue remodeling
Cervical	Papillomavirus

(FROM BALKWILL & MANTOVANI, *THE LANCET* 2001)[27]

often ignored by oncologists.[28] The report describes in great detail the processes by which cancer cells manage to lead the body's healing mechanisms astray. Just like immune cells gearing up to repair lesions, cancer cells need to produce inflammation to sustain their growth. To this end, they begin an abundant production of the same highly inflammatory substances—cytokines, prostaglandins, and leukotrienes—seen in the natural reparation of wounds.* They act as chemical fertilizers promoting cell reproduction—in this case, cancer cell reproduction. Growing tumors use these substances to help themselves develop and to make the barriers surrounding them more permeable. The very process that enables the immune system to repair lesions and pursue enemies in all the body's recesses is diverted for the benefit of cancer cells. They exploit it to spread and reproduce. Thanks to the inflammation they create, they infiltrate neighboring tissues, slip into the bloodstream, migrate, and establish remote colonies called metastases.

---

* This happens through the initial production of Cox-2 by cancer cells themselves. This is a key enzyme necessary for the inflammatory process, and it is the target of several modern antiinflammatory drugs known as Cox-2 inhibitors.

The Vicious Circle at the Heart of Cancer

In the case of normally healing lesions, the production of inflammatory chemical substances stops when the tissue is restored. In the case of cancer, production of these substances occurs continuously. In turn, surplus inflammatory chemicals in neighboring tissues block a natural process called apoptosis—the suicide of cells. Apoptosis is genetically programmed into every cell to prevent anarchy due to overproduction of tissues. Cells naturally enter into apoptosis in response to signals indicating that enough cells have been created to form healthy tissue. Thus, at the same time that they stimulate their own growth, cancer cells are also protected from death. It is the combination of these factors that causes the tumor to gradually expand.

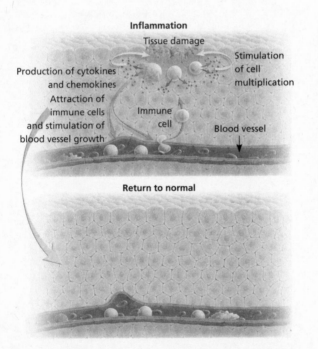

Figure 3. The normal inflammatory process. A lesion in tissue attracts immune cells. They track and destroy bacteria and stimulate the regrowth of cells and blood vessels in order to repair the breach. Once the repair is complete, the situation rapidly returns to normal.

By adding fuel to the fire of inflammation, tumors create yet another disruption. They "disarm" the immune cells in the vicinity. In simple terms, the overproduction of inflammatory factors throws neighboring white blood cells into disarray.[29, 30] The natural killer cells and other white blood cells are neutralized. They don't even try to fight the tumor, which prospers and grows in plain sight.[31]

To a large extent, the driving force behind a tumor is the vicious cycle cancer cells succeed in creating. By encouraging immune cells to produce inflammation, the tumor gets the body to make the fuel needed for its own growth and invasion of surrounding tissues. The larger the tumor, the more inflammation it causes and the better it sustains its own growth (see figure 4, page 46).

This hypothesis has been amply confirmed by recent research as reviewed in the journal *Science*. It has been proven that the more successful a cancer is in provoking local inflammation, the more aggressive the tumor and the better it is at spreading over long distances, ultimately reaching lymph nodes and creating metastases.[32]

Measuring Inflammation

The cancer-provoked inflammatory process is so crucial that measuring the production of inflammatory agents by tumors can predict survival time in many cancers (colon, breast, prostate, uterine, stomach, and brain).[33]

At the Glasgow Hospital in Scotland, oncologists have been measuring inflammation markers in the blood of patients with various cancers since the nineties. They have shown that patients with the lowest level of inflammation were twice as likely as the others to live through the next several years. These markers are easy to measure,* and to the astonishment of the Glasgow oncologists, they are a better indicator of the chances of survival than the patient's general state of health at the time of diagnosis.[34-36] It is as if the body's chronic underlying state of inflammation were a major determining factor of health. This is true even when the inflammation doesn't seem serious and gives no detectable signs such as joint pain or cardiovascular disease.

Several studies have been able to show that people who regularly take antiinflammatory medication (Advil, Nuprofen, ibuprofen, etc.) are less vulnerable to cancer than people who do not.[37-39] Unfortunately, these drugs have side effects; the risk of stomach ulcers and gastritis is significant. New antiinflammatory medications, such as Vioxx and Celebrex, initially inspired new hope. They are inhibitors of the calamitous COX-2—the very enzyme tumors produce to speed up their expansion. Several research projects explored these drugs' protective effects against cancer, with very encouraging results. However, in 2004 the demonstration of increased cardiovascular risks greatly dampened the early enthusiasm, and these drugs are not used clinically against cancer.

---

* The Glasgow researchers have developed a very simple formula for evaluating an individual's risk. It is based on two blood tests showing the level of inflammation: C-reactive protein < 10 mg/l and albumin > 35 g/l = minimum risk; CRP > 10 mg/l *or* albumin < 35 g = moderate risk; CRP > 10 mg/l *and* albumin < 35 g/l = high risk.

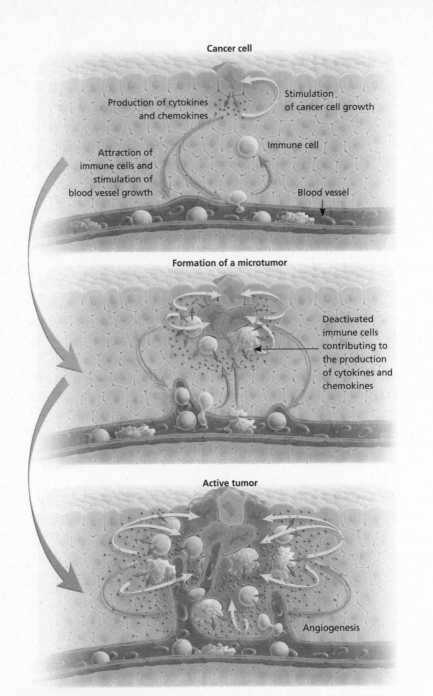

Figure 4. The vicious cycle of cancer. Cancer cells act as a wound that does not heal: They produce inflammatory factors (cytokines and chemokines). These stimulate local tumor growth and the development of new blood vessels (angiogenesis) and attract "deactivated" immune cells that, in turn, produce more inflammatory factors.

The Black Knight of Cancer

Thanks to the ongoing efforts of researchers, the Achilles' heel of cancer's mechanism for promoting inflammation is clearly identified today. In the laboratory of Michael Karin, PhD, professor of pharmacology at the University of California at San Diego, researchers working with a major German foundation* have demonstrated it in mice. The growth and spread of cancer cells relies to a large extent on a single proinflammatory factor secreted by the tumor cells—a sort of black knight without which tumors become much more fragile. That factor is referred to as nuclear factor–kappa B (or NF-kappa B), and blocking its production makes most cancer cells "mortal" once again. It also prevents them from creating metastases.[40] The key role played by NF-kappa B in cancer is so well identified today that Albert Baldwin, PhD, a professor at the University of North Carolina, concluded in the journal *Science* that "almost every cancer preventive is an inhibitor of NF-kappa B."[41]

As a matter of fact, many natural approaches are capable of blocking the inflammatory action of this key substance. The same article in *Science* notes, not without irony, that the whole pharmaceutical industry today is looking for drugs inhibiting NF-kappa B, while the molecules known to act against it are already widely available. The article cites only two of these molecules, qualified as low-tech: catechins, found in green tea, and resveratrol, found in red wine.[42] Actually, there are a good many of these types of molecules found in food, and some are even more active. We will go over them in detail in the chapter describing anticancer foods.

Stress: Adding Fuel to the Fire

There is one cause of overproduction of inflammatory substances that is rarely mentioned when cancer is discussed: persistent feelings of helplessness, a despair that won't let up. This emotional state is accompanied by changes in the secretion of noradrenaline (known as the fight-or-flight hormone) and cortisol, the "stress hormone." These hormones prepare the body for a potential wound, in part by stimulating the inflammation factors needed to repair tissues. At the same time, these hormones are also fertilizer for cancerous tumors, latent or already established.[43, 44]

The discovery of the key role of inflammation in growing and spreading cancer is relatively recent. A search on the major database Medline for articles published in English on inflammation and cancer shows that scientific interest is only just warming up to this concept (two articles in 1990, thirty-seven in

* Deutsche Forschungsgemeinschaft.

2005). This is one of the reasons why steps we could take to control inflammation are rarely mentioned in the advice we receive on cancer prevention and treatment. In addition, antiinflammatory medication has too many side effects to offer a valid solution to the problem. However, through natural approaches available to everyone, we can act to reduce inflammation. It's simply a matter of eliminating proinflammatory toxins from our environment, adopting an anticancer diet, seeking emotional balance, and satisfying our body's need for physical exertion. We will return to these themes in future chapters.

There is little likelihood that our physicians will suggest these approaches. Changes in lifestyle cannot, by definition, be patented. Thus, they do not become medications and they do not require prescriptions. This means that

TABLE 3. THE PRINCIPAL INFLUENCES ON INFLAMMATION	
Aggravates	**Reduces**
Traditional Western diet	Mediterranean diet, Indian cuisine, Asian cuisine
Refined sugars, white flour	Multigrain flour
Red meat from industrially raised animals	At most three times a week: organic meat from animals fed grass or flax meal
Oils rich in omega-6 (corn, sunflower, safflower, soy)	Olive oil, flaxseed oil, canola oil
	Fatty fish, rich in omega-3
Dairy products from industrially raised livestock (especially if full fat)	Dairy products from animals fed on grass or flax meal
Eggs from industrially raised hens fed corn and soybeans	Omega-3 eggs or eggs from hens raised in a natural environment or fed flax meal
Persistent anger or despair	Laughter, lightheartedness, serenity
Less than twenty minutes of physical activity a day	A fifty-minute walk three times a week (or thirty minutes six times a week)
Cigarette smoke, atmospheric pollution, domestic pollutants	Clean environment

most physicians don't consider them within their realm, so it is up to each of us to make them our own.

PART THREE: CUTTING CANCER'S SUPPLY LINES
Like Zhukov's Victory at Stalingrad

Combat against cancer often evokes military metaphors. None seem more appropriate to me than the greatest European battle of World War II.

It is August 1942. In the approaches to Stalingrad on the banks of the Volga, Hitler amasses the largest force of destruction in human history. More than a million seasoned men no enemy power has yet resisted, a massive panzer division, ten thousand cannons, twelve hundred planes. Facing them is the exhausted and poorly equipped Russian army, partly made up of adolescents or even schoolgirls who have never used a firearm but who are defending their country, their homes, their families. In combat of unimaginable violence, the Russian troops, backed up by civilians, hold on throughout the fall. Despite their heroism, they are desperately outnumbered. The Nazis' victory seems merely a matter of time. Marshal Georgy Zhukov then switches strategies completely. Instead of continuing a frontal assault, which offers no hope of victory, he launches the remains of his army across Nazi-held territory, behind German lines. This is where the units responsible for supplying the Nazi troops are stationed. Romanian or Italian, much less disciplined and fierce, they don't resist the attack for long. In a few days, Zhukov changes what seemed the inevitable outcome of the battle of Stalingrad. Once its supply lines have been cut, General Paulus's Sixth Army is incapable of fighting and ends up capitulating.

In February 1943, the German invasion is pushed back for good. Stalingrad represented a major turning point in the Second World War. It marked the beginning of the retreat of the Nazi cancer everywhere in Europe.[45]

Soldiers are aware of the strategic importance of supplying armies at the front. But the relevance of this thinking to cancer treatments long seemed preposterous to cancer researchers. Perhaps it wasn't purely by chance that the idea first sprouted in the mind of a military surgeon.

A Navy Surgeon's Insight

A medical officer in the U.S. Navy in the sixties, Judah Folkman, MD, was in charge of inventing a means of preserving stocks of fresh blood needed for surgery during the many months at sea on the first nuclear aircraft carriers. In order to test his conservation system, Folkman set up an experiment to find out if the preserved blood could meet the needs of a small living organ. He isolated a rabbit thyroid in a glass chamber, i.e., in vitro, and perfused it with the preserved blood, which, he saw, managed to keep it alive. The question then was: Would his system work as well with cells that were reproducing rapidly, as occurs during the healing process? To find out, he injected into his isolated rabbit thyroid cancer cells known for their rapid reproduction cycle. A surprise awaited him.

The injected cancer cells developed into tumors, but none of them beyond the size of a pinhead. First he thought these cells were dead. But once rein-jected into mice, the cancer cells rapidly grew into massive, deadly tumors. What was the difference between the rabbit thyroid in vitro and the live mice? One difference was very obvious to Folkman: The tumors developing inside the mice were infiltrated with blood vessels. The tumors in the thyroid isolated in the glass chamber were not. This observation led to the possible conclu-sion that a cancerous tumor quite simply cannot grow if it doesn't succeed in diverting blood vessels for its own use.

Obsessed by this hypothesis, Folkman found a host of positive evidence in his surgical practice. The cancerous tumors he operated on all presented this same characteristic. They were abundantly irrigated by fragile and contorted blood vessels. It was as if they had been made too quickly.

It didn't take Folkman long to reason that no living cell can survive if it isn't in contact with tiny blood vessels, filaments as fine as a human hair, called capillaries. Capillaries bring the oxygen and nutrients cells need and carry away waste from cellular metabolism. Cancer cells must also have nour-ishment imported and waste exported. To survive, tumors thus need to be deeply infiltrated with capillaries. But since tumors grow at high speed, new blood vessels must be made to sprout quickly. Folkman named this phenom-enon "angiogenesis," from the Greek *angio* for vessel and *genesis* for birth.

Blood vessels are typically a stable infrastructure. Their wall cells don't multiply and, except in particular circumstances, they don't create new capil-laries. New blood vessels grow when there is a need to repair wounds and after menstruation. This mechanism of "normal" angiogenesis is self-limiting and firmly controlled. Limits naturally placed on it prevent the creation of fragile vessels that would bleed too easily. In order to grow, cancer cells hijack the body's capacity to create new vessels for their own use. Folkman rea-soned that one method of combating cancer cell growth would be to pre-vent this hijacking of blood vessels. Then the growth could never get bigger than the head of a pin. By attacking their blood vessels instead of the cancer cells themselves, we should be able to dry out a tumor and perhaps even get it to regress.

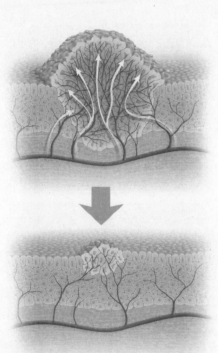

Figure 5. Angiogenesis, or neovascularization, involves the proliferation of new blood vessels. The process transforms a small, usually harmless cluster of abnormal cells (known as an in situ tumor) into a large mass that can spread to other organs. Intervention (dietary or other) that interferes with the making of new blood vessels can prevent the growth of tumors, maintaining them in a dormant state. Under some circumstances, it may even make an existing tumor regress.[46, 47]

Crossing the Desert

In the scientific community, nobody wanted to get involved in this "plumber's" theory thought up by a surgeon. Judah Folkman was just a manual worker used to dealing with drainage systems who probably didn't know anything about cancer biology. Still, he was a professor at Harvard Medical School and head of the surgery department at Children's Hospital, a renowned institution. So in 1971, the *New England Journal of Medicine* agreed to publish his eccentric hypothesis.[48]

Later, Folkman recounted a conversation he had during this time with his neighbor at the hospital lab, Professor John Enders, a Nobel laureate in medicine. Folkman wondered if he had talked too much about his ideas and if in publishing his article he had exposed his whole research program to copying by competing labs. Drawing on his pipe, Enders smiled and replied, "You are totally protected against intellectual theft. Nobody will believe you!"

In fact, Folkman's article got no response. Worse, his colleagues started showing their disapproval. They got up noisily and left the room when he spoke at conferences. They whispered that he was rigging his research results to back up his theories. Even worse for a physician, they called him a charlatan. After a brilliant career as a surgeon, they said, he had lost his way. Students, who are so necessary to the life of a research lab, started avoiding him. They didn't want their careers compromised by a connection to this crank. At the end of the seventies, he even lost his position as head of the surgery department.

Despite these snubs, Folkman's determination didn't weaken. Twenty years later, here is how he explained it: "I knew something that no one else knew, and I had been in the operating room. It wasn't the surgeons who were criticizing. It was basic scientists, and I knew that many of them had never seen cancer except in a dish. I knew that they had not experienced what I had experienced. The idea of tumors growing in three dimensions and needing blood vessels in the eye, in the peritoneal cavity, in the thyroid, and many other places, and the whole concept of *in situ* cancers and tumors waiting dormant—I had seen all that. So I kept saying, 'The ideas, I think, are right, and it will just take a long time for people to see them.' "[49]

Experiment by experiment, Judah Folkman built up the key concepts of his new theory of cancer:

1. Microtumors cannot change into dangerous cancers without creating a new network of blood vessels to feed them.
2. To do so, they produce a chemical substance called angiogenin that forces the vessels to approach them and to sprout new branches.
3. The new tumor cells that spread to the rest of the body—metastases—are dangerous only when they are able, in turn, to attract new blood vessels.
4. Large primary tumors send out metastases. But as in any colonial empire, they prevent these distant territories from becoming too important by producing another chemical substance that blocks the growth of new blood vessels—angiostatin. (This explains why metastases sometimes suddenly grow once the principal tumor has been surgically removed.)

It was all very well for the experiments to accumulate. Still, to most scientists the idea seemed too simple. It had to be heresy. Above all, as often happens in the scientific community, it couldn't be taken seriously as long as the *mechanism* by which tumors took control of blood vessels had not been elucidated. Proof was needed that there were such things as "angiogenin" and "angiostatin."

A Needle in a Haystack

Judah Folkman never let the critics get him down. He never lost confidence in his scientific colleagues' capacity to recognize the evidence once they had seen enough proof. He probably thought of Schopenhauer's saying: All great truth goes through three phases. First it is ridiculed, then violently attacked, and finally accepted as self-evident. He endeavored to prove the existence of the agents capable of preventing new vessels from growing.

But how could they be found among the thousands of different proteins produced by cancerous growths? It was like looking for a needle in a haystack. After many years and many setbacks, Folkman was on the point of giving up. Then, finally, luck was with him.

Michael O'Reilly was a young surgeon and researcher who had joined Folkman's laboratory. He thought of looking for angiostatin in the urine of mice resistant to metastases. O'Reilly's tenacity was as great as his boss's. He spent two years filtering hundreds of quarts of mouse urine. (He later commented on how foul smelling it was.) Finally, he found a protein that blocked the production of blood vessels when it was tested on a chicken embryo (in which blood vessels normally develop rapidly). The moment of truth had arrived. They could now test this potential angiostatin on live laboratory animals to see if it could prevent the development of cancer in a living body.

O'Reilly took twenty mice and grafted onto their backs a virulent cancer whose metastases spread aggressively and grow rapidly in the lungs once the principal tumor is removed. Immediately after removing the tumor, he injected angiostatin in half the mice and let the disease follow its course in the other half. A few days later, some of the mice showed signs of disease. The time had come to verify the theory.

Folkman knew that even if the results were positive, no one would believe him, so he invited all the researchers on the floor into his laboratory to watch the outcome. In the presence of the assembled witnesses, O'Reilly opened the thorax of the first mouse that had not received treatment. Its lungs were black, riddled with metastases. Then he opened the first mouse that had received angiostatin. Its lungs, a perfectly healthy rose color, showed no signs of cancer. He couldn't believe his eyes. One after the other, all the mice that had not been injected with angiostatin were shown to have been devoured by cancer. And all those that had received treatment were shown to have been completely cured. In 1994, after twenty years of scorn, the results were published in the periodical *Cell*.[50] Overnight, angiogenesis became one of the principal targets in cancer research.

An Exceptional Discovery

Later, Folkman was able to show that angiostatin could stop several types of cancer from growing, including three types of human cancer grafted onto mice. To the general surprise of the scientific and medical communities, preventing the creation of new blood vessels even brought about regression of existing cancers. Like the Nazis after Marshal Zhukov's attack on their supply lines, the tumors, once deprived of supplies, started shrinking. Reduced to microscopic size, they became totally inoffensive. In addition, it was shown that angiostatin attacked fast-growing blood vessels and didn't affect existing vessels in the least. Nor did it attack the body's healthy cells, in contrast to traditional cancer treatments such as chemotherapy and radiotherapy. In military terms, it didn't cause collateral damage. This made it a much less radical treatment than chemotherapy. As the article reporting these results in *Nature Medicine* concluded: "This regression of primary tumors without toxicity has not been previously described."[51] Beneath this laconic style peculiar to science quivers the excitement that signals exceptional discoveries.

With these two articles, Folkman and O'Reilly proved the role of angiogenesis in cancer metabolism. They also changed our conception of cancer treatment radically. If we can control the enemy by attacking its supply lines, then we can conceive of long-term treatments undermining the tumor's attempts to create new vessel growth. As in military strategy, these treatments can be combined with more precise strikes such as chemotherapy and radiotherapy. But planning for the long term calls for a "therapy of dormant tumors" to protect against the emergence of a first tumor, against relapses after early treatments, and against potential flare-ups of metastases after surgery.

Natural Defenses That Block Angiogenesis

Today many drugs similar to angiostatin (such as Avastin) are being developed by the pharmaceutical industry. But their effects on humans when used alone have turned out to be disappointing. While they have succeeded in slowing down the growth of certain cancers and have even brought on the spectacular regression of some tumors, the results have not been as consistent as those seen in mice. Besides, even if they are better tolerated than the usual chemotherapies, antiangiogenesis drugs have also produced more troublesome side effects than foreseen. As a result, they are probably not the long-hoped-for miracle drugs. But that isn't really surprising. Cancer is a multidimensional disease that rarely gives in to a single type of intervention. As with AIDS tritherapy, several approaches have to be combined to be effective.

The fact remains that the control of angiogenesis is a central concern in the treatment of cancer. As an alternative to waiting for the miracle drug, there are natural approaches that have a powerful effect on angiogenesis without side effects and that can be combined perfectly with conventional treatments:

1. Specific dietary practices (many natural antiangiogenesis foods have been discovered recently, including common edible mushrooms, certain green teas, spices, and herbs).[52-54]
2. Everything that contributes to reducing inflammation, the direct cause of the growth of new blood vessels (see chapter 8).[55, 56]

Cancer is a fascinating and perverse phenomenon. It borrows its disturbing intelligence from our vital functions to corrupt them and finally turn them against themselves. Recent studies have revealed how this corruption operates. Whether it is generating inflammation or fabricating blood vessels, cancer imitates our basic aptitude for regeneration, while aiming for the opposite outcome. It is the reverse of health, the negative of our vitality. But that doesn't mean that it is invulnerable. In fact, it is vulnerable in ways that our immune system naturally knows how to exploit. At the outposts of our defense system, our immune cells—including our NK cells—represent a powerful chemical armada that constantly nips cancers in the bud. All the facts bear out this conclusion; everything that strengthens our precious immune cells also impedes the growth of cancers. All in all, by stimulating our immune cells, fighting inflammation (with nutrition, physical exercise, and emotional balance), and fighting angiogenesis, we undercut cancer's spread. Acting in parallel with strictly conventional medical approaches, we can enhance our body's resources. The "price" to pay is to lead a more fully conscious, more balanced, and, in the end, more beautiful life.

CHAPTER 5

Breaking the News

Serious illness can be a terribly lonely journey. When danger hovers over a group of monkeys, arousing their anxiety, they instinctively huddle together and groom each other feverishly. This doesn't reduce the danger, but it relieves the loneliness. Our Western values, with their worship of concrete results, may blind us to our profound animal need for *presence* when facing danger and uncertainty. Gentle, constant, reliable presence is often the most beautiful gift our dear ones can give us. But not many of them know that.

I had a very good friend, who was also a physician, in Pittsburgh. He and I loved reinventing the world in interminable arguments. One morning I went to his office to break the bad news of my illness. As I spoke, the color drained from his face. Still, he showed no emotion. As a doctor, his instinct was to suggest a course of action or help me in some concrete way to make a decision. But I had already seen the oncologists. He had nothing to offer in this regard. Trying his best to give me advice, he made several practical suggestions. But he didn't express his feelings about what had happened to me.

When we talked about this conversation later, he explained with some embarrassment: "I didn't know what else to say." Perhaps saying something wasn't the point.

Sometimes circumstances force us to rediscover the power of presence. David Spiegel, MD, tells the story of one of his patients, a CEO married to the head of another company. Both were workaholics. They were used to keeping tabs on the most minute details of their lives. When she fell sick, they talked at length about the treatment options but very little about their inner feelings. One day she was so exhausted after chemotherapy that she collapsed on the living room rug. She couldn't get up. For the first time, she broke down in tears. Her husband recalls: "Everything I said just made her feel worse. I didn't know what to do, so I just got down on the floor and cried with her. I thought I was a complete failure because I couldn't make her feel better. But actually, that was what did make her feel better—when I stopped trying to fix it."

In our culture of control and action, the quality of mere presence has lost a lot of its value. Facing danger or suffering, an inner voice goads us on: "Don't just sit there. Do something!" In some situations, though, we would like to say to our loved ones, "Please stop trying to do something. Just sit there!"

Some people do find the words we want most to hear. I asked a patient who had suffered a lot during her long, harsh treatment for breast cancer what had sustained her most. She thought it over for several days before e-mailing me:

> My husband gave me a card early in my illness, which I pinned up in front of me on my bulletin board at work. I read it frequently. Here is what the card said:
>
> The cover read, "Open this card and hold it close to you. Now squeeze." Inside my husband wrote:
>
> "You are my everything—my joy in the morning (even on the days we don't make love!), my sexy and warm and laughing midmorning daydream, my phantom lunchmate, my building excitement at midafternoon, my soothing joy at seeing you when I get home, my workout decompressor, my sous-chef, my playmate, my lover, my all."
>
> The card continued, "It's going to be just fine." He wrote under that, "And I'll be there at your side, always.
> "Love,
> PJ"
>
> He was by my side every step of the way. His card meant so much to me and buoyed me throughout my journey.
>
> Since you asked,
> Mish

Usually, what's hardest is breaking the news to the people we love. For years, before finding myself in this situation, I had been giving a lecture to physicians in my hospital called "How to Break Bad News." I soon discovered that the exercise was a lot trickier when I had to apply it to myself.

In fact, I dreaded it so much that I kept putting it off. I was in Pittsburgh; my family was in Paris. I was about to give them a shock they would have to live with. First I talked to my three brothers, one after the other. To my great relief, they reacted in a simple, straightforward way. They didn't panic; they didn't try to reassure me, or themselves, with great, sweeping pronouncements.

They did not say, "It's not so bad. You'll see, you'll come out on top"—trite words that seem encouraging but are dreaded by anyone who is wondering what his chances of survival may be. My brothers found words to express their distress at what I was going through. They assured me of their loving support, and that was really all I needed.

When I called my parents, in spite of my "practice session" with my brothers, I had no idea how I was going to do it. I was terrified. My mother has always been a tower of strength in the face of adversity. But my father had aged. I sensed his vulnerability. Although I didn't have children yet, I knew that discovering a child's illness could be far more painful than learning of one's own.

When my father picked up the telephone on the other side of the Atlantic, I could hear his joy at getting my call. My heart sank. It was as if I was about to plant a dagger in his chest. Step by step, I followed the rules I had been teaching my colleagues: First, briefly state the facts, as they are: "Dad, I've found out I have a brain cancer. All the exams concur. It's fairly serious, but it's not the worst kind. There are good prospects of survival for several years. And it's not too painful."

Second, wait. Don't fill the silence with empty phrases. I heard him choke up. "Oh, David, this can't be. . . ." We didn't usually joke about subjects like this. I knew he had understood. I waited a little longer. I imagined him at his desk in the posture I knew so well, erect, getting ready to confront the matter at hand, as he had done all his life. He had never hesitated to put up a fight, even in the most difficult circumstances. But there wouldn't be any combat. There was no battle plan to draw up, no scathing article to write. I went on to step three: Talk about concrete steps. "I'm going to find a surgeon who'll operate as soon as possible. And depending on what they find during the operation, we'll decide whether to do chemotherapy or radiotherapy." He had heard and he had accepted.

Not long afterward, I realized the disease was letting me savor a new identity. This novel situation had its advantages. I had long been tortured by the fear of betraying the huge hopes that my father had placed in me. I was the eldest son of the eldest son. I knew he set his sights high for me, as they had been for him. Even though he never said it so clearly, I knew he was disappointed that I was "only a doctor." He would have liked me to go into politics as he had and perhaps succeed where he had not fully lived up to his own ambitions. No disappointment could have been more crushing to him than my falling seriously ill at thirty. But suddenly, through my illness, I regained a certain freedom. The obligations that had weighed me down since childhood were swept away. No more need to be at the top of the class or at the forefront of my field in research. I was exempt from the eternal race to test my excellence, prove my abilities, my intellectual worth. For the first time, I had the feeling I could lay down my weapons and breathe. That same week, Anna played a spiritual for me that moved me to tears, as if I had been waiting all my life for these words to ring:

> *I'm gonna lay down my heavy load*
> *Down by the riverside . . .*
> *Ain't gonna study war no more.*
> *I'm gonna lay down my sword and shield*
> *Down by the riverside . . .*
> *Ain't gonna study war no more.*

CHAPTER 6

The Anticancer
Environment

PART 1: A CANCER EPIDEMIC

After teaching at Yale, Michael Lerner, PhD, moved to California in
the seventies with a seemingly outlandish idea: He wanted to create
a center whose very lifestyle could help heal, both physically and
emotionally, people with serious illnesses. On this exceptionally peaceful site,
perched high above the Pacific just north of San Francisco, the food is exclusively organic. People practice yoga twice a day. They feel free to speak openly
to each other. Doctors with cancer sometimes come here looking for answers
they didn't learn in medical school.

Over the past thirty years, Lerner and his associate Rachel Naomi Remen,
MD, have helped a large number of patients—many of whom have become
friends. Some have left marvelously restored; some have been healed, others
have died. As the years have gone by, the center has seen a greater number
of young people among the dead. Cancer now affects people who have never
smoked and who have led a rather "well-balanced" life. A hidden, incomprehensible cause seems to doom thirty-year-old women to metastatic breast
cancer and young, seemingly healthy men to spreading lymphoma, colon, or
prostate cancer. There doesn't seem to be any logical reason why the patients
are younger.

What Michael and Rachel observe at their center is in fact a worldwide
phenomenon clearly identified by statisticians. Since 1940 the number of cancers has increased in all industrialized countries. This trend, which has picked
up speed since 1975, is particularly striking in the young. In the United States
between 1975 and 1994, the cancer rate in women under forty-five has risen
by 1.6 percent *a year* and even more in men (by 1.8 percent).[1] In some European countries—such as France—the cancer rate has increased by 60 percent

in the last twenty years.[2] As a result, we can't help wondering whether we are facing an epidemic.

When I asked an eminent professor of oncology this question three years ago, he came up with an array of answers meant to reassure the public. "There is nothing surprising about this phenomenon," he said. "As people are living longer today, compared to 1940, it's normal for the cancer rate to be higher. Besides, women give birth much later, so they are more likely to have breast cancer. Taking into account early screening, there are a greater number of cases recorded." His message was simple: We shouldn't be misled by alarmists invoking heaven knows what mysterious factors. To the contrary, we need to step up research to improve treatment and early detection, the two pillars of modern oncology. Like many of my colleagues, and like many other patients, I wanted to believe him. It was more comforting.

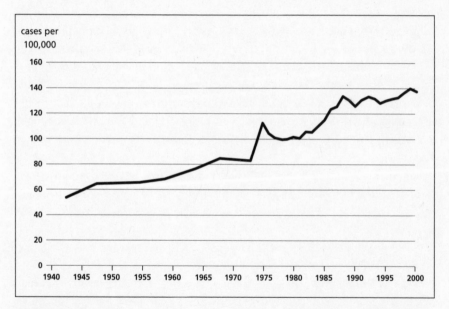

Figure 6. The rise in breast cancer cases in the United States between 1940 and 2000 (taking into account aging of the population).[3, 4]

But today even this archconservative oncologist has changed his view. The facts are indeed devastating. Annie Sasco, MD, PhD, who ran the unit of epidemiology for cancer prevention at the World Health Organization (WHO) for six years, points to the figures that have probably helped change the minds of those who refused to face reality. The rise in cancers clearly cannot be explained by population aging alone. WHO drew attention to this fact in *The Lancet* in 2004: Cancers in *children and adolescents* are among those that have risen the most since 1970.[5] True, there is a *slight* increase in risk among women who have their first child after thirty. But the age of procreation in women explains only a very small portion of the increase in cancers. The incidence of prostate cancer (which by definition affects only men) has risen still faster than that of breast cancer in Western countries.[6] It rose by 200 percent in several European countries between 1978 and 2000, by 258 percent in the United States over the same period.[7, 8] And finally, the argument concerning early screening is insufficient to explain these numbers: The increase in cancers that are not routinely screened for (pancreas, lung, brain, testicle, lymphoma) is equally striking, if not more so.[9–11]

There is indeed a cancer epidemic in the Western world.* It can even be dated, quite precisely, to World War II. A major study published in *Science* has shown, for example, that for women carrying high-risk genes (BRCA-1 or BRCA-2), the risk of developing breast cancer before age fifty has virtually *tripled* for women born after the war, compared to those born before the war.[12†]

Older physicians I have talked to are flabbergasted. In their time, cancer in a young person was very rare. One of them still remembers from medical school a thirty-five-year-old woman with breast cancer: All the medical students from the nearby departments had been invited to examine her. In the fifties, she was an exceptional case. Four or five decades later, I had cancer at thirty-one, and two of my cousins—one in Europe, the other in the United States—had cancer at forty. Forty—that was also the age at which the first childhood classmate whose bust I had noticed died. She died because of a tumor in those breasts we giggled about together in the school yard when they first started to show. Alas, the epidemiologists' figures are not just abstract numbers.

The Rich People's Disease

Gifted with impressive foresight, General de Gaulle founded the first international center at WHO "to determine the causes of cancer." It was set up in Lyon in 1964 and named the International Agency for Research on Cancer (IARC). Today it is the world's largest epidemiological center devoted to

---

* Technically, the word "epidemic" is used when there is a rapid rise in the number of cases of an illness. This is not true of *all* types of cancer. In the last decades, there has been a considerable reduction in stomach and ear, nose, and throat cancers in the West. Yet the rise in cancers of the breast, lung, brain, skin (melanomas), and lymphatic system (lymphomas) clearly follows an epidemic pattern.

† Another study, in Europe, shows that the risk of malignant brain tumors has also tripled for people born after the war.[13]

cancer. Epidemiology is real detective work. By association and deduction it tries to identify the causes of diseases and their progression. The science of epidemics emerged at a time when cities in Europe and America were devastated by cholera. In the middle of the nineteenth century, microbes had not yet been discovered; there was no explanation for cholera, making it all the more terrifying.

When epidemiologists have not yet identified the cause of a disease, health authorities may invent reassuring arguments to inspire confidence in whatever measures are being offered. In 1832 Americans faced a new epidemic of cholera, and the Medical Board of New York City was helpless. It published a bulletin stating that cholera victims were "either intemperate, imprudent, or prone to injury by the consumption of improper medicines." To avoid catching the disease, the board recommended not drinking alcoholic beverages, avoiding drafts, not eating salads, and "maintaining regular habits."[14] The discovery of the cholera bacillus by Robert Koch in 1883 did in fact confirm the role of raw salad in cholera's transmission. The rest was, in essence, quackery.*

Annie Sasco remembers that at twelve she wrote in her diary that someday she would be a doctor and work for WHO. Perhaps it was partly to show her father, a police sergeant and former member of the French Resistance, that she too would be capable of fighting for great causes. After medical school in France and a doctorate in epidemiology from Harvard, she spent twenty-two years at WHO's International Agency for Cancer Research. Her search for reliable data took her into the field, to China, Brazil, Central America, and Africa. The cancer maps resulting from these investigations provide the best clues to the rapid spread of the disease. She brings up maps on her computer screen showing the occurrence of various cancers and comparing the most affected with the least affected countries. The first map is stunningly clear: For the same age groups, breast, prostate, and colon cancers are diseases of the industrialized world, and particularly *Western* countries. There are nine times more such cancers in the United States and in Northern Europe than in China, Laos, or Korea, and four times more than in Japan.

After examining these maps, we can't help wondering whether Asian

---

* I am grateful to Sandra Steingraber, PhD, for this historical example. She introduces it in her book *Living Downstream*—essential reading on the connection between environmental pollution and the increase in cancers.[15] In another brilliant book on cancer and the environment, Devra Lee Davis, PhD, MPH, points out that authorities in the nineteenth century did not wait for a final proof to start putting in place basic improvements in hygiene and sanitation. These saved many lives, well before the cholera vibrio was finally identified.[16]

genes play a protective role against these cancers. But genes are not the answer here. When she was conducting her survey in China, Sasco asked a Chinese colleague how he explained the low incidence of breast cancer there. With an amused smile he answered: "It's a disease of rich women. You'll find it in Hong Kong but not here."

In fact, the cancer rate among the Chinese and Japanese in Hawaii and in San Francisco's Chinatown is fast approaching that of Westerners.[17, 18] And in the past decade, breast cancer rates in major cities of China, along with Hong Kong, have tripled.[19]

In his introduction to the report of the International Agency for Cancer Research, the general director of WHO concluded, "Up to 80% of cancers may be influenced by external factors, such as lifestyle and the environment." Indeed, the greatest success of Western medicine in the war against cancer is the quasi disappearance of cancer of the stomach in industrialized countries.

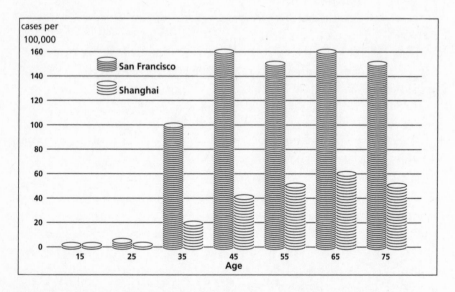

Figure 7. Breast cancer (per 100,000 women) among Chinese immigrants in San Francisco, compared to Chinese women who remained in China.[20] Cancer is a disease of the Western lifestyle.

Whereas all medical students of the 1960s were painfully familiar with this serious and common illness, which was present on every internal medicine ward, it is a disease barely discussed today in medical schools. The disappearance of gastric cancers in a matter of forty years is attributed to better refrigeration of food and less reliance on nitrates and salt for preservation: a purely "environmental" intervention.[21]

The Anticancer Environment • 65

Today it is widely recognized in biology and medicine that many toxic substances present in the environment play roles in the appearance of the first cancer cells in an organism, and then in their transformation into a more aggressive tumor. This process is referred to as carcinogenesis. In a recent report, experts at the U.S. National Cancer Institute emphasized that the process of carcinogenesis doesn't just trigger the disease. *It goes on after the disease has started.*[22] Thus, it is essential to seek protection against toxins that encourage tumor growth, whether we are healthy or already affected by the disease. Detoxification is a fundamental concept in most ancient medical traditions, from Hippocrates to Ayurveda, and is absolutely necessary today.*

Like everyone else, once diagnosed with cancer, I wanted to know what I could have done to prevent it and what I now had to do so that it wouldn't come back. To my great surprise, all the answers I got were evasive and noncommittal: "We don't really know for sure the cause of your illness. Don't smoke. That's all we can advise you." It's true: Except for tobacco or asbestos and lung cancer, there are few certainties that one particular food or one particular feature of our lifestyle or profession sparks a particular cancer. But, as we shall see further on, there are enough strong suggestions to justify starting to protect ourselves right away—all the more so because it doesn't require such a great effort.

A Watershed in the Twentieth Century

Cancer is more widespread today in the West and has been increasing since 1940. Hence, we must examine what has changed in our countries since World War II. Three major factors have drastically disrupted our environment over the last fifty years:

1. The addition of large quantities of highly refined sugar to our diet
2. Changes in methods of farming and raising animals and, as a result, in our food
3. Exposure to a large number of chemical products that didn't exist before 1940

These are not minor changes. There is every reason to believe that these three phenomena play a major role in the spread of cancer. To protect ourselves, we first must try to understand them.

---

* The concept of detoxification usually includes two notions—an end to accumulation as well as active elimination. I use it here principally to refer to ending accumulation of toxins.

PART 2: RETURNING TO THE FOOD OF YESTERYEAR

Our genes still bear the marks of having developed several hundred thousand years ago, when we were hunters and gatherers. They were adapted over time to our ancestors' environment and especially to their food sources, and they haven't changed much since.[23] Today our bodies still expect a diet similar to the one we had when we ate the products of hunting and gathering. That diet consisted of a lot of vegetables and fruit and occasionally the meat or eggs of wild animals. It provided a balance between essential fatty acids (omega-6 and omega-3) and very little sugar and didn't include flour. (The only source of refined sugar for our ancestors was honey. They did not eat cereals.)

Today Western surveys of nutrition reveal that 56 percent of our calories come from three sources that *were nonexistent* when our genes were developing:[24]

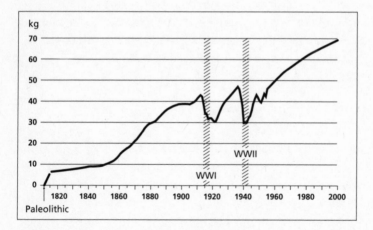

Figure 8. Changes in the consumption of refined sugar: 2 kilograms (4 pounds) a year per person during the Paleolithic (when our genetic makeup developed); 5 kilograms (11 pounds) a year in 1830; 70 kilograms (150 pounds) a year in 2000.[25]

- refined sugars (cane and beet sugar, corn syrup, etc.)
- bleached flour (white bread, white pasta, etc.)
- vegetable oils (soybean, sunflower, corn, trans fats)

It so happens these three sources contain none of the proteins, vitamins, minerals, or omega-3 fatty acids needed to keep our bodies functioning. On the other hand, they *directly* fuel the growth of cancer.

Cancer Feeds on Sugar

Consumption of refined sugar has skyrocketed. Whereas our genes developed in an environment where one person consumed at most 2 kilograms (4 pounds) of honey a year, human sugar consumption rose to 5 kilograms (11 pounds) a year in 1830 and a shocking 70 kilograms (150 pounds) a year at the end of the twentieth century.

The German biologist Otto Heinrich Warburg won the Nobel Prize in medicine for his discovery that the metabolism of malignant tumors is largely dependent on glucose consumption. (Glucose is the form of digested sugar in the body.) In fact, the PET scan commonly used to detect cancer simply measures the areas in the body that consume the most glucose. If a particular area stands out because it consumes too much sugar, cancer is very likely the cause.

When we eat sugar or white flour—foods with a high "glycemic index"—blood levels of glucose rise rapidly. The body immediately releases a dose of insulin to enable the glucose to enter cells. The secretion of insulin is accompanied by the release of another molecule, called IGF (insulinlike growth factor), whose role is to stimulate cell growth. In short, sugar nourishes tissues and makes them grow faster. Furthermore, insulin and IGF have another effect in common: They promote the factors of inflammation, which, as we saw in chapter 4, also stimulate cell growth and act, in turn, as fertilizer for tumors.

Today we know that the peaks of insulin and the secretion of IGF directly stimulate not only the growth of cancer cells,[26] but also their capacity to invade neighboring tissues.[27] Moreover, after injecting breast cancer cells into mice, researchers have shown that the cancer cells are less susceptible to chemotherapy when the mouse's insulin system has been stimulated by the presence of sugar.[28] The researchers concluded that a new class of medications is needed now to fight cancer: medicines that reduce insulin peaks and IGF in the blood.

Without waiting for these new medicines, each of us can already cut back on the amount of refined sugar and white flour we consume in our diets. It has been shown that simply reducing these two dietary factors has a rapid effect on the levels of insulin and IGF in the blood. This reduction has secondary effects, such as healthier skin.

The link between blood sugar levels and inflammation may seem far-fetched. How could candy, a lump of sugar in a cup of coffee, or a slice of white bread with jam affect physiology? Yet this link is patently obvious when it comes to pimples on the skin.

Loren Cordain, PhD, is a researcher in nutrition at the University of

Colorado. When he was told that certain population groups whose way of life is very different from ours had no experience of acne (which is caused by an inflammation of the epidermis, among other mechanisms), he wanted to find out how this could occur. The claim sounded preposterous. Acne is a rite of passage that affects 80 percent to 95 percent of Western adolescents. In order to investigate, Cordain accompanied a team of dermatologists to examine the skin of 1,200 adolescents cut off from the rest of the world in the Kitavan Islands of New Guinea, and 130 Ache Indians living in isolation in Paraguay. In these two groups they found *no trace whatsoever* of acne. In their article in *Archives of Dermatology,* the researchers attributed their amazing discovery to the adolescents' nutrition. The diets of these contemporary sheltered groups resemble those of our distant ancestors: no refined sugar or white flour, thus no peaks of insulin or IGF in the blood.[29]

In Australia, researchers convinced Western adolescents to try a diet restricting sugar and white flour for three months. In a few weeks, their insulin and IGF levels diminished. So did their acne.[30, 31]

In the second half of the twentieth century, a new ingredient took root and spread like a weed in Western diets: high-fructose syrup extracted from corn (a mix of fructose and glucose). Our bodies already had trouble tolerating the refined sugar we were loading up on. Now they were totally overwhelmed by this sugar syrup ubiquitous in processed foods. Removed from its natural matrix (there is fructose in all fruits) and mixed with glucose, it can no longer be handled by the insulin our bodies produce, at least not without collateral damage. It then becomes toxic.

There is good reason to believe that the sugar boom contributes to the cancer epidemic, as it is linked to an explosion of insulin and IGF in our bodies. Mice inoculated with breast cancer cells have been used to compare the effect on tumor growth of different foods of varying glycemic indices. After two and a half months, two thirds (sixteen) of the twenty-four mice whose blood sugar peaked frequently were dead, compared to only one of the twenty that had been on a low-glycemic-index diet.[32] For obvious reasons, it would be impossible to carry out such an experiment in humans. But a study comparing Asian with Western populations suggests the same thing: Those who eat low-sugar Asian diets tend to have five to ten times fewer hormonally driven cancers than those with diets high in sugar and refined foods, as is typical in most industrial nations.[33]

In addition, people with diabetes (characterized by high blood sugar levels) are known to be at above-average risk for cancer.[34] In a joint American-Canadian study, Susan Hankinson, ScD, of Harvard Medical

School, has shown that in a group of women under fifty, those with the highest level of IGF were *seven times* more likely to develop breast cancer than those with the lowest.[35] Another team, composed of researchers from Harvard and the University of California at San Francisco in the United States and McGill in Canada, demonstrated the same phenomenon for prostate cancer: In their group of men, the risk was as much as *nine times* greater for those with the highest levels of IGF.[36, 37] Additional studies have shown that a high glycemic index is likewise associated with cancer of the pancreas, colon, and ovaries.[38-41]

In 2009, two years after this book was first published, the massive Women's Health Initiative study of almost one hundred thousand postmenopausal women in the United States confirmed a link between increased insulin in the body stemming from a diet high in sugar and white flour and an elevated risk of breast cancer. Researchers observed these women at forty different academic centers in the United States for an average of six years *before* they became ill. They had drawn blood samples when the women first entered the study and were able to compare the risk of developing breast cancer several years later of those with high and low insulin levels at baseline. The study, published in the *Journal of the National Cancer Institute,* concludes that it is not obesity per se that is a risk factor for breast cancer, but rather high insulin levels that tend to be associated with excessive body weight. The women with the higher insulin levels (and who were not diabetic or taking hormone replacement therapy) had almost twice the risk of developing breast cancer during the follow-up period compared to those whose insulin levels were the lowest.[42]

All the scientific literature points in the same direction: People who want to protect themselves from cancer should seriously reduce their consumption of processed sugar and bleached flour. This means getting used to drinking coffee without sugar. (It's easier to give up sugar in tea.) It also means making do with two or three desserts a week. (There is no limit on fruit, as long as it is not sweetened with sugar or syrup.) Another option is to use natural substitutes for sugar that don't cause a sharp rise in blood glucose or insulin (see table 4).

Eating multigrain bread (made from wheat mixed with at least three other cereals, such as oatmeal, rye, flaxseeds, etc.) is also essential in order to slow down assimilation of the sugars coming from wheat. You can also choose bread made with traditional leaven ("sourdough") instead of the more common chemical baker's yeast, which raises the glycemic index of bread. For the same reason, ordinary white rice should be avoided and replaced by

TABLE 4. CHOOSE FOOD ACCORDING TO ITS GLYCEMIC INDEX[43]	
High Glycemic Index (avoid)	Low Glycemic Index (use liberally)
Sugar (white or brown), honey, syrups (maple, fructose, dextrose)	Natural sweeteners: agave nectar, stevia (a Pacific plant), xylitol, dark chocolate (>70% cocoa)
White/bleached flours: white bread, white rice, overcooked white pasta, muffins, bagels, croissants, puffed rice cakes	Mixed whole-grain cereals: multigrain bread (not just wheat); leavened ("sourdough") bread; Basmati or Thai rice; pasta (preferably multigrain) and noodles cooked al dente; quinoa, oats, millet, buckwheat
Potatoes, especially mashed potatoes (except for the rare Nicola variety)	Lentils, peas, beans, sweet potatoes, yams
Cornflakes, Rice Krispies, and most of the other bleached or sweetened breakfast cereals	Oatmeal (porridge), muesli, All-Bran, Special K
Jams and jellies, fruit cooked in sugar, fruit in syrup	Fruit in its natural state, particularly blueberries, cherries, and raspberries, which help to regulate blood sugar levels (use agave nectar for sweetening if necessary)
Sweetened drinks: industrial fruit juices, sodas	Water flavored with lemon, thyme, or sage
	Green tea (without sugar, or with agave nectar), which combats cancer directly (see chapter 8)
Alcohol (except during meals)	One glass of red wine a day with a meal
	Garlic, onions, shallots (when mixed with other food, they help lower insulin peaks)
(SOURCE: McMillan et al. (2006)	

AGAVE NECTAR, ACACIA HONEY, COCONUT SUGAR, AND XYLITOL

Recently, the team at the University of Sydney that introduced the concept of "glycemic index" pointed out a natural substitute for white sugar with a very low glycemic index: agave nectar. An extract from cactus sap (used to make tequila), it tastes delicious, comparable to a light honey. It is three times sweeter than white sugar, but its glycemic index is four to five times lower than that of honey. (The glycemic index is considered "low" if it is under 55; glucose has an index of 100. The glycemic index of agave nectar is between 15 and 21, and between 60 and 80 for most kinds of honey.) Agave nectar can be used instead of sugar or the usual syrups to sweeten tea, coffee, fruits, and desserts. Among the various kinds of honey, acacia honey, which is also very light in color, has a low glycemic index (roughly 30).

Another natural sweetener, coconut sugar, has a glycemic index of about 35. It has the further advantage of a crystalline presentation, similar to the sugar we're accustomed to using.

Be careful, however, not to abuse these three natural sugars. Despite their low glycemic indexes, they remain high-calorie foods. Overconsumption will result in both weight increase and elevated triglyceride levels in the blood.

Xylitol, a birch-bark extract, is highly sweetening but contains only one third of the calories of other sugars. It does not cause blood sugar or insulin levels to rise, and it is the only sugar that has been linked to a *decrease* in the risk of dental cavities. Xylitol can be found in organic stores and specialized shops, but it remains expensive.

brown or white basmati rice, for which the glycemic index is lower. Above all, it's much better, as we shall see in the chapter on cancer-fighting foods, to eat vegetables and legumes (beans, peas, lentils). Not only are their glycemic indexes low, but the potent phytochemicals they contain fight cancer growth every inch of the way.

Avoiding candies and snacks *between meals* is essential. When cookies (or other sugar) are consumed between meals, there is nothing to block a rise in insulin. Only their combination with other foods—especially vegetable, fruit fibers, or good fats, such as olive oil, canola oil, or organic butter—slows the assimilation of sugar and reduces insulin peaks. In the same way, some foods, such as onions or garlic, blueberries, cherries, raspberries, or spices like cinnamon, reduce the rise in blood sugar.*

The Food Chain Imperiled

Everybody has a friend who is overweight. Ever since childhood, she has been chubby. Despite diets of all kinds and regular physical exercise, her figure has never been "normal." She worries about her heavy hips, which won't slim down. Even when she manages to stick to her diet, she doesn't lose much weight. She gains it back as soon as she stops an active diet. Yet she is very careful about avoiding butter (for the last twenty years she has used only margarine). She may even use the "balanced" and "polyunsaturated" oils (usually based on sunflower oil) often recommended by nutritionists.

One of the great mysteries of modern epidemiology, apart from cancer, is the epidemic of obesity. Obesity is one of the highest risk factors for cancer. The link between obesity and cancer is becoming increasingly clearer. Only now are we beginning to understand how they share a common origin—not only the secretion of insulin, as the Women's Health Inititative study showed, but also the changing nature of the fats we consume. Let's look first at the riddle of obesity.

Between 1976 and 2000, Americans lowered their consumption of fats considerably (by 11 percent) and even their total calorie intake (by 4 percent). Still, obesity has gone on rising at breakneck speed. It has gone up 31 percent in this same period.[45] The head of the largest department of epidemiology and nutrition in the world, Walter Willett, MD, PhD, of Harvard, summed up the situation in his resounding article "Dietary Fat Plays a Major Role in Obesity: No."[46] This phenomenon of rising obesity alongside lowered fat comsumption, known as the American paradox, in fact now affects all of Europe, and Israel even more.[47]

A team of French researchers was the first to solve the mystery of the American paradox. Gérard Ailhaud, in his sixties, a bit overweight himself, eyes sparkling with intelligence and curiosity, set out with a simple observation. While everyone else was blaming the epidemic of obesity on junk food and lack of physical exercise, he exposed a flaw in the argument. In the United States, the mass of fatty tissue *in children under one* doubled between 1970 and 1990. In a fascinating book that tells the story of their discoveries, Pierre Weill, a biochemist and a farming engineer, as well as a fellow researcher,

---

* A diet based on foods with low glycemic indexes not only reduces the chances that a cancer will progress; it has also been shown by a research team from the Hôtel-Dieu Hospital in Paris to promote a reduction in fat tissue in favor of muscle tissue.[44]

recalls a remark by his friend Ailhaud: "Between 6 and 11 months of age, you can't blame McDonald's, snacking, TV, and lack of physical exercise!"[48]

No, infants are not overfed. They are still given the same quantity of milk, be it mother's milk or baby formula. Ailhaud and his colleague Philippe Guesnet demonstrated that the change in the *character* of milk since 1950 is responsible for infant obesity.[49, 50] This new imbalance in the very nature of milk acts on the growth of both adipose tissue (fat) and cancer cells.

Junk Food for Cows and Chickens

In the natural cycle, cows give birth in spring, when the grass is most luxuriant, and produce milk for several months until summer's end. Spring grass is an especially rich source of omega-3 fatty acids; these fatty acids are therefore concentrated in the milk from cows raised in pastures and in the milk's derivatives—butter, cream, yogurt, and cheese. Omega-3s are likewise found in beef from grass-fed cattle and in eggs from free-range chickens fed with forage (rather than grain).

Starting in the fifties, the demand for milk products and beef went up so much that farmers had to look for shortcuts in the natural cycle of milk production and reduce the grazing area needed to feed a 750-kilogram (1,600-pound) cow. Pastures were thus abandoned and replaced by battery farming. Corn, soy, and wheat, which have become the principal diet for cattle, contain practically no omega-3 fatty acids. To the contrary, these food sources are rich in omega-6s. Omega-3 and omega-6 fatty acids are called "essential" because the human body cannot make them. As a result, the quantity of omega-3s and omega-6s in our bodies stems directly from the content of the food we eat. In turn, the amounts of omega-3 and omega-6 fatty acids in our food depend on what the cows and chickens we eat have consumed in *their* feed. If they eat grass, then the meat, milk, and eggs they provide are perfectly balanced in omega-3s and omega-6s (a balance close to 1/1). If they eat corn and soy, the resulting imbalance in our bodies is as much as 1/15, even 1/40.[51]

The omega-3s and omega-6s present in our bodies constantly compete to control our body functions. Omega-6s help stock fats and promote rigidity in cells as well as coagulation and inflammation in response to outside aggression. They stimulate the production of fatty cells from birth onward. Omega-3s are involved in developing the nervous system, making cell membranes more flexible, and reducing inflammation. They also limit the production of adipose cells.[52, 53] Our physiological balance depends very much on the balance between omega-3s and omega-6s in our body, and therefore in our diet. It turns out that it is this dietary balance that has changed the most in the last fifty years.

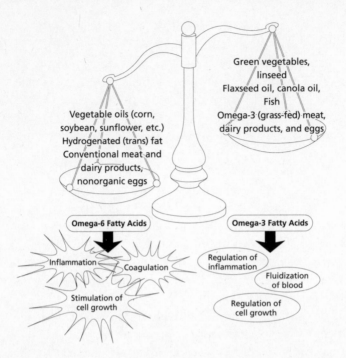

Figure 9. The imbalance between omega-6 and omega-3 fatty acids in our diets increases inflammation, coagulation, and the growth of adipose and cancer cells.

Cows are not the only farm animals affected by this change. Chicken diets have changed radically as well. Eggs—the embodiment of a natural food—no longer contain the same essential fatty acids they did fifty years ago. Artemis Simopoulos, MD, is a prominent American nutritionist who ran the department of nutrition research at the National Institutes of Health. In an unusual study published in the *New England Journal of Medicine*, she shows that eggs from chickens raised on corn (a nearly universal practice today) contain twenty times more omega-6s than omega-3s. Eggs taken from the Greek farm she grew up on retain a balance of virtually 1/1.[54]

While their diets have been radically overhauled, farm animals have sometimes been treated with hormones like estradiol and zeranol to fatten them even faster.* These hormones build up in fatty tissues and are excreted in milk. Recently a new hormone has been introduced on cattle farms to stimulate milk production: rBGH (recombinant bovine growth hormone, also called bovine somatotropin, or BST). It acts on the cow's mammary glands

---

* A European law forbids this use in EU countries, but it may be repealed.

and can boost milk production significantly. Widely used in the United States, rBGH is still banned in Europe and Canada. Because of trade agreements, however, this hormone is likely to find its way onto dinner plates anywhere in the world through imported ingredients derived from American milk. The effects of rBGH on humans are still unknown. But we do know it promotes IGF production in cows, that this IGF is found in milk, and that it is not destroyed by pasteurization. As we have seen, IGF is a major factor in the stimulation of growth of fatty cells and also accelerates growth in malignant tumors.

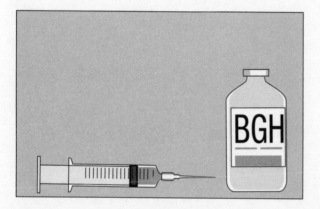

Figure 10. rBGH, the hormone injected into dairy cows in the United States to stimulate milk production. It is found in conventional (nonorganic) milk. It may stimulate the production of insulin growth factor and the growth of cancer cells in humans.

Finally, the switch from grass to the corn-soy combination has another inconvenient side effect. One of the very rare components of our diets that is from an *animal* source and that has possible anticancer benefits is a fatty acid called CLA (conjugated linoleic acid).[55] Among the first to bring to light the role of CLA in fighting the growth of cancer cells was Philippe Bougnoux, MD, and his team at INRA (the National Institute for Agricultural Research in Tours, France).[56, 57] CLA is primarily found in cheese, but only if the cheese comes from grass-fed animals. Thus, by disrupting the diets of cows, goats, and sheep, we have eliminated the only anticancer benefit they might have provided.

Margarine—A Lot More Dangerous Than Butter

The last factor that has changed our diets for the worse since the sixties is the emergence of margarine and "hydrogenated" or "partially hydroge-nated" trans fats. In the fifties, when a connection between animal fats and cardiovascular disease became apparent, many nutritionists and the food industry used their power of persuasion to encourage the use of industrial "vegetable" margarine instead of butter. But they overlooked the fact that these margarines are usually based on sunflower oil (which has seventy times more omega-6s than omega-3s), soybean oil (with seven times more), and canola oil (the least unbalanced, with only three times more omega-6s than omega-3s).* While this change helped lower cholesterol levels, it provoked a sudden rise in inflammatory disorders and even, in some countries, heart attacks. In Israel, for example, religious proscriptions forbid consumption of meat and milk products in the same meal. Thus, butter is virtually excluded, and cooking techniques rely heavily on vegetable margarine (rich in omega-6s) and sunflower oil, which is much cheaper than olive oil. An "Israeli paradox"—distinct from the "American paradox"—has emerged: Israel is marked by one of the *lowest* cholesterol levels in Western countries, combined with one of the *highest* rates of myocardial infarction and obesity.[58]

In Jerusalem, Elliot Berry, MD, professor of nutrition at the Hadassah University, identified the link between cardiovascular disease, obesity, and the high omega-6 levels in Israelis. When Pierre Weill visited him to examine the links between diet and health, Berry, a practicing Jew, assured him with a grin, "You know, I don't believe in much besides God, of course, and the importance of the Omega-6/Omega-3 ratio!"[59]

Processed Food: The Emergence of Trans Fats

We have been won over not just by margarine but also to a large extent by processed foods, such as cookies, crackers, pastries, pizza, or potato chips, containing "hydrogenated" or "partially hydrogenated" vegetable oils (trans fats). These are omega-6 oils (especially soy, sometimes palm or canola oil) altered to become solid at room temperature (whereas these oils are usually fluid, even in the refrigerator). This change makes them both *less* digestible and even *more* inflammatory than omega-6s in their natural state. But these oils have a practical advantage: They do not grow stale.

That's why they are used in almost all the processed foods destined to spend weeks or months on supermarket shelves. Thus, it is for purely industrial and commercial motives that these harmful oils have taken over. They didn't exist before World War II, yet their production and consumption have exploded since 1940.

In its 2004 report, Holland's Ministry of Health estimated that consumption of trans fats leads to over a thousand deaths per year.[60] In comparison,

---

* Omega-3s and omega-6s are better balanced in some newer brands.

880 people died in Holland in 2004 in motor vehicle accidents.[61] Hydrogenated oils are thus *more deadly* than car accidents. As Professor Frits Muskiet, a Dutch public health specialist and medical chemist, says, "We spend millions to force people to wear safety belts and respect speed limits so they can drive safely to the restaurant where they'll stuff themselves with trans fats."

These processed oils have been shown to be linked specifically to cancer. A new study of almost twenty-five thousand European women by the French National Institute for Health and Medical Research confirmed that the risk of breast cancer almost doubles in women who have high levels of trans fats in their blood.[62] This increased risk is at least as significant as the risk associated with postmenopausal hormone replacement therapy.

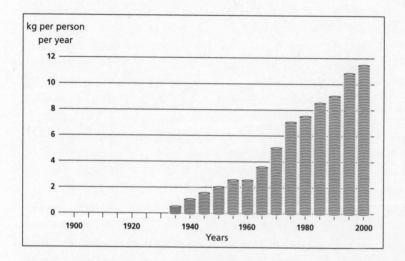

Figure 11. Increase in the production of omega-6 vegetable oils for human consumption in the twentieth century.[63]

Despite the now clearly established risks of trans fats, any food label you read will show you that these oils remain ubiquitous. How about a single serving of a common pepperoni and cheese pizza? It weighs 192 grams (8 ounces) and contains 490 calories—more than a quarter of one person's daily needs—and 39 percent of one person's daily fat allowance. And this in a single serving of a single dish in just one meal. Coming from cheese and from corn-fed pork, these fats are rich in omega-6 fatty acids and deprived of omega-3s. In addition, almost one fifth (4.5 grams) are trans fats. Then come 48 grams (2 ounces) of carbohydrates (one eighth of total recommended daily intake).

This single serving of pizza is not only high in calories, it also contains three times more fat than an ordinary steak. And these fats are among the worst for our health. In recognition of this danger, as of the summer of 2007, trans fats have been banned in restaurants in New York City and Philadelphia, and in January 2010 will be banned in restaurants in California too. They are also banned throughout the food industry in Denmark and Switzerland.

We finally have an explanation for the simultaneous epidemics of cancer and obesity. Changes in our diets over the last half century point to the culprit: a dietary imbalance in the ratio of essential fatty acids leading to the incredible overconsumption of omega-6s, together with the rise in insulin levels due to the higher and higher glycemic index of the modern Western diet. These imbalances are precisely the factors associated with certain cancers, or their dissemination as metastases, as Professor Bougnoux's team in France has shown.[64, 65]

A Simple Gastronomic Solution

The farm animals that feed us are raised under conditions worrisome for both our health and theirs. As Michael Pollan's brilliant investigation of U.S. cattle feedlots showed, they surely suffer still more than we do.[66-68] Amazingly, however, Gérard Ailhaud's research team has succeeded in demonstrating that the levels of omega-6s and omega-3s in the human body can be changed, not by altering our own diets, but by feeding differently the animals that supply our food. They simply need to have a balanced diet too!

Linseed (or "flaxseed"), a plant cultivated since ancient times, was an ingredient in the "Greek bread" Romans ate. It just so happens that linseed is the only seed in the entire plant kingdom that contains more omega-3s than omega-6s—three times more, in fact. When animals eat linseed (after appropriate cooking) it can greatly increase the omega-3 content in meat, butter, cheese, and eggs, even if it represents as little as 5 percent of the feed.[69]

After elucidating the "American paradox," the team started by Gérard Ailhaud, Pierre Weill, and Philippe Guesnet expanded to include more physicians, agronomists, biologists, and statisticians. The team split a group of animals of the same mix of species, raised under the same conditions, into two groups. Group A was fed with the usual "modern" ration of corn, soy, and wheat. Group B was simply fed the "old-fashioned" way: the same way as other animals but with an additional 5 percent of its feed coming from cooked linseed. Next, the team recruited two sets of volunteers. Each set received its meals at home for three months. All volunteers received similar quantities of the same products, but with one set receiving its food from Group A and the other from Group B. After three months, all the participants had blood tests. The volunteers who had received standard Group A products had a very unhealthy omega-3/omega 6 ratio (1/15) that was similar to that observed in all the other studies of the Western diet. In contrast, the ratio in those who had received the Group B (5 percent linseed) products was three times higher (1/5). In three months, the fatty acids in the blood of these Group B volunteers had become comparable to those of the much-vaunted Cretans, whose Mediterranean diet serves as a model of health in nutrition studies. What's reassuring for food lovers is that this result was achieved without restricting the quantity of animal products.[70]

When the experiment was carried out again two years later with diabetic patients who were significantly overweight, the researchers encountered another surprise. Patients fed an "old-fashioned" diet had lost weight—1.3 kilograms (3 pounds) on average—although they had eaten exactly the same quantity of animal products as the other group with its standard fare.[71]

The lesson is simple: When we respect the needs and bodies of the animals that feed us, our own bodies are better balanced. What's even more striking is that our bodies have the ability to sense this balance. The researchers commissioned an independent laboratory to conduct blind taste tests: Fifty volunteers, each in an isolated booth, tasted meat, cheese, and butter that was well balanced in omega-3s and omega-6s, thanks to the animals' diets. The volunteers compared the food they tasted to standard products commonly sold in supermarkets, without, of course, knowing their source. The great majority of the tasters preferred the products from animals that had been fed a healthy, balanced diet.[72] It's as if our taste buds recognize what is good for our bodies' cells and translate this message for us by reacting differently to healthy food.

Detoxifying Food

Dr. Annie Sasco is still puzzled by the mysteries contained in the world cancer map drawn up by WHO: "After all these years of work, we still aren't absolutely certain. But look at the strange case of Brazil," she says. "Its level of development is still low, but its breast cancer rate is as high as the most highly industrialized Western countries. Several of us wonder if this phenomenon isn't the result of their meat consumption—nearly three times a day—and widespread recourse, until recently, to all sorts of hormones to speed up the growth of farm animals."

Clearly, in every country there is a direct connection between the cancer rate and the consumption of meat, cold cuts, and milk products. Conversely, the richer a country's diet in vegetables and legumes (peas, beans, lentils), the lower the cancer rate.

Although studies in animals and epidemiological surveys in humans do not constitute proof, they provide strong suggestive evidence. They suggest that by upsetting the balance in our diets, we have created optimal conditions in our bodies for the development of cancer. If we accept that cancer growth is stimulated to a large extent by toxins from the environment, then in order to combat cancer, we have to begin by detoxifying what we eat.

In the face of this overwhelming body of evidence, here are simple recommendations to slow the spread of cancer:

1. Eat sugar and white flour sparingly. Replace them with agave nectar, acacia honey, or coconut sugar for sweetening and multigrain flour for pastas and breads (or sourdough bread made with traditional leaven).
2. Reduce consumption of red meat and avoid processed pork products. The World Cancer Research Fund recommends limiting consumption to no more than 18 ounces (500 grams) of red meat and pork products every week—in other words, at most four or five steaks. Their ideal recommended goal is 11 ounces (300 grams) or less.[73]
3. Avoid all hydrogenated vegetable fats—"trans fats"—(found in croissants and pastries that are not made with butter) and all animal fats loaded with omega-6s. Olive oil and canola oil are excellent vegetable fats that don't promote inflammation. Butter (not margarine) and cheese that are well balanced in omega-3s may not contribute to inflammation either.

Omega-3s are found in organic products from grass-fed animals or from animals with linseed in their feed. We should systematically favor these lipids to help our bodies fight disease. In doing so, we will also help restore much healthier diets in animals that are part of our own food chain. As a collateral benefit, we will help reduce our dependence on the fields of corn and soy needed for animal feed. Corn and soy use up more water, fertilizers, and herbicides that contaminate the environment than most other crops.[74, 75*]

Finally, to complete a detoxification program, we need to protect ourselves against the second harmful phenomenon linked to the spread of cancer in the West: the buildup of carcinogenic chemicals in our immediate surroundings.

---

* Two thirds of agricultural calories grown on the planet today come from just four crops. Corn and soy are the main two (the other two are wheat and rice).

CAUTION: "Organic" meats or eggs contain few or no pesticides, hormones, and antibiotics, but they are not necessarily balanced in omega-3s. If the animals have simply been fed organic corn and soy but are not grass fed or free range, their meat and eggs remain excessively rich in proinflammatory omega-6s and deficient in omega-3s. To be sure that you're eating products of the same quality as what your grandparents ate, look for labels that specify "grass fed" or "rich in omega-3s." (Information on producers concerned with proper nutrition for animals is available from Web sites such as www.eatwild.com and www.americangrassfed.com, or from European associations grouped under the label "TradiLin.")

PART 3: YOU CAN'T BE HEALTHY ON A SICK PLANET

Polar bears live far from civilization. The broad expanses of snow and ice they need to survive don't lend themselves to urban development or industry. Yet of all the animals in the world, the polar bear is *the most contaminated* by toxic chemicals—to the point where its immune system and reproductive capacities are threatened. This large mammal eats seals and big fish, which in turn live on smaller fish, which eat even smaller fish, plankton, and seaweed.

The pollutants we pour into our rivers and streams all end up in the sea. Many are "persistent," which means that they won't decompose and be assimilated into the biomass of the earth or the oceans. They travel round the planet in a few years' time and accumulate at the bottom of the ocean. They also build up in the bodies of animals that ingest them (they are "bioaccumulative") and have a particular affinity for fats. They are what scientists call "fat soluble"; thus, they are found in animal fat. First they find their way into the fat of small fish, then into the larger fish that have eaten the smaller ones, then into the bodies of animals that eat the big fish. The higher you go in the food chain, the greater the quantity of "POP," or persistent organic pollutants, in animal fat.[76] The polar bear is at the top of a food chain that is contaminated from one end to the other. It is necessarily the most affected by the increasing concentration—the "biomagnification"—of pollutants in the environment.

There is another mammal that reigns at the top of its food chain, a mammal whose habitat is, moreover, distinctly less protected than the polar bear's: the human being.

Daniel Richard is the president of the French section of the largest environmental group in the world, the World Wildlife Fund (WWF). Richard has a passion for nature. For twelve years he has lived in Camargue on the edge of a well-protected natural reserve. When European WWF sections undertook an unusual campaign in 2004 to measure the amount of toxic chemicals people were carrying around in their bodies, he volunteered. He was shocked to find out that his body carried nearly half the substances tested (42 of 109)—almost as many as the polar bears'. Why? "I'm a meat eater," he says. In the same study, thirty-nine members of the European Parliament and fourteen ministers of the environment from several European countries were tested. They were all carrying significant doses of pollutants whose toxicity for humans is well established. Thirteen chemical waste products (phthalates and perfluoro compounds) were systematically detected in *all* the members of parliament. As for the ministers, they revealed traces of, among others, twenty-five identical chemical substances: a flame retardant, two pesticides, and twenty-two PCBs (polychlorinated biphenyls).[77] This pollution is restricted neither to elected officials nor to Europeans. In the United States, researchers at the Centers for Disease Control have identified the presence of 148 toxic chemicals in the blood and urine of Americans of all ages.[78]

Like the leap in sugar consumption and the rapid deterioration in the omega-6/omega-3 ratio, the emergence of these toxic substances in our environment and our bodies is a radically new phenomenon. It, too, dates from the Second World War. The annual production of synthetic chemicals has risen from a million tons in 1930 to two hundred million tons today.[79]

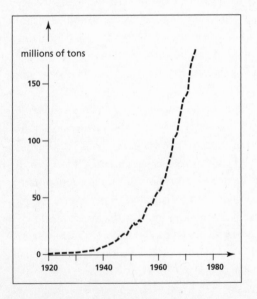

Figure 12. The production of synthetic chemicals, among them pesticides, is a new phenomenon marking the end of the twentieth century.[80]

When these figures were first published in 1979 by Devra Lee Davis, PhD, MPH, a brilliant and outspoken young epidemiologist, she was called a maverick. Courageously, she had entitled her article in *Science* "Cancer and Industrial Chemical Production." This was a topic nobody wanted to hear about, and the article threatened to put an end to her career. But Davis persisted. After the publication of many more articles and two widely influential books,[81, 82] Davis was eventually asked in 2005 to run the world's first Center for Environmental Oncology, created for her at the University of Pittsburgh. Today, the link between cancer and the environment is scarcely questioned anymore.

WHO's International Agency for Research on Cancer keeps a list of carcinogenic substances in the environment. In the past thirty years, it has tested nine hundred potential culprits (a tiny proportion of the over one hundred thousand substances released by industry since 1940, at a rate of several million tons a year).[83] Among these nine hundred products submitted to the IARC—usually by government organizations, medical societies, or consumer associations—*only one* has been recognized as *non*carcinogenic. Ninety-five have been identified as "known carcinogens" (meaning there have been enough epidemiological studies and research on animals to establish cause and effect). Three hundred and seven are "probable" or "possible" carcinogens (meaning studies on animals are convincing, but there has been *no research on humans, or else not enough to prove toxicity*). Four hundred and ninety-seven remain "unclassified" (which doesn't mean that they are safe, merely that their effects have not been sufficiently studied, often for lack of funding).

In many cases, these substances continue to be widely used. This is true of benzene, a known carcinogen found in gasoline, certain plastics, resins and glues, certain lubricants, dyes, detergents, and pesticides.[84] Industrialists defend this practice by arguing that the level consumers are usually exposed to is one hundredth of the toxic dose for animals. Sandra Steingraber, PhD, a biologist specializing in environmental questions, has pointed out that with a little arithmetic this argument becomes less convincing: In 1995 the National Toxicology Program carried out animal trials with four hundred chemicals. This was considered a "representative sample" of seventy-five thousand substances on the market at that time. The researchers' conclusion: 5 percent to 10 percent of the substances tested should be considered carcinogenic for humans. Five percent to 10 percent of the total number means we are regularly exposed to 3,750 to 7,500 carcinogens—so it is not exactly reassuring when we are told that each one may correspond to one hundredth of a toxic dose.[85] Combined, their total toxicity comes to thirty-seven to seventy-five times the dose considered toxic in animals. In Europe, a large group of physicians, researchers, and environmental organizations met at UNESCO and reached the same conclusions. They jointly signed the "Paris Appeal"—organized by Dominique Belpomme, MD, professor of oncology at the Georges Pompidou European Hospital. This document calls for the application of a precautionary principle before introduction of a new and potentially toxic chemical into the environment. It stresses that in devising policies about chemicals, as with many things in life, it is far better to be safe by acting now to reduce harm than to be sorry later for having failed to seek adequate protection. This is a principle that most of us spontaneously apply to ourselves and our children in everyday life, yet it has never been required of the chemical industry.[86, 87]

In 2008, a harshly critical report was presented to the European Parliament. Its author, Professor Andreas Kortenkamp, head of the Centre for Toxicology at the University of London, drew attention to the overwhelming role played by synthetic products—increasingly present in our environment—in the galloping epidemic of breast cancers. He noted that environmental factors have a greater causal impact than genetic predisposition and detailed the pseudoestrogen effect of pesticides and herbicides present in our food, as well as in certain cosmetics. (We'll return to this point.) The report highlighted the disturbing "cocktail effect" produced by the interaction of different substances that seem inoffensive when studied separately and at low doses in the lab but that become quite toxic when combined.[88] Like Professor Belpomme, Professor Kortenkamp wanted government authorities to improve the way they evaluate the toxicity of synthetic products.

Rick Relyea, a biologist from Pittsburgh University, recently provided confirmation of the harmfulness of this cocktail effect.[89] Relyea was surprised that researchers tasked with analyzing the toxicity of thousands of substances released into the environment almost always focus on each substance separately. He set up a protocol that mimicked real-life conditions: an aquatic environment where several species of plankton and tadpoles were exposed to a mixture of various pesticides. The result was devastating. Relyea demonstrated a combined effect that was considerably *more toxic* than the simple exposure to each substance alone. Taken in isolation and at its maximum permitted strength, each pesticide did not have any impact. But even at "acceptable" doses, when ten pesticides were combined they caused the death of 99 percent of the tadpoles.

Chemicals in our Foods

Many cancer-inducing substances accumulate in fat, including those from cigarette smoke—such as the highly toxic benzopyrene additive, one of the most aggressive carcinogenic substances known.[90] Among the cancers that have increased most in the West in the last fifty years are those in tissues that contain or are surrounded by fat: the breast, ovaries, prostate, colon, and lymphatic system.

A number of these cancers are sensitive to hormones circulating in the body. They are called hormono-dependent. That's why they are treated with hormone antagonists—such as tamoxifen for breast cancer or antiandrogens for prostate cancer. How do hormones act on cancer growth? By attaching themselves to certain receptors on the surface of cells, which has the effect of a key opening a lock. If the cells in question are cancerous, the hormone then sets off chain reactions sparking their destructive growth.

Many pollutants in the environment are "hormonal disruptors." This means that their structure imitates the structures of certain human hormones; they can thus get inside the locks and activate them abnormally. Several of them imitate estrogens. Devra Lee Davis named these "xenoestrogens" (from the Greek *xenos* for "stranger").[91] Found within certain herbicides and pesticides, they are attracted to and accumulate in the fat of farm animals. But some xenoestrogens simply come from certain plastics and some by-products of industrial waste disposal we are regularly exposed to. They are even widely found in beauty and household products.[92] (See the list of products to avoid at the end of this chapter.)

The xenoestrogen bisphenol A was the focus of a study published in 2008 by researchers at the University of Cincinnati, who confirmed the chemical's powerful toxicity. Bisphenol A (BPA) is one of the components of PVC (polyvinyl chloride), or hardened plastic. PVC is everywhere: in the inner lining of soda cans, plastic tubs of food, electric kettles, baby bottles, cups, microwavable bowls, and other plastic receptacles that have invaded our kitchens and cafeterias. It can also be found in the lining of many cans of food, particularly ravioli, tuna, green beans, fruit preserved in syrup, soup, and baby food. When PVC plastic is heated or enters into contact with hot liquids or food, it diffuses BPA.[93] This substance has for years been suspected of promoting the progression of certain cancers, and now there is clear proof that it is harmful. The Cincinnati researchers observed that even at very weak concentrations— comparable to those obtained by normal usage of a plastic cup in contact with a hot drink—BPA blocks the effect of several chemotherapy agents on human breast cancer cells. It seems, then, that BPA is a fundamental ally for tumors and makes them resistant to at least part of the arsenal that we use to fight cancer.[94]

Since publication of these studies, the government agency *Health Canada* has decided to ban baby bottles containing BPA and to limit the quantities of BPA discharged into the environment. In the United States, after a report was published by the National Toxicology Program in 2008, similar measures were recommended. However, it seems to me essential that people who suffer from cancer should not wait for government authorities to come to a decision on this point. They should try to avoid food and liquids that have been heated in plastic containers. They should also avoid, whenever possible, all foods from cans containing BPA. Canned food is generally heated to 110° during the sterilizing process, thus causing BPA to diffuse into the food. Personally, I have banned plastic containers for hot foods from my kitchen in favor of glass and ceramic bowls. Note that the problem does not occur to the same degree with plastics that have not been heated—plastic containers and bags kept in the fridge or freezer, for example. Yet it may be safer to avoid liquids that have been in prolonged contact with hard polycarbonate plastics (unfortunately, that includes most spring water "fountains" in office settings, as well as reusable sports bottles), as these have been found to leach BPA over time.[95] The softer plastic used for most mineral and spring water brands is normally made of recyclable polyethylene terephthalate (PET) and does not contain BPA (look for the number "1" on the bottom of the bottle that indicates the bottle is made of PET).

Chemicals find their way into our diets not only from pesticides and containers, but also directly through some industrial foods we eat. In 2008, researchers demonstrated that certain food additives commonly found in our modern diet had a growth-inducing effect on lung cancer in mice. A team from Seoul National University in South Korea focused on inorganic phosphate compounds, widely used in the food industry because they retain water and improve the texture of foods.[96] Mice genetically selected to develop lung cancer were divided into two groups, one fed with a normal diet and the other with a diet rich in phosphate additives. The team, led by Professor Myung-Haing Cho, discovered that after four weeks, tumor growth was much greater in mice who had been fed a diet rich in inorganic phosphates. And the levels of phosphates corresponded to those humans are commonly exposed to when eating a Western diet rich in industrial foods and sodas.

The authors of the study hypothesized that such excessive amounts of phosphates activate genetic pathways that stimulate the development of lung cancer cells. Such abnormal genetic signaling has indeed been linked to the predominant type of lung cancer, known as "non-small-cell" carcinoma.

Within the food industry, the use of phosphate additives has grown exponentially. We currently absorb an average of 1000 milligrams of phosphates every day, compared to 470 milligrams in the 1990s. They can now be found in meat and processed pork products (with preservatives), certain processed cheeses (particularly cheese spreads), processed pastries (the ones from the supermarket rather than the neighborhood bakery), almost all sodas (colas and other fizzy, sweet drinks), fruit syrups, food prepared with evaporated milk (including processed ice creams), and ready-made processed food (frozen pizza and frozen fish sticks in particular).

In the absence of more detailed studies, it seems to me that people who are being treated for non-small-cell lung cancer should avoid processed meats and all products whose listed ingredients include phosphate-based preservatives (calcium phosphate, disodium phosphate, phosphoric acid, sodium triphosphate, tricalcium phosphate, etc.).

In a long-range study of 91,000 nurses over twelve years, the Department of Epidemiology at Harvard showed that the risk of breast cancer in premenopausal women is twice as high in those who eat red meat more than once a day as in those who consume it less than three times a week.[97] The risk of breast cancer could therefore be halved simply by reducing consumption of red meat. In Europe the European Prospective Investigation into Cancer and Nutrition (EPIC), a major study that monitors more than 470,000 people in ten different countries, reached the same conclusion for colon cancer: The risk was twice as high for people who ate large quantities of meat as for those who consumed fewer than 20 grams (an ounce) a day. (With regular consumption of fish—rich in omega-3s—the risk went *down* by 50 percent.)[98]

It's not known whether the risk of eating meat is due to fat-stored organochlorine contaminants in the meat, since compounds used as preservatives in cold cuts are also known carcinogenic substances. Further complicating the picture are xenoestrogenic plastics in which meat is stored and packaged, and also the potential impact of how the meat is cooked. For example, molecules called heterocyclic amines are produced when meat is charred on a barbecue. It is also possible that the risk stems in part from the fact that big meat eaters consume a lot less anticancer food, almost all of which consists of vegetables.

What is already known for certain is that meat and dairy products (as well as large fish at the top of the food chain) furnish over 90 percent of human exposure to known contaminants. These include dioxin, PCBs, and certain pesticides that persist in the environment even though they have been banned for several years.* It is also clear that typical vegetables contain one hundredth the amount of contaminants found in meat and that organic milk is less contaminated than conventional milk.[102, 103]

Pesticides are a major source of environmental toxins. The United States

---

* Experts at the French Agency for Food Safety have shown, for example, that milk sold today contains dioxin and PCBs. Several European studies have shown it may also contain pesticides such as DDT and lindane, still present in the environment despite a ban several years ago.[99–101]

is the world's largest consumer of pesticides, Japan second, Brazil third, and France fourth.[104] Once again, these products were virtually nonexistent before 1930.

The European Union is the principal producer of pesticides in the world, and 72 percent of sales are for use in the EU. These products are not confined to farming and industry. Estimates are that 80 percent to 90 percent of the population is exposed to household pesticides from an average of three or four different products.[105] Like DDT forty years ago, atrazine is a pesticide with such economic benefits that its use was long thought to be an "acceptable" risk for the environment and for humans. But atrazine is also such a powerful xenoestrogen that it is capable of changing the sex of frogs in the rivers it ends up contaminating.[106, 107] Only in 2003, after a number of battles between scientists and industrialists, was atrazine finally forbidden in France and then, in 2006, in the European Union as a whole. It had been massively used in Europe and the United States for more than forty years, since 1962.

A significant number of brain tumors, such as mine, are sensitive to xenoestrogens.[108] A recent study found that wine-country workers who are regularly exposed to pesticides and fungicides have an increased risk of brain tumors.[109] Between 1963 and 1970, from age two to age nine, I played in cornfields sprayed with atrazine surrounding our country house in Normandy. All my life, until the day I was diagnosed with cancer, I drank milk and ate eggs, yogurt, and meat from animals fed with corn sprayed by pesticides. I ate unpeeled apples that had been sprayed fifteen times with pesticides before reaching the grocer's shelves. I drank tap water drawn from contaminated streams and water tables (atrazine isn't eliminated by most water purification systems). My two cousins who have had breast cancer played in those same fields, drank the same water, ate the same food with me in Normandy. We will never know the role atrazine or other agricultural chemicals may have played in our respective cancers. It's true that many other children from this region didn't get sick, but how do you decide whether the risk was "acceptable"?

And Organic Food?

In the Northwest of the United States, between the Pacific shore and a mountain chain, Washington is one of the most beautiful states in the great American West. As often happens when nature's beauty is overwhelming, the inhabitants are also the most progressive. Many organic co-ops and supermarkets flourish around Seattle. A large proportion of the inhabitants choose this food. As in Europe, the products labeled "organic" are grown with natural fertilizers, without chemical pesticides. However, organic foods are often criticized because they are more expensive and still sometimes partially contaminated with pesticides from neighboring fields. Can these foods really reduce our exposure to contaminants?

At the University of Washington, a young researcher, Cynthia Curl, PhD, questioned whether the organic food her friends gave their children was really healthier. She succeeded in organizing a study of forty-two children aged two to five by contacting families as they were leaving either a conventional supermarket or an organic co-op. For three days, the parents had to write down exactly what they gave their children to eat or drink. Their diet was considered "organic" if more than 75 percent of their food was labeled organic, and it was considered "conventional" if more than 75 percent of their food was not. Curl then measured the traces of organochlorine pesticides (the most common kind) in the children's urine. She found that the level of pesticides in the "organic" children's urine was distinctly below the maximum fixed by the Environmental Protection Agency. It was also one sixth that of the "conventional" children. For the children on the conventional diet, the level found was four times higher than the official safety limit.[110, 111] Clearly, organic food made a big difference, since toxicity levels were substantially lower.*

As reported by the *New York Times,* reactions to Curl's results were unfortunately typical. David Klurfeld, PhD, a reputable nutritionist at Wayne State University in Detroit, argued that there was no clear view of the impact of these amounts of pesticide on health: "I'm not saying there is no possible health hazard. But we have to be realistic and that means not to panic over any of this. I would not change any of my or my family's eating habits based on this study."

However, there are specialists who see things in a different light. In the Department of Environmental Studies at Yale, John Wargo, PhD, has been watching the impact of environmental changes on children's health for years. His reaction was just the opposite: "This justifies the importance of an 'organic' diet, and shows that organic foods lower a child's exposure. Industry people are saying 'show me the dead bodies.' I don't want them gambling with my kids that way."

Since then, a second study from the same university has backed up the original findings. Twenty-three children were first tested after following a conventional diet for several days. Their urine showed the presence of pesticides. These same children then consumed organic foods exclusively. In a few days,

---

* In Europe, Claude Aubert, an agronomist often called the godfather of European organic farming, carried out a similar demonstration. In a 1986 study, he showed that women who consumed conventional food during their pregnancy had three times more organochlorine pesticides in their milk than those whose diet during pregnancy was 90 percent "organic."[112]

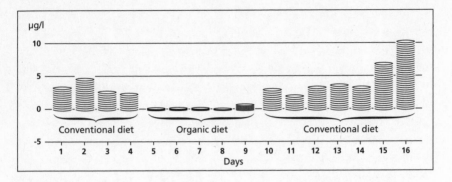

Figure 13. The quantity of organochlorine pesticide in the urine of twenty-three children aged three to eleven while they are given first a conventional diet, then an organic diet, then once again a conventional diet over a period of fifteen consecutive days. The pesticide traces disappeared almost immediately from the urine when they were eating an organic diet (days 5–9).

all traces of pesticides had vanished from their urine. When they resumed a conventional diet, the level of pesticides initially seen in their urine rapidly returned.[113]

Suppose there were a product you could simply sprinkle on a steak, on a fruit, or in a glass of milk. By changing color, a single drop of this product would reveal the presence of pesticides. Overnight, the food industry would have to change its practices radically to meet the most elementary precautionary principle in dealing with the questionable substances introduced in our food since 1940. But these toxic substances are odorless, colorless, and tasteless. Are they "acceptable" simply because they are hidden? Is this a concern only for those of us already affected once by cancer?

When Epidemiologists Will Be "Sure" . . .

Long the territory of green "activists," the connection between cancer and the environment is now a legitimate and active area of research. Alarmed by the data, experts at Inserm (France's medical research council) wrote in 2005: "It is generally recognized that environmental exposure is responsible for the majority of cancers." Tobacco represents around 30 percent of these cases.[114] As for most of the rest, there is no official explanation. Cancer usually takes five to forty years to develop in a human. Often the only available scientific studies were conducted on animals whose lifespan is much shorter. To some members of the scientific community—and their reasoning is legitimate— these animal studies do not provide definite proof that would allow us to blame cancer in humans on recent changes in the environment.

In 2002 in Victoria, Canada, victims of the breast cancer epidemic organized a conference with experts in epidemiology and biology. Dr. Annie Sasco explained her views. During her talk, she lined up, one after the other, the results of her work over twenty-five years as a world-class epidemiologist. Facing all these women seeking an explanation for their disease, she concluded: "If the data strongly suggest a connection between the rise in cancer and environmental change in the last fifty years, we still don't have the irrefutable scientific arguments to affirm a causal link." One of the women in the audience grabbed the microphone: "If we wait for epidemiologists to be sure before we do anything, we'll all be dead!" And Annie Sasco confided she had to agree.

Obstacles to Change

In 1950, 80 percent of Western men smoked tobacco. That habit was considered perfectly inoffensive, even by doctors. In medical journals there were ads for Winston and Marlboro. That year Drs. Evarts Graham and Richard Doll of Oxford University—smokers themselves, like most doctors at the time—showed beyond the shadow of a doubt that tobacco was the direct cause of the steep rise in lung cancer. In men who smoked over a pack a day, the risk was up to thirty times higher!* It took twenty-two years for the British government to pass the first measure against tobacco.† Today cigarette manufacturing, consumption, and exports are still perfectly legal everywhere.

The connection between cancer and animal fats—too rich in omega-6 and loaded with toxic chemicals—is not as firmly established as the link between cancer and tobacco. The increase in risk is about twenty to thirty times for tobacco users.[116, 117] The increase in risk arising from the imbalance and toxicity of animal fats is around 1.5 to 8, depending on the study and the degree of exposure. But in the realm of a life-threatening disease, this is certainly not negligible.

As with tobacco, there are very powerful economic reasons for not wanting to know more. Many politicians believe that pesticides promote agricultural productivity, although there is little hard data to support this belief.[118] Some argue that relying on conventional agricultural chemicals protects the economic activity and jobs in farming areas. It also preserves the interests of

---

* While the discovery of the link between tobacco and lung cancer is usually attributed to Dr. Richard Doll, for the sake of historical accuracy it should be mentioned that Dr. Ernst L. Wynder, a German Jewish epidemiologist who had emigrated to the United States, published a similar study reporting the same conclusions three months earlier in *JAMA*.[115]

† This was the increase in sales tax on cigarettes, decided by Denis Healey, chancellor of the exchequer, in 1972.

the chemical industry. Any changes in farming policy to promote practices that respect nature and human health have obvious, immediate downsides because they require changes in established practices. Thus, such changes require a real policy to support the development of organic farming. As with tobacco, some of the economic benefits stemming from this change, such as a notable reduction in health-care costs, will only be perceived in the long term. But others may be more immediate, such as improvements in water quality and worker health and safety.

In his documentary on global warming, *An Inconvenient Truth,* Al Gore quotes a well-known twentieth-century American journalist, Upton Sinclair: "It's difficult to get someone to understand something when his salary depends upon his not understanding it." We can't expect politicians or industrialists to make hard choices in our stead. The woman who seized the microphone in Victoria was right; if we wait for the epidemiologists to be "sure," we may well die first. On the other hand, we all have the power to take our own precautions. We can choose what we consume. When organic or farm-raised products are not available at our neighborhood grocer, it's often only a matter of asking before they are stocked. And when enough of us ask, prices will drop, as has already happened in a number of markets in the United States where organic prices are close to those of conventional goods.

Cell Phones: Be Careful

The mobile phone is a remarkable device and an instrument of communication that I, for one, would be loath to do without. But recent scientific data suggests that the electromagnetic fields of these little technological jewels are not without danger. True, the vast majority of current epidemiological studies have observed no link between cell phone use and cancer. However, most of these studies have focused on people using their phones for five years or less. In the case of tobacco, there is no effect on lung cancers in people who have smoked a pack a day for five years, or even ten. It takes fifteen or thirty years for the first cancers to appear. And indeed, the few studies that have measured the risks linked to daily use of a cell phone (one hour per day or more) for at least ten years observe that the risk *doubles* that such a person will develop a brain tumor *on the side on which they use their phone.* This is confirmed by the first results (published in 2008) of the massive international INTER-PHONE study. As Dr. Elisabeth Cardis, who coordinated the study, said in a television interview, "When we considered only tumors that developed on the side of the head on which phones were being used, the largest studies in terms of number of users showed an increased risk in long-term users."[119]

To summarize, there is not yet enough scientific proof to demand that preventive measures be taken, as they have been for tobacco or asbestos. But given the available evidence, I advise everyone who uses cell phones to take precautionary measures—particularly people who have cancer and who have every reason to want to reduce factors that may exacerbate their illness.

These are the precautionary measures that I currently advise, and that I use in my own daily life:

1) Except in rare cases, do not let children under twelve use cell phones. Growing organs, in children and in fetuses, are the most sensitive to the effects of electromagnetic fields.

2) During phone calls, try to stay as far as possible from the phone itself. At a distance of four inches (ten centimeters), the amplitude of the electromagnetic field is four times weaker; it is fifty times weaker three feet (one meter) away. As often as you can, use the "speaker" function, a regular headset, or even a Bluetooth headset, which will reduce the electromagnetic emissions of your cell phone by a factor of a hundred.

3) Keep away from people who are using their cell phones and avoid using yours in the subway, train, or bus: You'll be exposing your fellow travelers to the magnetic field of your phone.

4) Avoid keeping a cell phone constantly on your person, even if it is on standby. Do not keep it close to you at night (for example, under the pillow or on your nightstand), especially if you are pregnant. You can choose the "airplane" or "offline" mode, which stops electromagnetic emissions.

5) Restrict your cell phone use to short calls. The biological effects are directly linked to duration of use. And it's better to call back from a corded landline telephone: Cordless phones use microwave technology that is similar to that of cell phones and were recently incriminated in a Swedish study as possibly increasing cancer risk as well.[120]

6) When you use your phone, regularly change the ear you use. And before you put the phone to your ear, wait for the other person to pick up the call: The electromagnetic field will become less powerful.

7) Avoid using your phone when the signal is weak or during rapid travel, as in a train or a car. Because the phone is constantly searching to connect with a transmission antenna, its power output will be at maximum.

8) Use text messages rather than calls. This will limit the duration of exposure and reduce proximity with the body.

9) Choose a phone with the lowest possible SAR. (The "specific absorption rate" measures the level of radio frequencies emitted by the cell phone to the user.) Lists of the SAR levels of various brands of phones are available on a number of Web sites.

In addition to these individual precautions, manufacturers and service providers need to act responsibly. It is their job to provide users with equipment that reduces the risks to their health as much as possible and to constantly develop new technology to permit this. They should also encourage consumers to use their phones in the healthiest possible way.

Three Principles of Detox

When smokers give up tobacco, their risk of cancer drops sharply.[121, 122] If we stop promoting the growth of cancer cells in our bodies, the natural mechanisms of control over cancer can start to intervene and curb their spread.

To protect ourselves against cancer, we can limit our exposure to toxic factors in the environment. Among all those already identified or highly suspicious, I have selected three that seem to me the most deeply involved and the most easily changed:

1. Overconsumption of refined sugar and white flour, which stimulate inflammation and cell growth through insulin and IGF (insulinlike growth factor)
2. Overconsumption of omega-6s in margarine, vegetable oils (including trans fats), and animal fats (meat, dairy products, eggs) stemming from farming methods that have been out of balance since the Second World War
3. Exposure to chemical contaminants that have entered the environment since 1940, which accumulate in animal fats, and—though studies are not yet definitive—exposure to the electromagnetic fields of cell phones

The first two factors listed here are largely to blame for the inflammation that fosters the development of cancer. The first step in any process of detoxification therefore begins by eating a lot less sugar, white flour, and animal fat. Always choose animal products labeled "organic." Nonorganic foods don't have to be eliminated completely, but they should become only occasional foods, not the foundation of our diets. Instead of a steak with a bit of vegetables on the side, we need to imagine a little meat (well balanced in omega-3s) from time to time in a main dish of vegetables. This is the tradition in Mediterranean cooking. Think of Italian antipasti, with lots of vegetables and legumes and a little meat. This is also what the Vietnamese, Indians, and Chinese do, and their rates of cancer are far lower than those in the West.

"Whatever Befalls the Earth Befalls the Sons of the Earth"

If we all adopted this organic, balanced way of eating, we would not only help our bodies detoxify but also help the planet recover its balance. The 2006 United Nations report on food and agriculture concluded that current methods of raising animals for human consumption are one of the major causes of global warming. The contribution of animal farming to the greenhouse effect is *even larger* than that of transportation. Animal farming is responsible for 65 percent of emissions of nitrous oxide, a gas that contributes to global warming 296 times more than CO_2. Methane emitted by cows as a by-product of their poor digestion of corn contributes to warming twenty-three times more than CO_2. Thirty-seven percent of methane in the world comes from cattle. One third of arable land is devoted to growing corn and soy for animal feed. As there is still not enough arable land to meet the demand, forests are cut down, resulting in further reduction of the earth's capacity to absorb carbon dioxide. The UN report also concluded that raising animals is among the activities that harm water resources the most because of the massive dumping of fertilizers, pesticides, and animal excrement into rivers and streams.

An average Indian consumes 5 kilograms (11 pounds) of meat a year and lives in better health than a Westerner of a comparable age. It takes 123 kilograms (270 pounds) of meat a year to satisfy an American—twenty-five times more than that consumed by an Indian.[123, 124] Our modes of production and consumption of animal products are destroying the planet. Everything seems to suggest that they are helping destroy us at the same time.

At the end of every day, I write a few words in a diary to sum up what has given me the most joy. Usually, very simple things are involved. And I'm often surprised to note the pleasure I've felt if I've only eaten vegetables, peas, and fruit (and a little multigrain bread). I notice I've felt more alert and lighter all day long. I'm pleased to think that I weigh a little less on the planet that carries and sustains me.

After twenty years devoted to looking after cancer patients, Michael Lerner had had enough of seeing people aged thirty to forty who should never have participated in his program. Today the program continues, but Michael devotes most of his work to protecting the environment; he wants to prevent disease by getting to the root of the problem. He sums up the situation with simple words: "We can't live healthy on a sick planet."

In 1854, Chief Seattle of the Puget Sound Suquamish tribe solemnly handed over his territory and his people to the sovereignty of the United States. The speech he gave then serves as an inspiration to the ecological movement more than a century later, which has reinterpreted its particularly incisive words. It addresses us—the descendants of those white settlers—in ever more pressing terms:

> Teach your children what we have taught our children, that the earth is our mother. Whatever befalls the earth befalls the sons of the earth. If men spit upon the ground, they spit upon themselves.
> This we know: the earth does not belong to man—man belongs to the earth. This we know. All things are connected like the blood that unites one family. All things are connected.

TABLE 5. SUMMARY OF MAJOR STEPS TO TAKE TO PROTECT OUR EVERYDAY DIETS	
Reduce	**Replace With**
Foods with a high glycemic index (sugar, white flour, etc.) (see table 4 on page 64)	Fruit, flour, and starches with a low glycemic index (see table 4 on page 64)
Hydrogenated or partially hydrogenated (trans fat) oils Sunflower, soy, and corn oil Conventional dairy products (too rich in omega-6) and IGF Fried food, chips, fried appetizers	Olive oil, flaxseed oil, canola (rapeseed) oil Organic, grass-fed dairy products (balanced in omega-6s and omega-3s, free of rBGH), soy milk, soy yogurts* Hummus, olives, cherry tomatoes
Nonorganic red meat and eggs Poultry skin	Vegetables, legumes (peas, beans, lentils), tofu Organic poultry and eggs Organic, grass-fed red meat (maximum 200 grams/7 ounces a week) Fish (mackerel, sardines, salmon, even farmed)
Skins of nonorganic fruits and vegetables (since pesticides cling to their skin)	Fruits and vegetables, peeled or washed, or else labeled "organic"

Reduce	Replace With
Tap water in areas of intensive farming, because of the presence of nitrates and pesticides (A report on water content in nitrates, pesticides, and other contaminants can be obtained from local authorities.)	Improved local tap water Tap water filtered using a carbon filter or, better yet, through reverse osmosis (filter can be installed by kitchen sink) Mineral or spring water provided the plastic bottles haven't warmed up in the sun and the water doesn't smell of plastic, which would reveal the presence of polyvinyl chloride

* See the explanation of soy and breast cancer in chapter 8 (on nutrition and anticancer foods).

TABLE 6. THE MOST CONTAMINATED FRUITS AND VEGETABLES AND THOSE THAT ARE MUCH LESS CONTAMINATED

Most Contaminated (prefer organic)	Less Contaminated (growing methods less important)
Apples, pears, peaches, nectarines, strawberries, cherries, raspberries, grapes	Bananas, oranges, tangerines, pineapple, grapefruit, melons, watermelons, plums, kiwis, blueberries, mangoes, papayas
Peppers, celery, green beans, potatoes, spinach, lettuce, cucumbers, squash, pumpkin	Broccoli, cauliflower, cabbage, mushrooms, asparagus, tomatoes, onions, eggplant, peas, radishes, avocados

(SOURCE: THE ENVIRONMENTAL WORKING GROUP, WWW.FOODNEWS.ORG)[125]

TABLE 7. EVERYDAY HOUSEHOLD PRODUCTS TO AVOID AND TO PREFER	
Avoid as Much as Possible	**Alternatives**
Perchloroethylene/tetrachloroethylene used in dry cleaning	Air out dry-cleaned garments in fresh air for several hours before wearing, or employ wet cleaning, liquid CO_2, or silicone.
Deodorants and antiperspirants containing aluminum (especially for women who shave their armpits, which facilitates penetration of aluminum)	Use natural deodorants without aluminum.
Cosmetics, shampoo, lotions, gels, hair dye, nail polish, sunscreen containing estrogens or placental products (common in hair products for Afro hairstyles) or with parabens or phthalates. Phthalates to avoid include BBP and DEHP.* Parabens to avoid include methylparaben, polyparaben, isoparaben, butylparaben	Use natural and organic products free of parabens, phthalates, and estrogens. Many "organic" cosmetics are free of parabens and phthalates. Some companies, such as Body Shop or Aveda, make products without phthalates.
Perfumes containing phthalates (nearly all of them do)	Wear no perfume, or wear only toilet water (which contains fewer phthalates).
Chemical household pesticides and insecticides	Use pesticides made from essential oils, boric acid, or diatomaceous earth. (See complete list of alternatives to most suspect pesticides and insecticides at www.panna.org.)
Heating foods or liquids (coffee, tea, baby formula) in plastic containers made with PVCs (which are liberated into the food when heated), polystyrene, or Styrofoam	Use glass or ceramic containers (including when using a microwave oven).

Avoid as Much as Possible	Alternatives
Preparing food in scratched Teflon pans	Flawless Teflon, or else non-Teflon pans, such as stainless steel 18/10.
Common cleaning products such as liquid detergents, disinfectants, toilet bowl sanitizers with alkylphenols (nonoxynol, octoxynol, nonylphenol, octylphenol, etc.)	Use "green" or European Ecolabel products, or replace with white vinegar (for counters and floors), baking soda, or white soap.
Excessive exposure to electromagnetic fields of cell phones	Reduced use of cell phones with an air-tube headset.

* BBP = benzyl butyl phthalate; DEHP = di (2-ethylhexyl) phthalate.

CHAPTER 7

Lessons of a Relapse

I t was a few years after my first operation, and everything seemed to be back to normal. One afternoon I was having tea with one of the few friends who knew about my illness. We were talking about the future, when she said to me hesitatingly, "David, I have to ask you—what are you doing to treat your 'terrain'?" She knew I didn't share her enthusiasm for herbal medicine and homeopathy. To me, this concept of "terrain"—which I'd never heard of in medical school—was outside the confines of scientific medicine. I wasn't interested in it in the least. I told her that I had been very well looked after and nothing remained to be done other than hope that the tumor didn't return. And I changed the subject.

I remember my diet then. To save time at the hospital, I had learned to make do at lunchtime with a main course that could be easily eaten during a lecture or even in an elevator. I lunched almost daily on chili con carne, a plain bagel, and a can of Coke—an assortment that, in retrospect, strikes me as an explosive combination of white flour and sugar, together with animal fats loaded with omega-6s, hormones, and environmental toxins. Like most people who have had a first alert with cancer and who have pulled through, I chose to treat my illness like a bout of pneumonia or a broken bone. I had done what I had to, and it was already a thing of the past. Caught up in my work and the birth of my son, I had greatly reduced my physical exercise. I had also dropped my passing interest in meditation, originally aroused by reading Carl Jung. I had never considered the idea that if I'd had a cancer, it was probably because something in my "terrain" had enabled it to develop, and I needed to take charge of myself to limit the risk of a relapse.

Some months later, I accompanied a patient to a Native American cere- mony bringing together her family and close friends. A "medicine man" called on spirits to help her get through her illness. This shaman struck me as particu- larly humane, sincere, and sensitive. He found very simple words to describe each participant and get this patient to feel how much each of them contrib- uted to her desire to live and thus to her health. I didn't have the slightest doubt the shaman had, by his presence alone, an extraordinary therapeutic effect.

I was intrigued by the mysterious powers attributed to this man. After the ceremony I asked him to touch my skull and tell me if he felt something. He put his hand gently on my head, shut his eyes a few seconds, and then said, "There may have been something there, but it's gone. There is nothing left now." His words didn't impress me much. After all, I knew there was nothing left, because my annual exams had once again come up with normal results. He may well have detected that confidence in my attitude. But he added with a little mischief in his eyes: "You know, people always want to see me, but the real medicine man here is my mother."

The next day we went to see his mother. She was ninety years old, slight and frail. A tiny woman, she came up to my chin. Surprisingly sprightly for her age, she lived alone in a trailer. Her face was lined with wrinkles and she was practically toothless. But as soon as she smiled, her penetrating eyes seemed to light up with remarkable youth. She in turn put her hand on my head and concentrated for a moment. She said, smiling, "There is something amiss here. You've had something serious and it's come back. But don't worry, you'll be just fine." Then she said she was tired and ended the visit.

I didn't attach much importance to that divination. I was much more prone to trust the results of the scan from three months earlier. Still, something in me must have been sensitive to her warning, because I didn't wait as long as usual to have another examination. I found out then that the old medicine woman had been right: My cancer had come back, in exactly the same spot.

Finding out you have cancer is a shock. You feel betrayed by life and by your own body. But finding out you've had a relapse is crushing. It's as if you've suddenly discovered that the monster you thought you'd distanced was still there. It had gone on tracking you in the shadows and wound up catching you again. Would there never be a respite, then? After canceling my afternoon appointments, I set out on a walk alone. My head was buzzing. I still remember the tumult that gripped me. I would have liked to talk to God. But I didn't believe in him. I finally managed to concentrate on my breathing, calm the turmoil in my thoughts, and turn inward. In the end, it was a form of prayer: "O my body, my being, my life force, speak to me! Help me sense what's happening to you. Help me understand why you couldn't cope. Tell me what you need. Tell me what nourishes you, strengthens and protects you. Tell me how we are going to make our way together, because alone, with my head, I haven't succeeded, and I don't know what to do anymore." After a while, I found strength and took heart, ready, once again, to make the rounds of medical opinions.

Patients are often surprised that the different physicians they consult can recommend such different treatments. But cancer takes such extraordinarily different shapes that medicine strives to multiply the angles of attack. Faced with this complexity, each physician falls back on the approaches he or she has mastered best and has come to trust. As a result, physicians I know would never entrust themselves or a member of their family to the first advice that comes along; they would try to get the opinions of at least two or three colleagues. Depending on the medical culture they belong to, doctors differ substantially as to their preferred treatments. In the United States, for example, it was long thought that all breast cancers required an extensive operation consisting of removing not only the entire breast, but also the lymph nodes on the affected side and even muscles that help shape the armpit. This technique seemed indispensable to prevent a relapse. During the same period, French and Italian surgeons had begun to practice lumpectomies followed by radiotherapy, which involves removing the tumor in such a way that the rest of the breast and the body remain intact.[1] It turned out later that the results were exactly the same in the long term, with much less physical and psychological damage inflicted by the European approach.[2]

As is often the case with cancer, the surgeon I consulted told me an operation would be best, the radiologist said radiation would be a good approach, and the oncologist advised me to consider chemotherapy. There was also the option of various combinations of these treatments. But all of them had serious drawbacks.

Surgery required cutting into a broad swath of healthy tissue so as to leave as few cancer cells as possible—there are always some left behind with this type of cancer. With radiotherapy of the brain, there was a risk—small but significant—of developing dementia ten to fifteen years later. When chances of recovery are very poor, this is an option that one can often resign oneself to. But I preferred to count on a much longer survival. One of the most brilliant neuroscientists I had worked with had developed dementia some years after radiotherapy for a brain tumor that wasn't even malignant. The probability had been very slight, but he was unlucky. I didn't want to end up like him. As for chemotherapy, it is, by definition, a poison. Chemotherapy first kills the cells that reproduce rapidly—that is to say, cancer cells—but it also kills intestinal and immune cells, as well as hair follicles. It can also lead to sterility. I didn't find anything enticing in the thought of living with this poison in my body for several months. All the more so because there was no guarantee of success, given the unfortunate tendency of brain tumors to rapidly become resistant to chemotherapy.

Naturally, I received a lot of advice about "alternative" treatments that seemed too good to be true. Still, I understood how tempting it was to believe in the possibility of a complete cure while avoiding harsh treatments and their side effects.

AVOIDING CHARLATANS

There are a few simple rules to avoiding traps and charlatans. Avoid practitioners who:
- refuse to work in collaboration with an oncologist and recommend stopping conventional treatments
- suggest a treatment whose effectiveness has not been proven but that has proven risks
- suggest a treatment whose price is out of proportion to expected benefits
- promise that their approach is guaranteed to work, as long as you have a true desire to heal

---

Like most patients, the more information I got, the more confused I felt. Every physician who examined me, every scientific article I read, every Web site I looked at provided serious, convincing arguments in support of this or that approach. How could I choose? It was only by retreating into the depths of my inner self that I wound up "sensing" what sounded right for me. I decided against a state-of-the-art technique in which the surgeon's movements were computer guided. The surgeon who proposed it to me only talked about technology and seemed more interested in his robot than in my fears, doubts, and hopes. I preferred a surgeon whose direct gaze and warmhearted presence I liked. I felt cared for even before he examined me. This takes very little—a smile, a certain intonation, a few words. I liked what he said to me: "You never know what you're going to find inside, and I can't promise you anything. The only thing I can assure you of is I'll do everything in my power." And I felt it was sincere; he would do everything he could. That was the faith I needed. More than a state-of-the-art robot.

Finally, I decided to do a year of chemotherapy following the operation, to eliminate as many cancer cells as possible. It was at this point that I immersed myself in the scientific literature to try to overcome the statistics confronting me. This time I had gotten the message: I was going to have to look after my "terrain" seriously.

CHAPTER 8

The Anticancer Foods

PART 1: THE NEW NUTRITIONAL MEDICINE
The Tibetan Principle

My vision of medicine began to change in the streets of Dharamsala, the seat of the Dalai Lama's government in exile in India. During a humanitarian mission on behalf of Tibetan orphans, I learned that there were two health-care systems in Dharamsala. The first one was centered in the Dalac Hospital, a modern Western hospital with a surgery department, the usual apparatus for radiography and ultrasound examinations, and conventional medications. Around this hospital, physicians trained in Western medicine in India, Great Britain, and the United States had their private practices. In our discussions, we referred to the same textbooks I had used in medical school. We spoke the same language and understood each other perfectly.

But in the same city, there was a medical school that taught traditional Tibetan medicine, a factory for Tibetan plant remedies, and Tibetan doctors who treated their patients with totally different methods from those I knew. They examined bodies the way we look at garden soil. They didn't look for symptoms of disease, which are often obvious. Rather, they looked for failures in the terrain, for what the body needed to defend itself against disease. They wanted to understand how that particular body, that soil, should be reinforced so that it could, on its own, confront the problem that had led the patient to seek help.

I had never considered disease that way, and this approach threw me off. All the more so because to "strengthen" the body, my Tibetan colleagues called on remedies that to me seemed perfectly esoteric and probably ineffective. They talked about acupuncture, meditation, and herbal infusions, and a great deal about correcting diets. According to my system of reference, it was obvious that none of that could really be effective. At the most, these remedies could give patients a bit of comfort and something to keep them busy while lulling them into thinking they were doing themselves some good.

I wondered what I would have done if I had been Tibetan and had fallen ill. Given two parallel health systems, which one would I choose? While in Dharamsala, I put this question to everyone I worked with or had occasion to meet. I asked the minister of health, who had invited me there, and the Dalai Lama's brother, at whose home I stayed, and I asked the great lama physicians I was introduced to. I talked about it with ordinary people I encountered as I moved around the city on foot. I thought I was confronting them with a dilemma: Would they choose Western medicine—modern and effective—or their own ancient medicine, out of fondness for their tradition?

They looked at me as though I had asked an idiotic question. "But it's obvious," they invariably answered. "If it's an acute illness, like pneumonia or an infarction or appendicitis, you have to see Western doctors. They have fast, effective treatments for crises and accidents. But if it's a chronic disease, then you should see a Tibetan doctor. The treatments take longer to work, but they treat the terrain in depth. In the long term it's the only thing that really works."

And cancer? It is estimated that it takes five to forty years for a cancer cell to become a dangerous tumor. Is it an acute illness or a chronic disease? What do we do in the West to "treat the terrain"?

Fifty Researchers and "Nutraceuticals"

Richard Béliveau, PhD, a researcher in biochemistry and professor at the University of Montreal, runs one of the largest laboratories for molecular medicine in the world specializing in cancer biology. Over the past twenty years, he has worked with major pharmaceutical groups such as AstraZeneca, Novartis, Sandoz, Wyeth, and Merck to identify the mechanisms that make anticancer medicines work. The goal in understanding these mechanisms is to develop new medications with fewer side effects. Béliveau and his team focused on biochemical questions light-years away from the daily concerns of those who suffer from the disease. One day his laboratory moved to new premises, within the children's hospital of the University of Montreal. There, everything changed.

His new neighbor, the head of the Department of Hemo-oncology, asked him to look for complementary approaches capable of reducing the toxicity and improving the efficacy of chemotherapy and radiotherapy. "I am open to anything you can find to help us care for our children," he told Béliveau. "Anything than can be combined with existing treatments. Even if it were to involve diet."

Diet? The concept was foreign to the medical pharmacology that Béliveau had practiced for twenty years. But since his move, every day on his way to his laboratory, he walked through the department caring for children with leukemia. Parents often stopped him in the corridor and asked, "Is there something else we can do for our daughter? Something new that could be tried? We're ready to do anything for our child." The hardest part was being stopped by the children themselves with the same questions. He was profoundly shaken, and his mind was in turmoil. In the middle of the night he would get up with a new idea. Once he was more fully awake, he would realize it wasn't worth very much. The next day he would go back to combing through the scientific literature in search of a trail to follow. This is how he came across a revolutionary article one day, published in the prestigious journal *Nature*.

For some years, the entire pharmaceutical industry had been searching for new, synthetic molecules capable of blocking the development of the new blood vessels that tumors need to grow (see chapter 4 on angiogenesis). In this article, Yihai Cao, PhD, and Renhai Cao, PhD, two researchers at the Karolinska Institute in Stockholm, demonstrated for the first time that food as ordinary as tea (after water, the most widely consumed beverage in the world) was capable of blocking angiogenesis, using the same mechanisms as existing medications. Two or three cups of green tea a day were enough.[1]

The idea seemed brilliant to him. It meant searching in the realm of nutrition, of course! All the data in epidemiology actually confirmed it. The principal difference between populations with the highest cancer rates and those with the lowest was their food. When Asians developed breast or prostate cancer, their tumors were usually much less aggressive than a Westerner's. In fact, wherever green tea was drunk abundantly there was a lower incidence of cancer. For the first time, Béliveau wondered whether chemical molecules contained in certain foods were powerful anticancer agents. On top of that, with more than five thousand years of human experimentation, these foods would have already proven that they were harmless. He had finally hit on something that could be offered to children without exposing them to the slightest risk: anticancer foods or, as Béliveau liked to call them, nutraceuticals.

The laboratory of molecular medicine at the Sainte-Justine Children's Hospital in Montreal was one of the best equipped to analyze the effects of various molecules on cancer cell growth and on the angiogenesis of blood vessels needed to feed them. If Béliveau now decided to turn over his team of fifty researchers and twenty million dollars' worth of equipment to the search for anticancer foods, substantial progress could rapidly be made. But it was a risky decision. Given that there were no possible patents from foods, and therefore no real financial payoff, who would pay for all the research? Without more tangible proof of the validity of this approach, it didn't seem economically reasonable to pursue such a venture. It was life itself that led Béliveau to take the leap that no other laboratory in the world had yet risked.

A Cancer Without Disease

One Thursday evening, Richard Béliveau received a desperate call about a friend with a serious cancer of the pancreas. Lenny lived in New York. At Memorial Sloan-Kettering Hospital—one of the major cancer centers in the United States—Lenny had been told that he had only a few more months to live. Cancer of the pancreas is, in fact, one of the most ominous types of cancer.

Lenny was like a character out of a novel. A large man with a booming laugh and legendary fits of anger, he had always loved poker and gambling. He had been dealt a bad hand, but once more he was going to try his luck up to the end. Did Béliveau have anything to suggest? Lenny was ready to go to the ends of the earth to participate in any experimental protocol his friend might recommend.

On the telephone, Lenny's wife could hardly speak. She mumbled about having been together for thirty-two years, about having never been apart. She could not imagine that it was going to end like that, so suddenly. She pleaded for a little bit of time.

Béliveau had the medical file faxed to him, and the next morning he went through international databases for the most recent research trials. But there were very few on cancer of the pancreas, and the existing ones did not take patients at such an advanced stage. Heavyhearted, he called back Lenny's wife the same evening to announce his failure. She was in tears. She said she had heard about his interest in food and cancer. She was going to care for Lenny "from A to Z, every day till the end," she said. He would do anything she told him to, and if Béliveau had any suggestions, they'd try them all. They had nothing to lose.

There was indeed nothing to lose. If his ideas were right, this was the moment to give someone in need a chance to benefit from them. Throughout the weekend, Béliveau went over the Medline database.* He gathered articles from wide-ranging sources about foods that had a demonstrated effect in fighting cancer. He calculated concentrations of phytochemicals that could be obtained with quantities used in cooking, evaluated their assimilation by the intestine and their bioavailability to tissue. After two days of intense work, he produced a first list of "foods that fight cancer," on which he would later base a book.[2, 3] The list included, among other things, various kinds of cabbage, broccoli, garlic, soy, green tea, turmeric, raspberries, blueberries, and dark chocolate. That Sunday night, he called Lenny's wife to give her the list,

---

* A computerized archive of all medical articles published worldwide, organized by the National Library of Medicine in Washington, D.C.

along with key instructions: "Cancer is like diabetes. You must look after it every day. You have a few months; foods from this list must be eaten at every meal over that period with no exceptions. They are not to be eaten only occasionally. You must not depart from this list." He also told her that all fats except olive, canola, or flaxseed oil were proscribed, so as to avoid inflammation-promoting omega-6s. He recommended some Japanese recipes he knew and particularly liked. Lenny's wife took notes and promised to prepare these every day. It was the one hope she could cling to.

In the beginning she called often. She scrupulously did what she had promised, but she was frightened. Over the telephone she still wept, "I don't want to lose him. . . . I don't want to lose him. . . . " After two weeks, her voice changed. "It's the first time he's gotten up in the last four months," she announced. "Today he ate with a good appetite." Day after day, the improvement was confirmed: "He's feeling better. . . . He's walking. . . . He went out. . . . " Béliveau couldn't believe his ears. After all, it was cancer of the pancreas, a cancer that strikes like lightning, one of the most aggressive. But there was no doubt that something was changing in Lenny's exhausted body.

Lenny survived four and a half years. For a long time, his tumor was stable and even regressed by almost a quarter. He went back to his usual occupations and to his travels. His oncologist in New York said he had never seen anything like it. For a while it was as if Lenny carried around his cancer without being sick, though his body eventually succumbed. When Béliveau tells the story, he almost blushes. "It was the first time that I'd made this sort of recommendation. Obviously, it was a single case. It was impossible to draw any conclusions. But all the same . . . what if it were possible?"

For a researcher who had devoted his life to the biology of chemotherapy, it was a shock. But, in fact, what's to prevent us from eating better during chemotherapy or afterward? There is no drawback to eating this way. After the experience with Lenny, Béliveau continued to wake up in the middle of the night. "What shall I do with this?" he wondered. "Do I have the right to overlook such an important contribution to public health? Is it acceptable *not* to explore this dietary approach systematically, scientifically?" Eventually came the moment when he decided to launch his laboratory on the largest research program ever undertaken on the biochemical effects of anticancer foods. Since then, the results are such that they have drastically changed ideas on the best methods of protection against cancer. Here is how.

The Seed and the Soil

T. Colin Campbell, PhD, a professor at Cornell University, is the author of the most far-ranging study ever carried out on the link between cancer and dietary habits. He spent his childhood on a farm, and perhaps his knowledge of the land has been useful, because he described the relationship between diet and the development of cancer in a particularly compelling way.[4] He compared the three stages of tumor growth—initiation, promotion, and progression—to the growth of weeds. *Initiation* is the phase when a seed settles in the soil. *Promotion* is the phase when the seed becomes a plant. *Progression* is the phase when the plant becomes a weed, developing beyond control, invading flower beds and garden paths, growing right up to the sidewalk. A plant that doesn't spread is not a weed.*

Initiation—the presence of a potentially dangerous seed—depends largely on our genes and toxins in our environment (radiation, carcinogenic chemicals, etc.). But the seed's growth (promotion) depends on the existence of the indispensable conditions for its survival: favorable soil, water, and sun.

In the book Campbell devoted to his thirty-five years of experimentation on the role of nutritional factors in cancer, he concluded: "Promotion is reversible, depending on whether the early cancer growth is given the right conditions in which to grow. This is where dietary factors are so important. These dietary factors, called promoters, feed cancer growth. Other dietary factors, called anti-promoters, slow cancer growth. Cancer flourishes when there are more promoters than anti-promoters. Cancer growth slows or stops when the anti-promoters prevail. It's a push-pull process. The profound importance of this reversibility cannot be overemphasized."[5]

Even when the nutritional conditions for maximum promotion are present—as is the case in Western diets—it is thought that fewer than one cancerous cell out of ten thousand manages to become a tumor capable of invading tissues.[6, 7] By acting on the soil in which these cancer seeds are deposited, it is thus possible to considerably reduce their chances of developing. This is probably what happens with Asians, who carry as many microtumors as Westerners in their bodies, but whose microtumors don't become aggressive, cancerous growths. As in an organic garden, we can learn to control weeds by controlling the mix of the soil: limiting what feeds them—the "promoters"—and abundantly supplying the nutrients that stop them from growing—"the antipromoters."

This is exactly what the great English surgeon Stephen Paget understood. In *The Lancet* in 1889 he published an article describing his hypothesis, which

---

* This is likewise true for tumors. Beauty spots, for example, are tumors. They can appear, grow, or go away, but they act in a civilized way. They do not invade neighboring tissue beyond a few millimeters (1/10 inch), and they never spread to other organs or areas of the body. They are not "weeds" and, like flowers, they even have an aesthetic value.

is still considered authoritative 120 years later. The name he gave it is worthy of an Aesop fable: "the seed and soil hypothesis."[8]

A century later in the journal *Nature,* researchers at the Cancer Research Institute of the University of California at San Francisco showed the pertinence of that idea, and with respect to very aggressive cancer cells. If the tumor's environment is deprived of the inflammatory factors needed for its growth, it will not succeed in spreading.[9] The fact is that these inflammatory factors, these fertilizers for cancer, are provided directly by our diet. Major dietary fertilizers are refined sugars, which drive up proinflammatory insulin and IGF; insufficient amounts of omega-3s and the corresponding excess of omega-6s, which change into inflammatory molecules; and growth hormones (present in meat and nonorganic dairy products), which also stimulate IGF. Conversely, diet may also furnish "antipromoters," such as all the phytochemical components of some vegetables or particular fruits, which directly counterbalance inflammatory mechanisms (see below).

When Richard Béliveau talks about Western diets in light of these findings, he is distressed. "With all I've learned over these years of research, if I were asked to design a diet today that *promoted* the development of cancer to the maximum, I couldn't improve on our present diet!"

Foods That Act Like Medications

If certain foods in our diet can act as fertilizers for tumors, others, to the contrary, harbor precious anticancer molecules. As recent discoveries show, these go far beyond the usual vitamins, minerals, and antioxidants.

In nature, when confronted with aggression, vegetables can neither fight nor flee. To survive, they must be armed with powerful molecules capable of defending them against bacteria, insects, and bad weather. These molecules are phytochemical compounds with antimicrobial, antifungal, and insecticide properties that act on the biological mechanisms of potential aggressors. They also have antioxidant properties that protect the plant's cells from dampness and the sun's rays (by preventing cellular "rust" from forming when the cell's fragile mechanisms are exposed to the corrosive effects of oxygen).

Green Tea Blocks Tissue Invasion and Angiogenesis

Green tea, for example, which grows in particularly humid climates, contains numerous polyphenols called catechins. One of these, epigallocatechin gallate or EGCG, is one of the most powerful nutritional molecules against the formation of new blood vessels by cancerous cells. It is destroyed during the fermentation required to make black tea but is found in large quantities in tea that hasn't undergone fermentation and thus remains "green." After two or three cups of green tea, EGCG is plentiful in the blood. It spreads throughout the body by means of capillary vessels. They surround and feed every cell in the body. EGCG settles on the surface of each cell and blocks the switches (the "receptors") whose function is to set off the signal that allows the penetration of neighboring tissue by foreign cells, such as cancer cells.[10] EGCG is also capable of blocking receptors that issue commands for the creation of new vessels.[11] Once the receptors are blocked by EGCG molecules, they no longer respond to the orders that cancer cells send through inflammation factors to invade tissue and to make the new vessels needed for tumor growth.

In their molecular medicine laboratory in Montreal, Richard Béliveau and his team tested the effects of EGCG isolated from green tea on several lines of cancer cells. They observed that it substantially slowed the growth of leukemia and breast, prostate, kidney, skin, and mouth cancer.[12]

Green tea also acts as a detoxifier for the body. It activates mechanisms in the liver that can then eliminate cancerous toxins from the body more rapidly. In mice, it has been shown to block the effects of chemical carcinogens responsible for breast, lung, esophageal, stomach, and colon cancer.[13]

Finally, the effect of EGCG is still more striking when it is combined with other molecules commonly found in Asian diets—for example, soy. The Laboratory of Nutrition and Metabolism at Harvard has shown that, when taken together, the combination of green tea and soy enhances the protective effects observed when each is taken separately. This is true for both prostate and breast cancer.[14, 15] In the conclusion of their article, the researchers wrote: "Our study suggests that soy phytochemicals plus green tea may be used as a potentially effective dietary regimen for inhibiting progression of estrogen dependent breast cancer." In the extremely cautious language that characterizes scientific articles on cancer (not to mention the reserved style of Harvard researchers) these words are highly significant.

HOW MANY CUPS OF GREEN TEA PER DAY?

This question is answered by two studies on patients in Japan, a country full of green tea drinkers. In a group of Japanese women suffering from breast tumors that had not yet metastasized, researchers discovered that those who consumed three cups of green tea a day had 57 percent fewer relapses than those who only drank one cup a day.[16] In men with prostate tumors, daily consumption of five cups of green tea reduced the risk that their cancer would progress to an advanced stage by 50 percent.[17] The effect of green tea is quite remarkable. So why deprive ourselves?

Is Olive Oil the Green Tea of the Mediterranean Diet?

Everyone has heard of the beneficial effects of the "Mediterranean diet." Epidemiological studies have shown that people who follow a Mediterranean diet are, on average, far less affected by degenerative illness, cardiac disease, and cancer, despite the significant presence of fats in their diet.[18-20] For a long time, the benefits of this diet were attributed to its combination of fiber, fish, fruit, and vegetables whose antioxidant potential and wealth of anticancer phytochemical agents have been demonstrated. Recently, researchers have realized that a determining factor in the etiology of some cancers is not only the quantity, but also the *type* of fats consumed. It's now time to pay closer attention to a central ingredient in Mediterranean cooking: olives, and the oil that we extract from them.

A study directed by Dr. Robert Owen of the German Cancer Research Center in Heidelberg has demonstrated that olives contain an abundance of antioxidants such as acteosides, hydroxytyrosol, tyrosol, and phenylpropionic acids.[21] The direct effect of such molecules is to limit the initial development of cancer.

Particularly when it is *virgin*, olive oil also contains secoiridoids and lignans, both known antioxidants that have been linked with slower progression of cancer.

Since all these chemicals are fat soluble, they are absorbed into fatty tissues, with a resulting known protective effect against breast cancer,[22] colon cancer,[23] and uterine cancer.[24]

At the Catalan Oncology Institute, another group of researchers analyzed the effects of chemical agents contained in olive oil on certain genes.[25, 26] These Spanish researchers demonstrated that polyphenols and oleic acid can inhibit expression of the HER2 gene, which has been implicated in close to one fifth of breast cancers. The researchers emphasize, however, that to obtain this result, we would have to ingest olive oil in quantities difficult to achieve through normal consumption. I do not recommend using olive oil to replace Herceptin, a medication that is very effective in inhibiting the HER2 gene. On the other hand, I do recommend olive oil as part of a daily diet because continuous consumption over the course of months or years may have a small daily effect on these genes. In synergy with all the other foods in the Mediterranean diet, olive oil may contribute to slowing the progression of cancer. It is also possible that consumption of olive oil by women taking Herceptin may increase the efficacy of the medication.

Soy Blocks Dangerous Hormones

Soy, too, contains powerful phytochemical molecules that counteract the mechanisms essential to the survival and spread of cancer. These are the soy isoflavones—especially genistein, daidzein, and glycitein. They are called phytoestrogens because they are very similar to female estrogens. The abundance of natural and chemical estrogens in Western women is known to be one of the causes of the breast cancer epidemic.[27] This is why today hormone replacement therapy is prescribed to postmenopausal women only with great caution: It is associated with an increased risk of breast cancer.* Soy phytoestrogens are only *one hundredth* as biologically active as natural female estrogens. They act along the same lines as tamoxifen—a drug commonly used to prevent relapses in breast cancer. Their presence in the blood substantially lowers overstimulation of the body by estrogens and, as a consequence, *may slow* the growth of estrogen-dependent tumors. However, the protective action of soy against breast cancer has been formally demonstrated only for women who have consumed it since adolescence. Its protective effect against cancer has not been proven where consumption begins in adulthood. As one of the soy isoflavones, genistein, closely resembles male hormones that stimulate the growth of prostate cancers, the same protective mechanism is likewise at work in men who consume soy regularly.

Some breast cancer patients have been advised *not* to consume soy-based products. In reality, the consensus in the scientific literature on this subject suggests that there is no dangerous effect from soy in breast cancer, aside from in certain experiments with dietary supplements in high doses, which are not advisable. It seems that soy consumed regularly (every day) may reduce the dangerous effects of xenoestrogens, especially when the soy is part of a diet rich in anticancer ingredients (green tea, cruciferous vegetables, etc.) and is in normal quantities for food (avoid isoflavone supplements). While awaiting more specific scientific data, the French Agency for Food Safety (AFSSA) recommends that women who have had breast cancer restrict their consumption of soy to moderate amounts (no more than one soy yogurt or one glass of soy milk a day).[29] On the other hand, *concentrated extracts* of isoflavones sold as dietary supplements for use during menopause have been suspected of promoting tumor growth and should be avoided.

---

* In the United States, the breast cancer rate has *declined* for the first time in several years, and this followed a sharp reduction in prescriptions for hormone treatments in the preceding three years.[28]

Moreover, like EGCG in green tea, soy isoflavones also block angiogenesis. They thus play an important role in fighting a number of other cancers besides breast and prostate cancer. Different forms of soy (tofu, tempeh, miso, edamame, etc.) are therefore likely to be a useful part of an anticancer diet.

Turmeric Is a Powerful Antiinflammatory

Another remarkable culinary compound that is particularly effective also comes from Asia. This time it is a spice with astonishing properties—turmeric.

Indians consume on average 1.5 to 2 grams (1/4 to 1/2 teaspoon) a day of turmeric. The turmeric root yields a yellow powder that is the principal spice in yellow curry. It is also one of the most common ingredients used in ayurvedic medicine for its antiinflammatory properties. No other food ingredient has such a powerful antiinflammatory effect. The principal molecule responsible for that effect is curcumin. In the laboratory, curcumin inhibits growth in a large number of cancers: colon, prostate, lung, liver, stomach, breast, ovarian, brain, and leukemia, for example. It also inhibits angiogenesis and forces cancer cells to die (through the process of cell suicide known as apoptosis). In mice, curcumin prevents the development of several types of tumors caused by chemical carcinogens.[30] Additionally, curcumin inhibits the growth of human tumors when implanted in mice.

Perhaps, then, it's not surprising that Indians have one eighth as many lung cancers as Westerners of the same age, one ninth as many colon cancers, one fifth as many breast cancers, one tenth as many kidney cancers, and one fiftieth our rate of prostate cancer.[31] This is true despite Indians' exposure to numerous carcinogens in their environment, often on a worse scale than in the West.

At the M. D. Anderson Cancer Center in Houston, Professor Bharat Bhushan Aggarwal, PhD, is considered a brilliant iconoclast. One of the most cited cancer researchers in the world,[32] he is head of a section of the laboratory working on experimental cancer therapies. Like Béliveau in Montreal, his preeminence in biochemistry and pharmacology has not prevented him from keeping an open mind to anything that may help fight cancer. During Aggarwal's youth in Batala in Punjab, ayurvedic plant medicine was "the only medicine we had," he says. He has never forgotten just how effective it was.

After completing his PhD at the University of California at Berkeley, he was among the first biologists hired by Genentech, a famous genetic engineering firm, to identify new molecular treatments for cancer. In the eighties at Genentech, he discovered the role of inflammatory factors in the development of tumors, through the activation of the notorious NF-kappa B. Later he wrote that controlling the harmful effects of NF-kappa B in cancer is a "question of life or death."[33] Since then, he has continued to hunt for the means to counteract the carcinogenic mechanisms he discovered.

Turmeric has been mentioned in medical texts in India, China, Tibet, and the Middle East for more than two thousand years. Aggarwal remembers that the yellow powder was a constant feature of his mother's kitchen in India. As a researcher, he thought that turmeric's power to reduce inflammation with few or no side effects might be useful in controlling tumor growth. He went on to study this ancient yellow powder with the same scientific curiosity and rigor with which he had learned to approach any new molecule produced by the pharmaceutical industry.

Aggarwal first showed that curcumin is very active against cancer in cell cultures.[34] Then, in 2005, he proved that it was capable of acting on breast cancer tumors grafted onto mice, tumors that no longer responded to chemotherapy with Taxol.*

In these mice, the administration of dietary doses of curcumin reduced the spread of metastases impressively. Microtumors could still be found in the lungs, but in the majority of cases they could no longer grow and were no longer a significant threat.[35]

To oncologists at the highly orthodox M. D. Anderson Cancer Center, these unlikely experiments based on traditional folk remedies did not deserve much attention. When Aggarwal, excited by his findings, approached them to show his results, he was quickly disappointed. As soon as he mentioned that he had been studying a traditional ayurvedic medicine from India, he could see that he had lost their attention. The first three he tried to share his results with gently brushed him off before he even had a chance to present them with his data on the profound effects of turmeric on the cellular biology of cancer. Then he changed tack. Going into the office of the head of clinical research at M. D. Anderson, he announced, "I've been studying a new pharmaceutical compound that has properties I have never seen before." That got the physician's attention. He proceeded to show him the battery of lab tests he had run on this new compound, and the wide variety of anticancer effects he had observed. His colleague became very animated. "We need to launch a clinical trial right away with this drug, Bharat!" Still, after learning that the "drug" was a traditional remedy from India, his interest waned rapidly. Until an unexpected turn of events.

A few months later, John Mendelsohn, MD, president of the center and one of the most influential oncologists in the United States, was attending a conference with Aggarwal and stayed to listen to his presentation. Amazed, he immediately

---

* Taxol is one of the very few drugs that is still considered effective against metastatic breast cancer, but it works in less than 50 percent of cases.

went up to speak to him afterward. "I had no idea that the science behind your results was so solid," he said. On his return to Houston, Mendelsohn decided to launch several clinical trials with curcumin. The first trial concerns one of the most common cancers of the blood (multiple myeloma), the second involves pancreatic cancer (one of the most difficult to treat), a third investigates the potential for prevention of lung cancer in high-risk subjects, and a fourth involves a protocol to make colon cancer more responsive to treatment with radiotherapy. He has already accumulated a large number of animal experiments to support studies in the clinic with gynecological cancer, breast cancer, and bladder cancer, and the combination of curcumin with chemotherapy in pancreatic cancer. These human studies are currently in progress, and all the results are not yet known.

By 2008, a few years after Aggarwal's initial publications, the *Journal of the National Cancer Institute* printed an editorial titled "Curry Compound Fights Cancer in the Clinic." It highlighted the entrance of turmeric in cancer research and announced that by then more than twenty clinical trials were already under way.[36]

Turmeric magnificently illustrates the benefit of the great culinary traditions, in comparison to the consumption of isolated substances. When researchers in Taiwan tried treating cancerous tumors with turmeric delivered in capsules, they discovered that it was very poorly absorbed by the digestive system.[37] In fact, when it is not mixed with pepper or ginger—as it always has been in curry—turmeric does not pass the intestinal barrier. Pepper increases the body's absorption of turmeric *by 2,000 percent*.[38] Indian wisdom has thus been far ahead of modern science in the discovery of natural affinities between foods.

When I was researching information on my own cancer, I was astonished to find out that even brain tumors such as glioblastomas were more sensitive to chemotherapy when curcumin was prescribed at the same time.[39]

According to the Aggarwal team in Houston, turmeric's extraordinary effect seems to be due in large part to its capacity to interfere directly with the black knight of cancer we encountered in chapter 4, NF-kappa B, which protects cancer cells against the body's defense mechanisms. The entire pharmaceutical industry is looking for new, nontoxic molecules capable of fighting this mechanism of cancer promotion. It is now known that curcumin is a powerful NF-kappa B antagonist, while over two thousand years of daily use in Indian cooking has proved that it is totally innocuous. Turmeric can also be eaten with soy products that replace animal proteins and provide the genistein mentioned above, which detoxifies and helps check angiogenesis. Add a cup of green tea and imagine the powerful cocktail that, with no side effects, keeps in check three of the principal mechanisms of cancer growth.

Mushrooms That Stimulate the Immune System

In Japan the shiitake, maitake, kawaratake, and enokitake mushrooms are staple foods. They are now also found in hospitals, where they are provided to patients during chemotherapy treatment.[40-42] These mushrooms contain a molecule called lentinian, and this, along with other polysaccharides they contain in great quantities, stimulates the immune system directly. The rate of stomach cancer, for example, is as much as 50 percent lower among Japanese peasants who consume large amounts of these mushrooms than among those who do not.[43] In Japanese university studies, the number and activity of immune cells increase notably in patients who are given mushroom extracts, and immune cell activity increases even within the tumor itself.[44-48] Researchers at the University of Kyushu in Japan have shown that when these mushrooms are provided during or after chemotherapy, colon cancer patients live longer.[49] This is probably because activation of their immune system slows tumor growth.

In Béliveau's laboratory, various mushrooms have been tested for benefits in combating breast cancer cells. Asian mushrooms are not the only ones to have beneficial effects. Some, such as oyster mushrooms, can stop cancer growth in cell cultures almost completely.

Berries: Blackberries, Raspberries, Strawberries, Blueberries . . .

In its fight against cancer, the pharmaceutical industry is also actively pursuing leads to antiangiogenic drugs.

Richard Béliveau has also worked since the midnineties on antiangiogenic medications that the industry has asked him to test in his laboratory. His work consists of growing in vitro blood vessel cells stimulated by chemical growth "boosters" like those made by cancerous tumors. With a micropipette, a tiny dose of the test medication is applied to the boosted cells to measure their capacity to prevent the creation of new blood vessels. It takes several days before any effects, often relatively subtle, can be detected.

Béliveau remembers mornings when he arrived in his laboratory, impatient to find out if this or that new molecule had passed the test. Any time he observed a promising effect, his adrenaline would rise and he would call the pharmaceutical firm with a triumphant "We've got a hit!" These promising results would galvanize the firm to invest even more money in the work, and Dr. Béliveau would quickly find himself heading a large-scale research program. However, there was always a shadow over this rosy picture. In this type of research, 95 percent of these promising synthetic molecules end up rejected when they are evaluated on animals and then on humans. Even when they are effective against cancer cells in a test tube, they are usually too toxic to be prescribed. But today, in the laboratory of molecular medicine of the Sainte-Justine Children's Hospital, the atmosphere is no longer quite the same.

Instead of evaluating a new chemical molecule, Béliveau recently decided to examine the antiangiogenic potential of an extract of raspberry. Ellagic acid is a polyphenol found in large quantities in raspberries and strawberries (it is also found in hazelnuts and walnuts). In doses amounting to a normal dietary portion of raspberries or strawberries, ellagic acid had already shown it could slow tumor growth significantly in mice exposed to aggressive carcinogens.

Tested with the same rigor as that applied to any drug, Béliveau found, ellagic acid in raspberries is potentially just as effective as a medication proven to slow the growth of blood vessels. Indeed, ellagic acid was shown to act against the two most common mechanisms of stimulation of blood vessels (vascular endothelial growth factor, or VEGF, and platelet-derived growth factor, or PDGF).[50] Béliveau knew how important this discovery was. If it had been a pharmaceutical molecule, his fax machine would have been going all day and the grants would have poured in. All the more so in this case, then, since there was no risk of discovering later that the promising molecule was too toxic for use on humans: After all, hominids have been eating raspberries since prehistoric times. But whom should he call? There was no question of a patent on raspberries; thus, there was nobody on the other end of the line to share the excitement of the moment and no grant money to be won.

Small fruits such as strawberries and raspberries (or walnuts, hazelnuts, and pecans) are more promising still. Unlike classic antiangiogenic drugs, their action is not confined to this single mechanism. Ellagic acid also detoxifies cells: It blocks the transformation of environmental carcinogens into toxic substances and stimulates the elimination of toxins.[51] The toxins we are referring to here are dangerous because they interact with DNA and provoke potentially life-threatening genetic mutations. Hence, ellagic acid is a kind of supermolecule that acts on several fronts, and without side effects.

Another natural anticancer food is cherries, which contain glucaric acid, a substance that can detoxify the body by facilitating elimination of the xenoestrogens that come from environmental chemicals.[52] Blueberries contain anthocyanidins and proanthocyanidins, molecules that are capable of forcing cancer cells to commit suicide (apoptosis).[53] In the laboratory, these molecules act on several cancer lines and are particularly effective against colon cancer. Other rich sources of proanthocyanidins are cranberries, cinnamon, and dark chocolate.[54]

Recent studies in animals have confirmed these laboratory results. Researchers at Ohio State University showed that rats who consumed black raspberries from Canada experienced an inhibiting effect on cancers of the esophagus, mouth, and colon. A team led by Professor Gary Stoner obtained equivalent results with raspberry powder containing a high concentration of anthocyanins. In both cases, rats in the group that consumed the berries developed 50 percent fewer tumors than the control group.[55] This magical little fruit has already proven its effects in a small group of patients who genetically suffer from a particular kind of polyp that is known to aggravate the risk of breast cancer. Patients who took black raspberry extract had up to 59 percent fewer of these dangerous polyps than the group who were given a placebo.[56]

Plums, Peaches, and Nectarines: It's Time for Stone Fruit

Berries have recently found some competition: peaches, plums, nectarines, etc. (collectively known as stone fruit), whose anticancer virtues were previously unknown. According to a group of researchers in Texas who reviewed more than a hundred species, these fruits—particularly plums—are at least as rich in anticancer elements as small berries. In this time of economic recession, it's good to know that a single plum contains as many antioxidants as a handful of berries and costs far less. In laboratory tests, stone fruits have also demonstrated their efficacy against breast cancer cells and cholesterol.[57]

Spices and Herbs Acting on the Same Mechanisms as Medications

In 2001 the Food and Drug Administration broke all speed records in approving a new anticancer drug—Gleevec. This medication is effective in treating both a common form of leukemia and a very rare and typically fatal intestinal cancer. In an enthusiastic interview in the *New York Times,* Dr. Larry Norton, the former president of the American Society for Clinical Oncology and one of the principal oncologists at Memorial Sloan-Kettering Hospital in New York, did not mince his words. He called Gleevec's effects "a miracle."[58]

Indeed, to oncologists, Gleevec has inaugurated an entirely novel approach to treating cancer. Rather than trying to poison cancer cells (as chemotherapy does), Gleevec blocks the cellular mechanisms that day after day enable the cancer to grow. It acts on one of the genes that stimulate cancer growth, but it is now thought that another key function may be to block one of the switches that stimulate the creation of new blood vessels (the PDGF receptor). Administered daily, Gleevec can "contain" cancer growth, which then ceases to be dangerous. We have reached the stage of "cancer without disease," in the language of Judah Folkman, who discovered angiogenesis.[59]

It so happens that many herbs and spices act along some of the same lines as Gleevec. This is true of the labiate family, for example, which includes mint, thyme, marjoram, oregano, basil, and rosemary. They are rich in fatty acids of the terpene family, which makes them particularly fragrant. Terpenes have been shown to act on a wide variety of tumors by reducing the spread of cancer cells or by provoking their death.

One of these terpenes—carnosol in rosemary—affects the capacity of cancer cells to invade neighboring tissues. When it is incapable of spreading, cancer loses its virulence. Moreover, researchers at the National Cancer Institute have demonstrated that rosemary extracts help chemotherapy penetrate cancer cells. In tissue cultures, they lower the resistance of breast cancer cells to chemotherapy.[60]

In Richard Béliveau's experiments, apigenine—plentiful in parsley and celery—has demonstrated powerful inhibition of the creation of blood vessels, which tumors need to grow, and to a degree comparable to Gleevec. This effect occurs even with very small concentrations, similar to those observed in the blood after consumption of parsley.[61]

The Synergy of Foods

The list of foods whose molecules act against cancer is, fortunately, much longer than people often think. I provide one practical list (not exhaustive, of course) in the appendix at the end of this chapter.*

Here is a quick summary of a few of the main results of the research described so far:

1. Some foods are cancer "promoters" and feed into the mechanisms that fuel cancer growth. We talked about them in chapter 6.
2. Other foods are "antipromoters." They block the mechanisms necessary for cancer growth or force cancer cells to die.
3. Food acts every day, three times a day. It thus has a considerable influence on the biological mechanisms that speed up or slow down cancer growth.

Medications usually act on a single factor. The latest generation of anticancer medications prides itself on offering "targeted" treatments. This means these drugs intervene at a specific molecular stage, limiting (it is hoped) their side effects. Anticancer foods, to the contrary, act on several mechanisms at the same time. And they do it gently, without provoking any side effects. As

---

* Richard Béliveau and the biochemist Denis Gingras, who has collaborated with him for twenty years, have published a superbly illustrated book entirely devoted to these anticancer foods. I recommend it highly.[62]

for the *combinations* of foods we consume at meals, they enable us to act on an even larger number of mechanisms involved in cancer. That's what makes their examination in the laboratory so complicated: The number of possible combinations to test is astronomical. But this plethora of combinations is also the reason why they are so promising.

At the M. D. Anderson Cancer Center, Isaiah Fidler, DVM, PhD, chairman of cancer biology, investigates the conditions under which cancer cells manage to invade—or fail to invade—other tissues. He shows his colleagues a picture of pancreatic cancer under the microscope. His team has succeeded in coloring its cells according to the different growth factors, the "fertilizers," they respond to. Growth factors enable the tumor to settle in, grow, and resist the treatments it is subjected to. In this experiment, a tumor of the pancreas appears to be multicolored—green, red, and yellow for growth factors and blue stain for the nuclei. The presence of multiple colors indicates that most of the tumor's cells exploit several different growth factors. "What does that mean?" Fidler asks his audience, pointing his laser at the slide on which the colorful tumor is displayed. "Treat against the red, and the green will kill you. Treat against the green, and the red will kill you. The only answer is to attack them all."[63]

Researchers at the University College of Medical Sciences in New Delhi, no doubt influenced by the great medical tradition of Ayurveda, have shown to what extent certain combinations of food can act in synergy to protect the body from carcinogens.[64] Chronic exposure of female mice to a well-known carcinogen—dimethylbenzanthracene, or DMBA—provoked breast tumors in 100 percent of them. This held true unless they were given certain substances commonly found in healthy food. The nutritional substances tested were selenium (found primarily in organically grown cereals and vegetables, as well as in fish and shellfish); magnesium (found in spinach, nuts, hazelnuts, almonds, whole-grain cereals, and some mineral water); vitamin C (found in most fruits and vegetables, especially citrus fruit and green vegetables, and in cabbage and strawberries); and vitamin A (found in all bright-colored fruits and vegetables, as well as in eggs). Among the mice that received only *one* of these components along with the carcinogenic substance, 50 percent developed a tumor. Among those that received *two* of these substances at the same time, only a third developed cancer. If three components were combined, the proportion of sick mice went down to one in five, and to only one in ten among those that consumed all four substances. As the statistics show, simply by consuming a combination of ingredients found in common foods, these mice went from a 100 percent risk of developing cancer to a 90 percent chance of *escaping* it.[65] This striking difference is most likely the result of a synergy between the various nutritional compounds working to slow down or block mechanisms that promote cancer growth. This synergistic, combinatorial approach is exactly the kind of therapy suggested by Isaiah Fidler.

Professor John Erdman, the author of an interesting 2007 study on the virtues of certain food combinations,[66] is also interested in synergy. "When tomatoes and broccoli are consumed together, we can see a cumulative effect," he explains. "This is probably due to the fact that both these foods contain anticancer elements that act according to different mechanisms." Together with his team from the University of Illinois, Professor Erdman studied the effects of a diet including tomatoes and broccoli (at levels equivalent to human consumption) in rats with prostate cancer. Rats whose diet was enriched with a mixture of powdered tomato *and* powdered broccoli saw the weight of their tumors diminish by 52 percent—far more than those who received only powdered tomato (34 percent reduction) or powdered broccoli (42 percent reduction). Those who received only lycopene, which is widely considered to be the protective component in tomatoes, saw their tumors diminish by no more than 18 percent. "Real" foods are thus more effective than supplements, and they are more effective in combination than when eaten separately.

"Tomatoes contain a whole series of bioactive elements, such as vitamins C, K and E; fibers; folates; polyphenols like quercetin; and carotenoids like phytoene and phytofluene, all of which may have anticancer potential," the researchers explain. The same is true of broccoli, whose effect cannot be reduced to any one of its constituent elements. Eating a complete food means that we absorb a combination of several phytonutrients, and eating a varied meal further multiplies this effect.

Professor Erdman calls it "reductionist" to study these specific elements one at a time in isolation, in the hope of finding *the* active component. He insists that we need to do much more research on food *synergy*. To date, no study has evaluated the effect of a diet that combines all variables—green tea, a lower glycemic index, reduction of omega-6 oils and increased consumption of omega-3s, turmeric, herbs, consumption of broccoli three times a week, olive oil, garlic/onions/leeks, berries, stone fruit, etc. Moreover, existing studies indicate that there is no reason to fear any negative interaction among these foods, whereby eating one would reduce the benefit of another. We can therefore reasonably conclude that a diet that combines numerous bioactive principles and pulls together a wide range of anticancer mechanisms most probably leads to a particularly strong synergy against a variety of cancer growth factors.

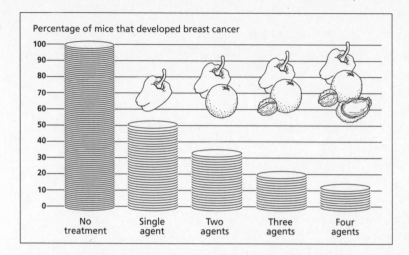

Figure 14. A combination of components in food has a much greater effect than a single component. Alone, one component reduces the risk of breast cancer by 50 percent in mice exposed to a powerful carcinogen. Four components administered together lowered the risk by 90 percent.[67]

DOES COOKING PRESERVE ANTICANCER PROPERTIES OF FOOD? CAN THEY BE FROZEN ?

Doesn't cooking cause the precious bioactive components of anticancer foods and herbs to go up in smoke? A researcher from Kingston University in Britain has studied this very question.[68] Her conclusions are clear: Most methods of cooking preserve the beneficial properties (at least, the antioxidant power) of foods. In the case of tomatoes, they actually *need* to be cooked in oil in order to release their precious anticancer phytochemicals, such as lycopene. Teas/infusions, soups, and stocks are the most effective preparation methods to get the best of herbs, and although grilling or sautéing food does reduce its nutritional properties slightly, it retains most. Boiling broccoli and other cruciform vegetables destroys their precious ingredients, though. As for food storage, the beneficial properties of anticancer agents are preserved when foods are frozen to −20°C. One notable exception to this concerns omega-3 fatty acids from seafood. Grilling, sautéing, or freezing fish or other seafood actually destroys about 30 percent of its omega-3s. The most appropriate cooking methods for fish are steaming and slow oven baking on low heat. And it is always best to eat seafood fresh rather than frozen.

A Vegetable Cocktail That Fights Cancer

If Béliveau's hypothesis is correct, the synergy among anticancer foods consumed daily ought to significantly slow down the development of cancers. Thus, it makes sense to combine all these components in a vegetable cocktail.

In their laboratory at Sainte-Justine Children's Hospital, Béliveau's team has evaluated the effect of this cocktail on seriously ill mice. "Nude" mice have a genetic flaw depriving them of both their immune system and their fur. They are defenseless against infection and do not reject grafts from human cancer cells. When human lung cancer cells are injected underneath their skin, they develop enormous tumors representing as much as 5 percent of their weight— the equivalent of a 3- to 4-kilogram (6- to 9-pound) tumor in a human.

Béliveau's colleagues recall that brewing the cocktail given to the mice produced an appetizing aroma that was a pleasant contrast to the typical laboratory smell of chemical compounds and other detergents. The mixture contained brussels sprouts, broccoli, garlic, scallions, turmeric, black pepper, cranberries, grapefruit, and even a bit of green tea. Its proportions were calculated so that they matched what a human could take in during an ordinary day: 100 grams (4 ounces) of cabbage, 50 grams (2 ounces) of blueberries, 2 grams (0.07 ounces) of tea, etc.

Wearing sterile masks and gloves to protect these vulnerable mice from infection, the researchers fed and weighed them daily. After a scant week, the mice that had not been fed the soup developed misshapen tumors under the skin. Those fed anticancer vegetables seemed in much better shape; they moved around more, were more curious, and had better appetites. Above all, although these mice lacked an immune system and had cancer cells under their

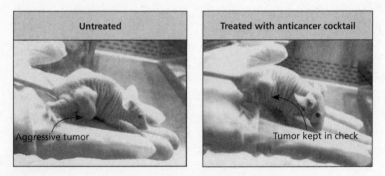

Figure 15. Mice that are deprived of an immune system and that consume an "anticancer" vegetable cocktail every day (as well as their usual diet) are in better health (right) and develop malignant tumors that are much less serious than those of mice that are fed only their customary diet (left).[69]

skin, the tumors they developed took much more time to emerge and grew much more slowly.

Is this how Lenny survived for so many years with such a typically aggressive cancer? Was it the food specially prepared by his wife that held the cancer at bay, by simultaneously blocking the various growth factors of his pancreatic cancer? We can't be sure, but what is certain is that he couldn't possibly have endangered his health by following that diet.

Every day, at every meal, we can choose food that will defend our bodies against the invasion of cancer by

- detoxifying carcinogenic substances;
- supporting our immune system;
- blocking the development of new vessels needed for tumor growth;
- preventing tumors from creating the inflammation that serves as their fertilizer;
- blocking the mechanisms that will enable them to invade neighboring tissues; and
- promoting the suicide of cancer cells.

FOODS: MORE IMPORTANT THAN CONTAMINANTS

The fact that anticancer foods are able to detoxify bodies by eliminating many carcinogens is particularly important. It follows, for example, that even if certain nonorganic fruits and vegetables are contaminated by pesticides, *the positive impact of anticancer molecules wins out over the negative effect of carcinogens.* As T. Colin Campbell of Cornell argues, as far as cancer is concerned, "foods trump contaminants every time."[70]

What About Wine?

In early 2009, in rapid succession, a major research study by the University of Oxford in Britain and a report by the French National Cancer Institute both concluded that alcohol is carcinogenic—including just one glass of alcohol, *even if it is a glass of red wine.*

A few days after these two papers were published, another massive study—the Color cohort, which followed almost one hundred thousand people in France over twenty-five years—concluded that although alcohol in general is indeed a risk factor for many cancers, moderate consumption of red wine actually *protects* against some cancers.[71] Indeed, centuries of common wisdom and numerous research studies have linked moderate consumption of red wine with good health.

Together with my colleagues Professor Richard Béliveau and Dr. Michel de Lorgeril, we decided to evaluate these contradictory reports.[72] Although existing studies do indicate that alcohol significantly increases the risk of developing cancer, we do not have sufficient data to say whether this holds true for red wine, consumed in moderation and during meals. On the contrary, the cardiac benefit of such consumption is well known, and in our opinion a similar benefit is likely against cancer too.

I would like to try to explain the current confusion over the risks and benefits of alcohol and the reasons for our recommendations on the basis of the existing literature. To begin, it is a fact that excessive consumption of alcohol poses serious health risks. This is particularly true for the most dangerous pattern of consumption: binge drinking—and all studies are in agreement on this point. Furthermore, I certainly do not consider wine drinking to be an essential part of an effective anticancer diet and would not want to appear to be encouraging nondrinkers to pick up a wine-drinking habit.

However, it is clear that the dietary context in which alcohol is consumed can considerably modify the body's response. For example, it has been documented that a deficit in omega-3 fatty acids and an excess of omega-6s—a pattern that is typical of contemporary American and British diets—increases by a factor of five or ten the quantity of carcinogenic free radicals produced upon consumption of alcohol.[73] Similarly, several studies have shown that only women whose diet is low in green vegetables (less than 400 micrograms of folates per day) see their risk of breast cancer increase with alcohol consumption—the same is not true of women eating diets rich in folates.[74-76]

The reported protective effect of red wine in particular is significantly enhanced when it is consumed in one particular context: during meals, especially as part of a Mediterranean diet. This diet includes numerous vegetables rich in polyphenols, flavonoids, beta-carotenes, and folates (among other phytochemical compounds beneficial to health), and it provides a favorable balance of omega-3 and omega-6 fatty acids.

In Britain, a large proportion of the population doesn't eat a healthy amount of vegetables, consumes between fifteen and thirty times more omega-6s than omega-3s, and is physically inactive and overweight. The University of Oxford study cited earlier was conducted on this population—in other words, on women whose lifestyles likely put them at a high risk of developing cancer.

In a different context, studies are likely to report completely different results, as was demonstrated in a major American study published in 2008.[77]

This analysis of 84,170 California men showed that the number of lung cancers was significantly lower among those who regularly consumed red wine than among those who preferred to drink beer or hard liquor. This protective effect was even more significant in smokers—a fact that clearly indicates a need for more research into ways of blocking the harmful effects of tobacco. In California, consumption of wine is also linked to a healthier lifestyle: fewer cigarettes, less meat, lower consumption of fats, and more fruits and vegetables.

Although none of this research should be taken lightly, we may easily grasp the current bottom line by simply looking at the numbers: The potential for preventing cancer through a few lifestyle modifications is far greater (48 percent) than the increase in risk noted by the Oxford study (11 percent).

PART 2: WHY IS ADVICE ON NUTRITION STILL MISSING FROM THE CONVENTIONAL TREATMENT OF CANCER?

For the last five thousand years, all the great medical traditions have used diet to influence the course of disease. Ours is no exception. In the fifth century B.C. Hippocrates said, "Let food be thy medicine and thy medicine thy food."[78] In 2003 *Nature* published a long article that concluded—in a more modern style—"Chemoprevention by edible phytochemicals is now considered to be an inexpensive, readily applicable, acceptable and accessible approach to cancer control and management."[79]

Nevertheless, while diet continues to be a pillar of ayurvedic, Chinese, and Arabic medicine, what Western doctor refers to it in his practice?

When I went back to see my oncologist after the second operation that followed the relapse in my brain tumor, I was getting ready to start a year of chemotherapy. I asked him if I ought to change my diet to make the most of the treatment and avoid another relapse. In spite of the devotion he had shown in looking after me, despite his patience and kindness fostered by years of dealing with distraught patients, his answer was perfectly stereotypical: "Eat what you like. It won't make much difference. But whatever you do, keep up your weight."

I looked at oncology textbooks that serve as the foundation for many of my colleagues' training. The best example is *Cancer: Principles & Practice of Oncology.*[80] It is essential reading for future oncologists, cowritten by Professor Vincent T. DeVita, former director of the National Cancer Institute, famous for discovering the cure for Hodgkin's disease by combined chemotherapy. In the latest edition of this remarkable book, which sets the tone for oncology all over the world, there is not a single chapter on the role of nutrition in the treatment of cancer or the prevention of relapses.

Like everybody who has had cancer, every six months I go through the ritual of making sure that my body continues to keep in check the cancer cells that inevitably escaped surgery and chemotherapy. In the waiting room of the large university medical center where I go for my followup exams, booklets of all sorts are at the patient's disposal. During my last examination, I carefully read a pamphlet called "Nutrition for the Person with Cancer: A Guide for Patients and Families."[81] I found a number of sensible ideas, such as the recommendation to eat more fruits and vegetables and "some meals without meat every week," as well as advice to lower consumption of fatty food and alcohol. And then, in the section on "nutrition after treatment," I found the uninspiring statement: "There is very little research to show that the food you eat can prevent your cancer from coming back."*

My oncologist colleagues saved my life, and I have a profound admiration for their daily commitment to patients with this particularly trying disease. Yet I must ask, how can these exceptional doctors go on promoting such a false idea? After talking to some of them, whom I count among my friends, I have managed to find an answer to that question. In fact, there are several answers.

"If It Were True, We'd Know About It"

Like all physicians, oncologists are constantly looking for scientific advances that may help their patients. They participate in conventions every year to keep abreast of new treatments. They subscribe to scientific journals where new studies are published, as well as to professional journals of a more commercial sort that provide journalistic coverage of current medical opinion. Several times a month they see sales representatives from the pharmaceutical industry, who show them the latest drugs available on the market. They feel they are aware of everything going on in their field, and in general, they are.

But in medical culture, changes in recommendations given to patients are allowable in only one case and one alone: when there has been a series of "double-blind" studies demonstrating the effectiveness of a treatment in humans. This is called, legitimately, "evidence-based medicine."

Compared to these experimental studies with humans, epidemiology is

---

* In the same brochure, I also found a list of "nutritive snacks" intended to sustain me during chemotherapy. That list recommended a mix of cookies, ice cream, white bread, pretzels, muffins, milkshakes, and even eggnog—in other words, foods with a high glycemic index and heavy in unbalanced animal fats that directly stimulate the inflammatory process. On none of the ninety-seven pages was there any mention of turmeric, green tea, soy, raspberries, or immune-stimulating mushrooms.

looked on merely as a source of hypotheses. At the same time, to an oncologist who spends his days in contact with patients, studies carried out in laboratories on cancer cells or on mice are not taken into consideration either. Until they have been confirmed by large-scale studies in humans, they do not constitute "evidence." Even when these studies are published in *Nature* or *Science*, they usually don't even appear on the radar screens of these specialists, who simply do not have the time to explore the huge volume of work being carried out in laboratories. Unless they hear about these results from their typical sources, they tend to think "it can't be true, or I'd know about it."

The validation of an anticancer drug up through the stage of adequate experimentation on humans costs between five hundred million and a billion dollars. This kind of investment seems justified when one considers that even a relatively minor anticancer medicine such as Taxol brings in a billion dollars a *year* to the company that holds the patent. On the other hand, it is not financially feasible to invest such sums in demonstrating the usefulness of broccoli, raspberries, or green tea, because they can't be patented and their sale will never cover the cost of the original investment. Even when they exist, human studies of the anticancer benefits of food will simply never match the caliber of those for drugs. Animal studies are more common and financially reasonable and can help point us in the right direction. Unfortunately, the commonly held notion that studies on mice don't prove anything about humans is true.

This is why it is so essential to encourage public institutions and foundations to finance human studies on the anticancer benefits of food. Still, I am convinced there is no need to wait for such large-scale results before beginning to include anticancer food in one's diet. It is clearly established that the type of diet I have adopted myself and recommend here does not expose those who follow it to any risks and leads, rather, to health benefits that go far beyond its effect on cancer. This sort of diet has beneficial effects on arthritis, cardiovascular diseases, and Alzheimer's disease, to name a few.[82–88]

"Stop Boring Us Stiff with Your Diet!"

More serious, perhaps, is the fact that nutrition is barely taught in medical schools. In most schools, concepts of nutrition are sprinkled throughout other disciplines, such as biochemistry and epidemiology. My knowledge of nutrition prior to my experience in Tibet was considerably less than that of an average reader of *Cosmopolitan*. With only minor exaggeration, the following sums up the extent of what I'd been taught:

- Foods are composed of carbohydrates, lipids, proteins, vitamins, and minerals.

- People who suffer from obesity need to eat fewer calories.
- If diabetic, people must eat less sugar; if hypertensive, less salt; with cardiac disease, less cholesterol.

My ignorance of nutrition long led me to assume a contemptuous attitude toward the therapeutic role of food. I too preferred treatments from the noble branch of pharmaceutical medicine. I well remember a cardiologists' dinner in the nineties where I had been invited to give a lecture on the link between depression and cardiac disease. To persuade these busy physicians to attend, the pharmaceutical company organizing the event invited us to one of the best steak restaurants in Pittsburgh. It was entirely dedicated to devotion to American beef. When the time came to order, one of the cardiologists turned down the maître d'hôtel's suggestion of a superb 700-gram (1.5-pound) Chateaubriand steak. She informed him diplomatically that she was watching her cholesterol and asked if she could have fish instead. She was immediately teased by the others at the table: "Take your Lipitor and stop boring us stiff with your diet."*

That reaction didn't even strike me particularly at the time. It's a perfect illustration of the state of mind in which we doctors live and breathe: If there's a problem, there's a drug. Even in the case of cardiologists, who willingly acknowledge that the risk of cardiac disease can be lowered by changing one's eating habits, our medical culture encourages us to neglect that approach and prefer a pharmaceutical solution.

"The Experts Don't Agree Among Themselves"

In 1977, I accompanied my father to meet Senator George McGovern in his office in the Senate in Washington. As I recall, his office seemed very small to me for a senator who had been the Democratic candidate for the presidency of the United States. I also remember the peculiar map of South Dakota, the state he represented, that covered the wall behind his chair. It consisted of a large, nearly empty rectangle with a handful of small towns whose names I'd never heard of. McGovern was downcast and worried. He was facing a revolt far more devastating than Nixon's attacks on his Watergate headquarters during the 1972 presidential race. "I've just made the biggest mistake of my political career," he said. He had agreed to preside over the congressional committee responsible for drawing up public health recommendations on nutrition. The experts who had testified for the committee had presented straightforward

---

* The drug Lipitor is the pharmaceutical industry's biggest moneymaker. At its sales peak, it brought in a million dollars an hour, 365 days a year (nine billion dollars a year).

results. They reported that the rate of coronary diseases had risen sharply since World War II, while in countries where diets were richer in vegetables than in animal products these diseases were almost nonexistent. The epidemiologists had also observed that during the war, when meat and dairy products were rationed, the rate of cardiac disease had fallen substantially.

With the best of intentions, the committee had published a report that seemed grounded in common sense. In its "Dietary Goals for the United States," it naively recommended "lowering the consumption of meat and dairy products."

Ever since that announcement, McGovern had been caught up in a political storm that he couldn't quell. He had sparked the fury of the entire beef and dairy cattle industry of the United States. On its vast, empty prairies, South Dakota didn't have many more human inhabitants than head of cattle. That day in his office, McGovern explained there were issues that were better left alone.

Three years later, the subsidies from the powerful cattle industry went to his political opponent, ending his career as a senator. McGovern's sad demeanor suggested that he already knew what was in store. Experts of all ilks, financed by the industry, affirmed that it would be a grievous error to incriminate one food in particular. The "saturated fats" that were being incriminated by the report were found not only in meat and dairy products, they explained in learned terms, but also in fish (which is true, but in much smaller quantities!). The industry thus managed to get the recommendations changed so that reducing the consumption of one specific food was never explicitly recommended. In doing so, the commission left the public in confusion, perhaps for decades. What should have been a clear and simple message became an unintelligible hodgepodge that finally had no impact. As Michael Pollan, a professor of journalism at Berkeley, emphasized in an article in the *New York Times Magazine,* the only message the public received was the one the industry sends when it doesn't want anything to change: "The experts don't agree."[89]

Like patients, doctors are caught in a pincer between two powerful industries. On one side, they have the pharmaceutical industry with its obvious logic, offering easy pharmacological solutions rather than encouraging patients to take themselves in hand. On the other side, they have the food industry, protecting its interests jealously by discouraging the dissemination of overly explicit recommendations on the links between food and illness. And what they have in common is a most profound desire for nothing to change.

For those who, like me, want to protect themselves against cancer, it is unacceptable to continue to be the passive victim of these economic forces.

There is no choice but to arm oneself with all the available information on what might help control the disease without harming one's body. The good news is that there is already enough data on the anticancer effects of food for everyone to begin applying this treatment to themselves.

"People Don't Want to Change"

Are we really ready to help ourselves? I remember a conversation with a fellow physician at a convention where I had presented data on the decline of dietary habits in the West since World War II. I had insisted on the urgency of correcting these habits. "You may be right, David, but people don't want to change," he said. "It's useless to tell them all that. All they want is to take a medication and forget about it."

I don't know whether he's right. I know that it isn't true in my own case. I prefer to believe that I'm not alone in thinking this way.

What's certain is that institutions find it hard to change. After my last screening at the university's cancer center, I stopped at the cafeteria pleasantly located under a glass roof near the entrance to the building. I discovered eight different types of tea and infusions: Darjeeling, Earl Grey, chamomile, and several fruit-flavored herbal teas. This was certainly a large variety of teas for a hospital cafeteria, but there was no green tea.

APPENDIX TO CHAPTER 8:
ANTICANCER FOODS IN DAILY PRACTICE

A New Standard Plate

The anticancer diet is principally composed of vegetables (and legumes) accompanied by olive (or canola or flaxseed) oil or organic butter, garlic, herbs, and spices. Meat and eggs are optional. They don't represent the main ingredient of the plate. They are there primarily for added taste.* This is exactly the contrary of a typical Western dish (a large slice of meat in the middle with a few vegetables on the side).

A List of Recommended Foods

Green Tea

Rich in polyphenols, including catechins (and particularly epigallocatechin gallate-3, or EGCG), which reduce the growth of the new vessels needed for tumor growth and metastases. It is also a powerful antioxidant and detoxifier

---

* The 2007 report of the World Cancer Research Fund recommends not more than 500 grams (18 ounces) of red meat per week.[90]

Grains	Fats	Herbs and spices
multigrain bread,	olive, canola, or	turmeric, mint,
whole-grain rice,	flaxseed oil,	thyme, rosemary,
quinoa, bulgur ...	omega-3 butter	garlic ...

Animal proteins (optional)

fish, organic meat, omega-3 eggs, organic dairy products

Vegetables and fruits and vegetable proteins

lentils, peas, beans, tofu ...

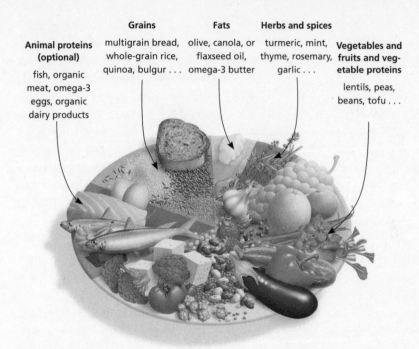

Figure 16. The Anticancer Plate

(activating enzymes in the liver that eliminate toxins from the body), and it facilitates the death of cancer cells by apoptosis. In the laboratory, it enhances the effects of radiotherapy on cancer cells.

Note that black tea is fermented, a process that destroys a large proportion of its polyphenols. Oolong tea has undergone a kind of fermentation midway between green tea and black tea. Decaffeinated green tea still contains all its polyphenols.

Japanese green tea (sencha, gyokuro, matcha, etc.) is even richer in EGCG than common varieties of Chinese green tea.

Green tea must be steeped for at least five to eight minutes—ideally ten minutes—to release its catechins.

Recommendations for use: Steep 2 grams (0.07 ounce) of green tea for ten minutes in a teapot and drink within an hour. Drink two to three cups a day. Do not store green tea after steeping, as it loses its beneficial polyphenols after an hour or two.

Take further note: Some people are sensitive to the caffeine in green tea and may lose sleep if they drink it after 4 P.M. In this case, use decaffeinated green tea.

Olives and Olive Oil

Olives and olive oil contain particularly high concentrations of phenolic anti-oxidants. They are ideal health foods. Black olives seem to be richer in antioxidants than green, especially when they have not been subjected to the Spanish method of brining. Similarly, olive oil should preferably be cold-pressed, extra-virgin oil, a product that has considerably higher concentrations of bio-active components than refined oil.

The recommended consumption is between one half and one tablespoon of oil daily, used in cooking (fish, tofu, meat, vegetables), in salad dressings, or as an accompaniment to pasta, rice, or quinoa.

Be careful, however. Olive oil is very good for your health, but it is still oil. Excessive quantities will make you gain weight.

Turmeric and Curry

Turmeric (the yellow powder that is one of the components of yellow curry) is the most powerful natural antiinflammatory identified today. It also helps stimulate apoptosis in cancer cells and inhibit angiogenesis. In the laboratory, it enhances the effectiveness of chemotherapy and reduces tumor growth.

Take note: To be assimilated by the body, turmeric must be mixed with black pepper (not simply with peppers). Ideally, it must also be dissolved in oil (olive, canola, or linseed oil, preferably). In store-bought curry mixes, turmeric represents only 20 percent of the total. So it's better to obtain turmeric powder directly.

Recommendations for use: Mix ¼ teaspoon of turmeric powder with ½ tablespoon of olive oil and a generous pinch of black pepper. Add to vegetables, soups, and salad dressings. A few drops of agave nectar can remove the slightly bitter taste.

Ginger

Ginger root also acts as a powerful antiinflammatory and an antioxidant (more effective than vitamin E, for example) and has protective effects. It acts against certain cancer cells. Moreover, it helps reduce the creation of new blood vessels. A ginger infusion tea also helps alleviate nausea from chemotherapy or radiotherapy.[91-93]

Recommendations for use: Add grated ginger to a vegetable mix while it is cooking in a wok or frying pan. Or marinate fruits in lime juice and grated ginger (a touch of agave nectar may be added for those who prefer more sweetness). Make an infusion by cutting a small piece of ginger (about an inch) into slices and steeping in boiling water for ten to fifteen minutes. Can be drunk hot or cold.

Cruciform Vegetables

Cabbages (brussels sprouts, bok choy, Chinese cabbage, broccoli, cauliflower, etc.) contain sulforaphane and indole-3-carbinols (I3Cs), which are powerful anticancer molecules. Sulforaphane and I3Cs are capable of detoxifying certain carcinogenic substances. They prevent precancerous cells from developing into malignant tumors. They also promote the suicide of cancer cells and block angiogenesis.[94-96] In 2009, at the Cancer Research Center of the University of Pittsburgh, biologist Dr. Shivendra Singh and his team studied the impact of sulforaphane—an antioxidant contained in cruciform vegetables—on prostate cancer in mice. They made two radical new discoveries. First, consumption of sulforaphane three times a week considerably increases the action of NK cells against tumors (by more than 50 percent). Second, tumor-carrying rats that consumed sulforaphane were shown to have *half* as much risk of developing metastases as those that did not.[97]*

Take note: Avoid boiling cabbage and broccoli. Boiling risks destroying sulforaphane and I3Cs.

Recommendations for use: Cover and steam briefly or stir-fry rapidly in a wok with a little olive oil.

Garlic, Onions, Leeks, Shallots, Chives

Garlic is one of the oldest medicinal herbs (prescriptions for garlic are found on Sumerian tablets from 3000 B.C.). Louis Pasteur observed its antibacterial properties in 1858. During World War I, garlic was widely used in bandages to prevent infections, and it was used later by Russian soldiers in World War II. When they suffered from a shortage of antibiotics, they used it to such an extent that garlic was called "the Russian penicillin."

The sulfur compounds of this family (the "alliaceous" family) reduce the carcinogenic effects of nitrosamines and N-nitroso compounds, which are created in overgrilled meat and during tobacco combustion. They promote

---

* Dr. Singh's team used a concentrated extract of sulforaphane corresponding to a consumption of broccoli that would be impossible to achieve in a normal diet—twenty bowls of broccoli three times a week. However, as discussed earlier, we know that one nutrient component alone is less powerful than when the whole food is consumed.[98] In addition, we know that the anticancer effects of foods are multiplied when they are combined. It is thus probable that, even when consumed at levels one twentieth as high as in the Pittsburgh study, broccoli may still have a powerful immune-stimulating and antimetastasis effect when combined with other anticancer foods such as garlic, onions, tomatoes, and olive oil. Unfortunately, scientific studies require simplicity and experimental purity, and they rarely address the benefits of such combinations. Studies that have addressed them almost invariably observe that in nutrition, as with lifestyle, the effect of a combination of factors is far superior to the effect of a single element.[99-107]

apoptosis (cell death) in colon, breast, lung, and prostate cancer, as well as in leukemia.

Epidemiological studies suggest a reduction in kidney and prostate cancer in people who consume the most garlic.[108]

Moreover, all the herbs in this family help to regulate blood sugar levels. This, in turn, reduces insulin secretion and IGF, and thus the growth of cancer cells.

Take note: Active molecules of garlic are released when a garlic clove is crushed and are much more easily assimilated if they are dissolved in a little oil.

Recommendations for use: Chopped garlic and onions can be gently fried in a little olive oil, mixed with steamed or stir-fried vegetables, and combined with curry or turmeric. They can also be consumed raw, mixed in salads, or eaten in a sandwich of multigrain bread and organic butter (or olive oil).

Vegetables and Fruits Rich in Carotenoids

Carrots, yams, sweet potatoes, squash, pumpkins, certain varieties of poti-marron squash (also known as Hokkaido squash), tomatoes, persimmons, apricots, beets, and all the bright-colored (orange, red, yellow, green) fruits and vegetables contain vitamin A and lycopene, which have the proven capacity to inhibit the growth of cells of several cancer lines, including brain gliomas.

Lutein, lycopene, phytoene, and canthaxanthin stimulate the growth of immune cells and increase their capacity to attack tumor cells. They make NK cells more aggressive.

A study that tracked breast cancer patients for six years showed that those who consumed the most foods rich in carotenoids lived longer than those who consumed less.[109]

Tomatoes and Tomato Sauce

It has been concluded that lycopene in tomatoes leads to longer survival for prostate cancer patients (men in the study consumed tomato sauce in at least two meals a week).[110] Tomatoes also contain a whole series of antican-cer nutrients whose combined action is more effective than lycopene on its own.[111] Take note: Tomatoes must be cooked in order to release these nutri-ents. Moreover, olive oil improves their assimilation.

Recommendations for use: Use canned tomato sauce with olive oil and with no sugar added. Or prepare homemade tomato sauce: Cook the tomatoes in a frying pan with a little olive oil over low heat. Add onions, garlic, tofu, or eggs rich in omega-3s, along with cumin, turmeric, pepper, and seasonings.

If you are using canned tomato sauce, be careful to avoid brands that have a plastic lining, as this is a source of bisphenol A, or, to be safe, choose a brand sold in a glass jar.

Soy

Soy isoflavones (including genistein, daidzein, and glycitein) block the stimulation of cancer cells by sex hormones (such as estrogens and testosterone). They also intervene by blocking angiogenesis. There are significantly fewer breast cancer cases among Asian women who have eaten soy since adolescence. When they do have breast cancer, their tumors are usually less aggressive with higher survival rates.

Take note: Isoflavone supplements (in pill form) have been associated with an *aggravation* of certain breast cancers, but this is not the case for soy taken in as food.

INTERACTION BETWEEN SOY AND TAXOL

It seems that the genistein in soy can interfere with Taxol. While awaiting confirmation of this interaction from human studies, it is advisable not to consume soy-based foods during chemotherapy with Taxol. (Stop several days before, and start again several days after treatment.)

Recommendations for use: Replace conventional milk products with soy milk or soy yogurts for breakfast. Also, use tofu, tempeh, and miso. Tofu can be eaten raw or cooked; it takes on the taste of other ingredients—onions, garlic, curry, etc.—and the sauces it is cooked with in a wok or frying pan. It can also easily be added to soups. It is an excellent source of complete proteins that can be used to replace meat.

Mushrooms

Shiitake, maitake, enokidake, cremini, portobello, oyster, and thistle oyster mushrooms all contain polysaccharides and lentinian, which stimulate the reproduction and activity of immune cells. These mushrooms are often used in Japan as a complement to chemotherapy to support the immune system. (Maitake probably has the most pronounced effect on the immune system.) Under laboratory conditions, pleurotus mushrooms have been shown to be among the most effective against breast cancer cells.

In one 2009 study, Australian researchers demonstrated that Chinese women who consumed 10 grams of mushrooms per day reduced their risk of developing breast cancer by 64 percent. If they also drank green tea (1 gram of leaves infused per day—a more precise measurement than number of cups), their risk was reduced by a whopping 89 percent. This represents a degree of risk reduction not observed with any other dietary or lifestyle factor I know of.[112]

Recommendations for use: in soups, vegetables, or chicken broth, oven-grilled, or stir-fried in a wok with other vegetables.

Herbs and Spices

Cooking herbs such as rosemary, thyme, oregano, basil, and mint are very rich in essential oils of the terpene family, to which they owe their fragrance. They promote apoptosis in cancer cells and reduce their spread by blocking the enzymes they need to invade neighboring tissues. Carnosol in rosemary is also a powerful antioxidant and antiinflammatory. Its capacity to enhance the effectiveness of certain chemotherapies has been demonstrated.

Parsley and celery contain apigenin, an antiinflammatory that promotes apoptosis and blocks angiogenesis.

Seaweed

Several varieties of seaweed commonly eaten in Asia contain molecules that slow cancer growth, especially that of breast, prostate, skin, and colon cancer. Brown seaweed lengthens the menstrual cycle, thanks to an antiestrogen effect. Fucoidan, found in kombu and wakame seaweed, helps provoke cell death by apoptosis and stimulate immune cells, including NK cells.[113, 114] Fucoxanthin is the ingredient in certain varieties of seaweed that makes them brown. It's a carotenoid (from the same family as lycopene in tomatoes) even more effective than its cousin lycopene in its capacity to inhibit cell growth in prostate cancer.

The principal edible seaweeds are nori, kombu, wakame, arame, and dulse.

Nori is one of the extremely rare vegetable species that contain long-chain omega-3 fatty acids—the most effective against inflammation and indispensable to the proper functioning of neurons.

Recommendations for use: Seaweed can be used in soups or salads or can be added to pulses such as beans and lentils. (In particular, kombu is reputed to shorten cooking time for legumes and to make them more digestible.)

Berries

Strawberries, raspberries, blueberries, blackberries, and cranberries contain ellagic acid and a large number of polyphenols. They stimulate the mechanisms of elimination of carcinogenic substances and inhibit angiogenesis. Anthocyanidins and proanthocyanidins also promote apoptosis in cancer cells.

Recommendations for use: At breakfast, mix fruit with soy milk and multigrain cereals, which, in contrast to standard breakfast cereals such as cornflakes, do not raise the level of blood sugar, insulin, and IGF. (The best cereals are muesli or combinations of oats, bran, flaxseed, rye, barley, spelt, etc.)

In fruit salads or snacks between meals, berries provide a fresh, sweet flavor that does not set off a glycemic peak in the blood. Freezing does not damage the anticancer molecules in these berries, so in winter frozen berries can replace fresh ones.

Plums, Peaches, and Nectarines

Researchers have recently discovered that peaches, nectarines, and other stone fruit—and especially plums—contain as many anticancer agents as berries, and at far lower cost. In particular, a study at the University of Texas observed that plum extracts had a powerful effect against the growth of breast cancer.[115]

Citrus Fruit

Oranges, tangerines, lemons, and grapefruit contain antiinflammatory flavonoids. They also stimulate the detoxification of carcinogenics by the liver.

It has even been shown that flavonoids in the skin of tangerines—tangeritin and nobiletin—penetrate brain cancer cells, facilitate their death by apoptosis, and lower their potential for invading neighboring tissues. (Be sure to choose organic tangerines if you use the skin.)[116, 117]

Recommendations for use: Grated citrus fruit skins can be sprinkled over salad dressings or breakfast cereals. Skins can also be steeped in tea or hot water.

Pomegranate Juice

Pomegranate juice has been used in Persian medicine for thousands of years. Its antiinflammatory and antioxidant properties have already been confirmed, as well as its capacity to substantially reduce the development of prostate cancer (among others), even in its most aggressive forms. In humans, daily consumption of pomegranate juice slows the spread of an established prostate cancer by 67 percent.[118]

Recommendations for use: one glass (225 milliliters or 8 ounces or 1 cup) a day of pomegranate juice with breakfast.

Red Wine

Red wine contains many polyphenols, including the celebrated resveratrol. These polyphenols are extracted by fermentation; hence, their concentration is much greater in wine than in grape juice. Since they come from the skin and seeds of the grape, there are not nearly as many in white wine. The methods used for preserving wine protect it from oxygen, which means resveratrol is not exposed to rapid oxidation as it is in grape juice or raisins, which have lost most of their polyphenols.

Resveratrol acts on genes (called sirtuines) that are known to protect healthy cells against aging. It can also slow the three stages of cancer development—initiation, promotion, and progression—by blocking the action of NF-kappa B.[119, 120]

Because resveratrol also acts as an antiangiogenic, like thalidomide it can interfere with fetal development. This is one more reason to avoid alcohol (even red wine) during pregnancy. Resveratrol supplements should also be avoided by women who may become pregnant.

Recommendations for use: These results are observed with concentrations similar to those obtained after consumption of one glass of red wine a day. (More than one glass daily should be avoided, since it may lead to an increase in cancer.) Pinot noir, originally from the damp climate of Burgundy, is particularly rich in resveratrol.

Dark Chocolate

Dark chocolate (more than 70 percent cocoa) contains a number of antioxidants, proanthocyanidins, and many polyphenols (a square of chocolate contains twice as many as a glass of red wine and almost as many as a cup of green tea properly steeped). These molecules slow the growth of cancer cells and limit angiogenesis.

Consumption of 20 grams a day (one fifth of a bar) represents an acceptable number of calories. The satisfaction it produces is often greater than that of a candy or dessert, and it takes the edge off one's appetite more effectively. Its glycemic index (its capacity to raise the blood sugar level and provoke harmful peaks of insulin and IGF) is moderate, distinctly lower than that of white bread.

Take note: Mixing dairy products with chocolate cancels the beneficial effects of the molecules of cocoa. Avoid milk chocolate.

Recommendations for use: Eat a few squares of dark chocolate instead of dessert at the end of a meal (with green tea). Or melt dark chocolate in a double boiler, then pour it over pears or any fruit combination. It is also delicious with grated ginger or grated tangerine peels.

Vitamin D

Skin cells produce vitamin D when they are exposed directly to the sun. People who live away from the equator produce less vitamin D and can sometimes be deficient. This is the reason why a spoonful of cod liver oil was long recommended for children living at northern latitudes to avoid rickets. It has recently been shown that a significant supply of vitamin D reduces considerably the risk of several cancers (by more than 75 percent with a daily intake of 1,000 international units [IUs] of the 25-hydroxyvitamin D form), in a Creighton University study published in 2007.[121] In a Canadian pilot study of fifteen patients with prostate cancer, researchers reported on the effects of taking just 2,000 IUs of vitamin D3 daily over a median of eight months (up to sixty-five months for one of the patients). Fourteen of them saw a slowing of progression of their PSA levels (the most common marker of prostate cancer, used to follow its growth over time). And these levels actually dropped significantly in nine of the patients compared to their levels at the start of treatment.[122]

Other studies published recently have shown positive effects of vitamin D3 on breast cancer, non-small-cell lung cancer, colon cancer, and prostate cancer. Many researchers now believe that vitamin D3 contributes to slowing down *all* forms of cancer, at least in the early stages. Moreover, we now know that vitamin D3 very likely protects us from colds and flu and contributes to maintaining a positive mental outlook—a precious antidote to lower energy levels during the dark, cold months of winter.[123]

The Canadian Cancer Association now recommends a daily intake of 1,000 IUs of vitamin D during the fall and winter months (because of Canada's limited access to sunlight) and all year long to people over sixty-five years of age and those who get very limited exposure to the sun because of lifestyle or religious reasons.[124] The first step is to discuss with your doctor whether you might benefit from measuring the levels of vitamin D3 in your blood (some doctors do this regularly, and others do not) and to add supplements to your diet if necessary. Specialists recommend either a daily intake of 1,000 to 5,000 IUs or a single dose of 100,000 IUs twice a month. Take care: Vitamin D2, or ergocalciferol, should be avoided, since some specialists have reported potential toxicity from hypercalcemia.

Remember that twenty minutes of noonday sun exposure to the entire body provides between 8,000 and 10,000 IUs. (But beware of the risk of sun overexposure, which is clearly related to skin cancer. The skin should never be exposed to the point of burning.)

Foods that contain the most vitamin D are cod liver oil (1,460 IUs in a tablespoon), salmon (360 IUs in 100 grams), mackerel (345 IUs in 100 grams), sardines (270 IUs in 100 grams), and eel (200 IUs in 100 grams). Milk enriched with vitamin D contains only 98 IUs per glass, an egg 25 IUs, and calf liver 20 IUs per 100 grams.

Though rare, there are possible risks associated with excessive intake of vitamin D3. Kidney stones may develop, due to excessive calcium in the urine, and hypercalcemia (excessive levels of calcium in the bloodstream) may develop, which, in some very rare cases, can be lethal to people with cancer. I therefore recommend that you measure blood levels of vitamin D3 and calcium levels in blood and urine under your doctor's supervision before you begin supplements and roughly every three months subsequently.

Omega-3s

Long-chain omega-3s found in fatty fish (or in high-quality purified fish oil supplements) reduce inflammation. In cell cultures, they reduce cancer cell growth in a large number of tumors (lung, breast, colon, prostate, kidney, etc.). They also act to reduce the spread of tumors in the form of metastases. Several human studies show that the risk of several cancers is significantly lower in people who eat fish at least twice a week.[125–132]*

Take note: The bigger the fish (for example, tuna, but especially dogfish, shark, and swordfish), the higher it is in the food chain and the more contaminated it is by mercury, PCBs, and dioxin, all of which pollute the ocean floor. The best sources of fatty fish are small fish, such as whole anchovies, small mackerel, and sardines (including canned sardines, provided they are preserved in olive oil and not in sunflower oil, which is too rich in omega-6s). Salmon is also a good source of omega-3s, and the level of contamination is still acceptable. Frozen fish progressively loses some of its omega-3 content over the course of conservation.

Flaxseeds are rich in short-chain vegetal omega-3s and also in lignans. These phytoestrogens allay the harmful effects of hormones that promote cancer growth. They have also been linked to lower cholesterol and attenu-

---

* Two important articles published in 2006 raised doubts about such a reduction in cancer risk with greater fish consumption.[133, 134] However, these analyses have been contested because, among other reasons, they did not include very recent large studies, such as the European EPIC study— with 475,000 participants—which largely confirmed the protection conferred by more frequent fish consumption—up to a 54 percent reduction in risk for colon cancer, for example.[135]

ation of spikes in blood sugar levels. For example, 50 grams (1.75 ounces) of flaxseed-enriched bread produces an increase in blood sugar levels that is 30 percent less than that seen in response to the same quantity of white bread. In a recent study at Duke University, daily intake of 30 grams of ground flaxseeds slowed the growth of existing prostate tumors by 30 percent to 40 percent.[136] In France, researchers working with Professor Philippe Bougnoux, an oncologist specializing in omega-3 research, reported that women with breast cancer whose tissue samples were richer in omega-3 fatty acids derived from plants (such as flaxseeds, nuts, and canola oil) had a significantly lower risk of developing metastatic tumors.[137]

Flaxseeds may lead to digestive problems comparable to those observed with other foods rich in fiber, especially in persons whose colons are particularly sensitive. In this case, daily consumption should be limited to no more than 45 grams.

Recommendations for use: Grind the seeds in a coffee grinder and mix the powder with organic milk or soy milk (or an organic or soy yogurt). The powder can also be mixed with breakfast cereals. Or stir the powder into a fruit salad to give it a nutty flavor. Ground flaxseed can be replaced by flaxseed oil, which is easier to use (though it doesn't contain as many lignans), but be sure to keep this oil in the refrigerator in a lightproof bottle to avoid oxidation (as well as a rancid smell). It is advisable not to store it more than three months.

Probiotics

The intestines ordinarily contain "friendly" bacteria, which help digestion and facilitate regular bowel movements. They also play an important stabilizing role for the immune system. Among the most common of these bacteria are *Lactobacillus acidophilus* and *Lactobacillus bifidus*.

It has been demonstrated that these probiotics inhibit the growth of colon cancer cells. Their effect on the facilitation of bowel movements also lowers the risk of colon cancer by reducing the time the intestines are exposed to carcinogenic substances in food. Probiotics thus also play a role in detoxification.[138] In addition, according to a 2006 Korean study, probiotics improve the performance of the immune system, as well as increasing the number of NK cells.[139]

Organic yogurts and kefir are good sources of probiotics. Soy yogurts are usually enriched with probiotics. These precious bacteria are also found in sauerkraut and kimchi.

Finally, certain foods are *prebiotics*, which means they contain polymers of fructose, which stimulate the growth of probiotic bacteria. Examples are garlic, onions, tomatoes, asparagus, bananas, and wheat.

Foods Rich in Selenium

Selenium is an oligoelement found in the soil. Vegetables and cereals grown organically contain large quantities of selenium. (Intensive agriculture depletes farmland of its selenium content, so selenium has now become rare in European-grown vegetables and cereals.)[140] This mineral is also found in fish, shellfish, and giblets and offal. Selenium stimulates immune cells and particularly NK cells (an increase as great as 80 percent, according to one study).[141] Selenium also boosts the effects of antioxidant mechanisms on the body.

TABLE 8. OMEGA-3 CONTENT IN FISH AND SEAFOOD	
Type of Fish	Amount Required to Provide the Recommended Daily 1 g of EPA + DHA*[142] (oz fish or g capsule)

Capsules
  cod-liver oil
  standard fish body oil
  omega-3 fatty-acid concentrate
	
	5.0
	3.0
	1.0–2.0

Catfish
  farmed
  wild
	
	20.0
	15.0

Clams	12.5

Cod
  Pacific
  Atlantic
	
	23.0
	12.5

Crab, Alaskan king	8.5
Flounder/Sole	7.0
Haddock	15.0
Halibut	3.0–7.5

Type of Fish	Amount Required to Provide the Recommended Daily 1 g of EPA + DHA* (oz fish or g capsule)

Herring
  Pacific
  Atlantic
	
	1.5
	2.0

Lobster	7.5–42.5
Mackerel	2.0–8.5

Salmon
  chum
  sockeye
  pink
  chinook
  Atlantic, farmed[†]
  Atlantic, wild[†]
	
	4.5
	4.5
	2.5
	2.0
	1.5–2.5
	2.0–3.5

Sardines	2.0–3.0
Scallops	17.5
Shrimp, mixed species	11.0

Trout, rainbow
  farmed
  wild
	
	3.0
	3.5

Tuna
  light, in water, drained
  white, in water, drained
  fresh
	
	12.0
	4.0
	2.5–12.0

*EPA = eicosapentaenoic acid and DHA = docasahexaenoic acid.
Fish and seafood represent a principal source of long-chain omega-3 (EPA and DHA). The levels vary depending on the type, the source, the raising, and the season in which they are fished.
[†]Farm-raised salmon, which aren't as active as wild, have more fat and, therefore, a higher omega-3 content than wild.

CHAPTER 9

The Anticancer Mind*

PART ONE: THE MIND-BODY CONNECTION

The Mind-Body Link

It was the 1980s, and an audience of physicians from an American university hospital had gathered to listen to a prominent psychologist talk about his research into the link between cancer and stress. The psychologist was excitedly discussing his latest results, which suggested that psychological factors have an unquestionable effect on the progression of tumors. But he had scarcely begun to address the question when a rather irritable surgeon sitting in the front row burst out, "You don't seriously believe all this bullshit, do you?" The surgeon's outburst perfectly illustrates the general attitude at the time. Until very recently, no one understood how purely psychological factors could have the slightest impact on the body's biology, and consequently on disease.

Today, more than twenty years after this incident, the existence of such an effect continues to be contested by some scientists, including psychiatrists who specialize in psycho-oncology. For some, the very idea that the psyche could influence cancer resembles a hope, a fantasy, even a mystical belief. A recent review in this vein recognized that a patient's quality of life benefits from receiving psychotherapy, but it nonetheless affirmed that "we have no proof today that links exist between the psychic processes, psychotherapeutic work, and the progression of tumors."[1]

It is true that the relationship between psychology and cancer has always given rise to interpretations that, though often based on sound observation, depended more on intuition than on rigorous proof. Two thousand years ago, the Greek physician Galen observed that depressed people were particularly

---

* I am especially grateful to Michael Lerner, Rachel Naomi Remen, David Spiegel, Francine Shapiro, and Jon Kabat-Zinn for the ideas presented in this chapter, which are largely inspired by my encounters with them and their writings.

prone to develop the illness. In 1759 an English surgeon wrote that cancer went along with "disasters in life, as occasion much trouble and grief."[2] In 1846 British medical authorities considered that "mental misery, sudden reverses in fortune, and habitual gloominess of temper . . . constitute the most powerful cause of the disease." The author of that article, Dr. Walter Hyle Walshe, a great surgeon and the most prominent authority on cancer in the middle of the nineteenth century, added his personal observation: "I have myself met with cases in which the connection appeared so clear that I have decided questioning its reality would seem a struggle against reason."[3]

Studies show that a large proportion of women diagnosed with breast cancer are convinced that their disease results from a major life stress, such as an abortion, a divorce, a child's illness, or the loss of a job they cared a great deal about.[4] What should we believe? Is there a causal link between the inevitable dramas of life and the onset of illness? Can we really "give ourselves cancer"?

I have thought about this a great deal, partly in the context of my own case. And after much thinking, reading, and discussion with specialists, I have come to conclusions that I would like to share with you here, because I believe they can help us all avoid illness or to be better equipped to confront it.

We should note first that it usually takes anywhere from five to forty years for the bad "seed" of cancer in the form of a cellular anomaly to become a detectable cancerous tumor. During this process, cells that were initially healthy become seriously malfunctional, due to abnormal genes or, much more commonly, exposure to radiation, environmental toxins, or other carcinogens such as benzopyrene from cigarette smoke. I must insist on one point: *No psychological factor by itself has ever been identified as being capable of creating that bad seed.* In other words, nothing permits us to state that psychic trauma can be the sole cause of cancer.

However, as with nutrition, exercise, or the quality of our air and water, certain psychological states can profoundly influence *the soil in which the seed develops.* Most patients I've known remember a period of particular stress in the months or years preceding the diagnosis of their cancer. Usually it was an ordeal that created a terrible feeling of helplessness. Many of us have been confronted with a chronic conflict that seems insoluble, or with overwhelming obligations that create a feeling of suffocation. These situations, I must insist, don't spark cancer, but, as an article published in *Nature Reviews Cancer* in 2006 observed, we know today that they can give it an opportunity to grow faster.[5] The factors contributing to cancer are so numerous and varied that no one should ever blame themselves or feel guilty for developing this disease. If your cat developed cancer, you would never dream of saying it was the cat's fault. However, anyone who has been diagnosed with cancer has the opportunity to learn to live differently, with the likely benefit of aiding in recovery. That is what I too had to do.

Stifled Emotions

I was born the eldest son of the eldest son. Scarcely had I been born when I was taken from my mother's arms and breast because they were considered inadequate. I was handed over to the nursery, to nursing assistants and baby formula, a system considered "more modern," more effective at protecting the child who was going to carry on the family line. I cried a great deal, partly, I imagine, because like all infants I would have liked to be in my mother's arms, rather than in a sort of incubator behind a soundproof window. My mother was twenty-two years old when she gave birth to me. Despite her intelligence and her character, she was only a child compared to her thirty-seven-year-old husband, who ran the country's most prominent news magazine. Very soon my paternal grandmother decreed that my mother wasn't competent enough to look after her grandson, and I was entrusted to a live-in nursemaid. My mother suffered terribly from the separation. She remembers her breasts leaking milk during the night when she was prevented from coming to me. During the years that followed, we never managed to heal our relationship; there had been too much suffering and privation.

I soon had three brothers, and she attached herself to them. Throughout my childhood, I suffered from my mother's absence. Still today, when I hear someone speak with emotion of everything his mother was to him, I know that I can't understand him completely. My body preserves the memory of the painful void I experienced as an infant. As I grew up, I managed to find emotional balance, to a great extent thanks to the nanny who looked after me from the time I was three months old. Her love, though sometimes awkward (after all, she was only eighteen years old!), was constant and sincere and gave me the oxygen I needed in the emotional emptiness that filled me. But I've never forgotten that to get me to obey, she would often remind me that if I wasn't good she would leave. These threats put me in a terrible state of powerlessness and despair. Quickly, I learned to give what was expected of me and of a firstborn. No temper tantrums, no outbursts. Instead, discipline and an attention to appearances. I think I played my role well, covering up my feelings to keep my place.

When I met Anna, thirty years later, I had still never managed to completely trust a woman. I certainly did not trust in her capacity to tolerate my faults without threatening to leave. Yet Anna didn't leave when we found out that I had a potentially fatal disease. I thought I found in her face—so calm and beautiful—that maternal, total, unconditional love that I had never known. She became the rock on which I built my life as a young adult. When I was alone and shut my eyes, her image appeared in front of me and I felt her presence. Part of her entered me and lived in my body. To say "I love you," Yanomami Indians of the Amazon say, "Ya pihi irakema," meaning "I have been contaminated by your being"—a part of you has entered me, and it lives and grows. That's exactly what I felt with Anna. Something of her lived in me. When I had barely emerged from my first surgery, with my shaved head sporting a broad, L-shaped scar, I asked her timidly if she would marry me. Her direct, unhesitating, deeply felt answer was one of the most beautiful moments of my life. My rational mind couldn't understand how this woman—so brilliant, so strong, so full of life—could agree to be tied to the frail and not very attractive person I was at that moment. But my heart knew that she had said yes with all her being, and that we were bound by something stronger than death itself. Love, our love, swept away all fear.

I remember our honeymoon on a riverboat in the estuary of Cape Fear. I wasn't a very skillful navigator. We spent a good part of those few days short of electricity, water, and fuel. But Anna was so playful and we were so in love that each of these upsets was a chance to share a laugh, cook, make love, or look at the stars when we ran aground a long way from everything, awaiting help that would arrive only the next day. After that, our whole life together seemed inspired by this same lightheartedness. Our "honeymoon" went on for two years. I felt invincible. As long as we were together, we could deal with anything. For the first time, I had the impression I was living the good life. And then Anna wanted to have a child. I would never have dared to ask her. I didn't want her to find herself raising a child alone. Nor did I want that child to grow up with the recollection of a father he or she had hardly known. I was thus profoundly touched when Anna said she was ready, she wasn't afraid, and she wanted a child from me whatever happened. Anna wasn't impulsive, and I knew that she had given it a lot of thought, and I also knew that she had the strength to raise a child alone. She immediately became pregnant. The birth of my son was the second most beautiful day of my life. Anna wanted to give birth as naturally as possible, and I watched her do it as one watches an Olympic athlete win a marathon. She was perfectly concentrated on the immense and triumphant task of giving life. Sometimes, between contractions, she looked at me briefly or grasped my hand. Sacha was born that night at the very beginning of spring, when the pear trees lining the streets of Pittsburgh had opened their first white blooms. She held him on her chest all night long. I didn't know then that this love I found so beautiful announced the end of ours.

Sacha slept very badly. We took him into our bed at night, and Anna didn't want him to leave it. During the day, he only napped in her arms. She refused to have him looked after by a babysitter. In five years we did not spend a single weekend alone. A part of me admired Anna's unbelievable devotion to this maternal love. But another part couldn't tolerate the intensity of this new relationship that was driving us apart. Very soon, I found myself as alone as I had been before meeting her. Exhausted by her day, she would wait for me to come home in the evening to share a little of her workload; but she asked me to give Sacha more attention than I was capable of. I felt myself disconnected from her and deprived of the energy that our relationship had given me. I was also falling seriously behind in my research work. More and more frequently, I slept alone in my office, next to the dog. It was an impossible situation. I was losing everything that had given meaning to my life: professional success, my wife's love, and the connection with my own son. For several years, I forced myself to do what was expected of me, even though I no longer got any satisfaction from it. I had lost all hope of restoring our relationship as a couple. In a certain way, my life had reverted to the childhood pattern I'd known before: getting just enough love to survive, and doing my best to fulfill obligations and keep up appearances. It was at the very moment when I couldn't go on— only two weeks after deciding to leave home and this marriage that no longer was one—that I learned my cancer had returned. It almost wasn't a surprise.

A Cancer-Prone Personality?

In the psychology department at the University of California at San Francisco, Lydia Temoshok, PhD, and Andrew Kneier, PhD, compared the emotional reactions of cancer patients with those of patients with heart disease. They subjected them to mild electric shocks and measured their physiological reactions. They then asked both groups of patients to explain how they had felt during the experiment. According to physiological measures, cancer patients reacted to the shocks more strongly than those with heart disease. But it was the cancer patients who later tended to minimize their professed discomfort when they answered the researchers' questions.[6] Temoshok suggested the concept of a "type C personality" for cancer patients (in contrast to the impatient, aggressive tendencies of the "type A personality" often found in cardiac patients).[7] Most psychotherapists—such as Drs. O. Carl and Stephanie Simonton, Dr. Lawrence LeShan, and Ian Gawler—who have worked with people with cancer have observed psychological characteristics similar to this personality type.[8–10]

Those exhibiting this type C personality are often people who, rightly or wrongly, never felt fully welcome in their childhood. Their parents may have been violent or irascible, or simply cold, distant, and demanding. Often these children received little encouragement and developed a feeling of vulnerability and weakness. Later, to be sure of being loved, they decided to conform to the best of their ability to what was expected of them rather than follow their own desires. Rarely angry (sometimes never!) they become "really nice" people as adults ... "always ready to help others" ... "saints!" They avoid conflict and put their needs and aspirations on the back burner, sometimes for the rest of their lives. In order to safeguard the emotional security that they so value, they may overinvest in a single aspect of their lives: their profession, their marriage, or their children. When this investment is suddenly threatened or lost—by a professional setback, a divorce, or retirement, or simply when children leave the nest—the childhood grief returns. Often it is more devastating still because it elicits the feeling that whatever one does, emotional suffering is inescapable.

As seductive as it may seem, in reality the concept of a type C personality lacks scientific rigor, and today it has been abandoned. I introduce it here, however, because it drew attention to the role of an important factor in cancer development—the feeling of helplessness, which has since attracted great interest and been the subject of a large number of scientific studies.

Whatever the personality type, certain ordeals are experienced as "second traumas" that reopen poorly healed wounds and inspire feelings of helplessness, despair, and abandonment. We know today that these feelings—helplessness in particular—can weigh heavily on psychological and biological balance. One of my therapist colleagues calls this the "hit and sink" phenomenon, referring to the children's game Battleship. The first wound, from childhood, is difficult but manageable. When a second "hit" strikes exactly the same spot, the entire psychological and even the physical structure may collapse.* At Emory University in Atlanta, the laboratory of Charles B. Nemeroff, MD, PhD, published a recent study that fits with this model of "hit and sink." In depressed adult patients with a history of trauma in early childhood, inflammation factors—those that contribute to the development of cancer—react particularly strongly to laboratory-induced stress.[12] Indeed, a team led by Professor Spiegel at Stanford University has observed that women suffering from advanced breast cancer who reported enduring severe trauma in their lives showed less resistance to their illness in the form of shorter disease-free survival periods following treatment.[13]

---

* Freud, being the pioneer he was, had already described a similar phenomenon relating to psychological trauma, which he called the "shock/aftershock" (machträglich) phenomenon.[11]

Feelings of Helplessness Feed Cancer

In humans, it is not a straightforward matter to investigate whether feeling helpless—never expressing one's emotions and almost *never* enjoying deep inner calm—can affect the growth of a tumor or the benefits gained from chemotherapy. It is obviously out of the question to subject patients to devastating situations in order to examine the consequences on their cancer. However, we can observe how the physiology of laboratory animals responds to situations of helplessness. One very clever experiment measured precisely how helplessness generated by experimental manipulation modified the growth and spread of cancer in rats.

At the University of Pennsylvania, in the laboratory of Martin Seligman, PhD, rats were grafted with the exact quantity of cancer cells known to induce a fatal tumor in 50 percent of them. In this experiment, the rats were divided into three groups. In the first group, the control group, the animals received the graft but were then left to live their lives as usual in the laboratory cage. In the second group, the rats were given small, random electric shocks which they had no control over. The animals in the third group were given the same random shocks but were provided with a lever that they quickly learned to press to avoid getting *extra* shocks.

The results, published in *Science,* were very clear. One month after the graft, 54 percent of control rats had successfully rejected their tumor. The rats subjected to shocks with no means of escape had become despondent. They would not fight against intrusions into their cage, and lost their appetite for food and for sexual partners. Only 23 percent of these rats managed to overcome their cancer. The most interesting group was the third one. Though they were submitted to the intense stress of the same number of frequent electric shocks, having learned that they could avoid receiving extra shocks by pressing a lever, these animals did not become despondent. They remained feisty when intruded upon, ate well, and copulated as frequently as rats do in a normal environment. And in that group, 63 percent successfully rejected the tumor, more than the rats left alone. It seems that the helplessness was capable of hastening the tumor's spread, not the shocks themselves.[14]

The lesson of this study is crucial. It isn't stress itself—the "electric shocks" life inevitably gives—that promotes cancer development; it is the persistent perception of helplessness we may have in the face of stress that affects the body's reaction to the disease.* Perhaps there may even be a "good

---

* Three other studies on rodents published since have confirmed the effect of unmanageable stress—which induces feelings of helplessness—on the immune system and the progression of tumors.[15–17]

stress," one that challenges us to reach for our inner resources, and that may stimulate our natural defenses to do their work more effectively. Yet many of us often feel that we just don't have a lever that would allow us to regain some semblance of control—at least over ourselves, if not always over the situation. Regaining this control is what the remainder of this chapter is about.

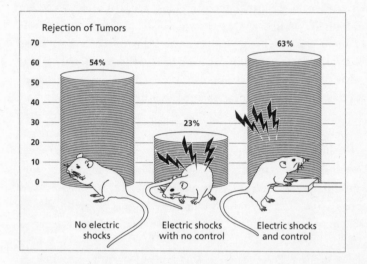

Figure 17. Rats subjected to electric shocks they can't control develop aggressive tumors. Those that learn how to evade the shocks reject the tumors much more effectively.[18]

Ian Gawler's Great Calm

If the experience of helplessness and despair promotes cancerous growth, will a state of serenity, on the contrary, slow it down? Certain exceptional cases suggest this may be so. In Melbourne, Australia, Ian Gawler, a young veterinarian who had just finished training, found out that he had a dangerous osteosarcoma (cancer of the bone) that had affected his leg. Amputation, followed by a year of conventional treatments, was unsuccessful in halting tumor growth. It spread to his hip and thorax, where it created visible deformities. His oncologist expected him to live no more than a few weeks, perhaps less than a month. With nothing to lose and with his wife's full support, Ian threw himself into an intensive practice of meditation. He wanted to enjoy in his remaining days the calm he had discovered practicing yoga. His physician, Dr. Meares, had been initiated into meditation in India, where he had encountered great mystics. He was particularly impressed by the calm his young patient succeeded in experiencing. He attributed it to the characteristic serenity of the dying in their final days. But after a few weeks of this regimen, to the astonishment of all, Ian seemed to be getting better. After several months of intensive meditation (an hour, three times a day!), along with a strict diet, Ian recovered his strength. The hideous bone deformities that had marked his chest started to dissolve. A few months later, they had completely vanished. Dr. Meares asked Ian how he explained his extraordinary remission. "I think it's our way of living, the way we experience our life," Ian answered, speaking of his wife and himself. As if, Dr. Meares explains, at every moment of his existence, this patient was filled with the peace he experienced in his intense periods of meditation.[19] Today, thirty years later, Ian Gawler is still alive. Since his recovery, he has devoted most of his time to working with groups of cancer patients, helping them integrate meditation and other healthy habits into their lives.*

Proof of the Mind-Body Link

Skeptics will object that Ian Gawler's story, however inspirational, may only be the exception that proves the rule. Until we have studied the effects of a calm psyche under a rigorous, scientific framework, we will never be able to dispel this doubt. However, just this kind of indisputable evidence is starting to emerge.

Almost despite himself, David Spiegel, MD, a psychiatrist from Stanford University, challenged conventional views on the relationship between stress and the chances of survival in the most serious cancers. As an undergraduate, he had studied philosophy at Yale University. A key idea that has guided him throughout his career: To be fully human, people ought to have as authentic a relationship as possible with others. They should know that in their deepest being they are intrinsically free to reconstruct and transform themselves, and they need to grant others this same powerful freedom.

After his medical and psychiatric studies at Harvard, Spiegel devoted his research to the conditions that enable an individual to attain this powerful authenticity and openness to others. Like Sartre, he firmly believed that in confronting the fear of death, human beings sometimes fully become themselves. As a young psychiatrist, he had the opportunity to work at Stanford University with the great psychotherapist Irvin Yalom, MD, who was testing this idea. Together they conducted weekly support groups of seriously ill women. These women,

---

* Ian Gawler tells the story of his extraordinary recovery in a very beautiful book, *You Can Conquer Cancer*. Meditation and a strictly natural diet were not the only resources he used. He also drew on a number of different natural treatments, both psychological and psychospiritual. However, he attributes his recovery principally to his inner calm.

all with metastatic breast cancer, had an expectation of survival ranging from a few months to a few years. If the psychiatrists' hypothesis was correct, this was a particularly auspicious time for them to grow into their full potential.

In the study, groups of eight to ten women met every week. They discussed their fear, their loneliness, and their anger, as well as their desires and their ways of dealing with the disease. They soon learned one of the most fundamental lessons in life: Everyone is wounded, to a greater or lesser degree, and has learned to be ashamed of it. In these support groups, everyone was seriously affected by disease. There was nothing left to hide. The women could speak out and share their innermost thoughts with one another.

For some of them, it was the first time in their lives they had experienced the reassuring peacefulness of such trust. Quite naturally, something of a miracle occurred then: These meetings were neither tragic nor pathetic, but tended to be filled with natural laughter and camaraderie. It was as if in accepting their own wounds, they had opened the way to positive emotions, to joy, to the desire to be alive, to the satisfaction of being together here and now.

Sometimes, of course, one of them was carried off by the disease. Then the women talked about the loss of their departed friend. They recalled her hearty laugh when she described her husband's blunders, her watchful gaze as another participant explained the difficulties of her last surgery, or the grace she maintained even when in pain. They yielded freely to their feelings of grief. These moments were very difficult, but everyone felt that the absent member would go on living in their hearts through these memories. Implicitly, they sensed that when their turn came, they too would be honored by such recollections and live on in their companions' hearts.

For a year the women met regularly before each went her own way. For the purposes of his study, Spiegel first compared the psychological state of the participants with that of women with the same diagnoses and the same medical treatments who had not participated in these group meetings. The women who had learned, thanks to the support group, to confront their fear, to express their inner feelings, and to experience relationships more authentically were less subject to depression, anxiety, and even physical pain.[20, 21]

Their entire emotional state had improved, just as Dr. Spiegel had expected. But he had never dared to imagine a possible effect on the course of the disease, and still less on the chances of survival. Spiegel was even certain of the contrary. He was convinced there was no link between a patient's mental state and the development of cancer. He was furious with those who attributed cancer to psychological conflict. He felt that this argument gave patients the painful feeling that their cancer was in part their own fault. To prove once and for all that this hypothesis was wrong, he wanted to show that the women who had participated in the support group and whose mental state had clearly improved had *not* lived longer than those in the control group. But when he followed up on his study, a major surprise awaited him.

First, when he called the families, three out of fifty of the original participants answered the telephone themselves, ten years after the discovery of their disease. Considering the seriousness of their condition, this was, quite simply, unbelievable. Not a single one of the thirty-six women in the control group had survived so long. Next, while questioning the families about the length of time the support group women had survived, he observed that they had lived on average twice as long as the others. A difference could even be observed between those who had attended the group regularly and those who had participated sporadically. The more regularly a woman had attended, the longer she had lived.* When these results were published in *The Lancet,* they startled the world medical establishment.[22] Thanks to this study, the link between mental state and the development of disease suddenly went from being a slightly harebrained "new age" concept to being a perfectly respectable scientific hypothesis.[†]

What Is the Feeling of Helplessness?

Since the publication of Spiegel's study, researchers have sought to measure more precisely the impact of psychology, and specifically the feeling of helplessness, on cancer. One of the most enlightening studies on this topic was published in 2006. Researchers at the University of California at Berkeley analyzed the results of a longitudinal study undertaken in Finland, in a region characterized by an abnormally high rate of mortality in relatively young men. Searching for the psychosocial causes of this pathology, the researchers

---

* It's important to stress that at the beginning of the study all the patients had similar diagnoses, and that the choice between those who joined the therapy group and those in the control group was random. This guaranteed that the longer survival of the therapy group members wasn't due to better health at the outset or to a different psychological disposition.

† Since then, several other studies have evaluated this hypothesis. Four of them found results comparable to Stanford's.[23-26] Six of them did not observe any effect. But in three of these there was no psychological improvement in the patients. Thus, an impact on survival time could not be expected. In all, there are therefore five studies that observe an improvement in survival time, and three that have not found an effect.[27-32] In a recent replication of his study—on 125 patients—David Spiegel and his research team observed a *tripling* of survival time in women participating in the group, but only in those who tested negative for estrogen receptors.[33] Those who were given Tamoxifen or other estrogen antagonists did not show a prolongation of survival (linked to participation in the group), suggesting that these drugs had already given them the protection that may be conferred by psychological treatment. (Antagonists to estrogen receptors did not exist at the time of the study published in 1989.)

discovered the particular importance of the feeling of helplessness, not just for cardiac disease but for all causes of mortality, and notably for cancer.[34] As this was a prospective study—in other words, a study of people who *were initially healthy*—the results are particularly striking.

The authors sought to evaluate precisely the intensity or extent of feelings of helplessness. Each participant was asked to respond "true" or "false" to two statements:

1. "I feel that it is impossible to reach the goals I would like to strive for."
2. "The future seems to me to be hopeless, and I can't believe that things are going to change for the better."

Six years later and all other factors being equal, the persons who had rated both statements as "true" had a mortality rate (from all causes combined) that was *three times higher* than that of persons characterized by the lowest level of helplessness (who didn't think either statement applied to them). They also developed 160 percent more fatal cancers.

These numbers are all the more significant because they measure the specific impact of the feeling of helplessness, independent of all other variables—biological state, tobacco or alcohol use, socioeconomic status, depression, or social isolation. Struck by the strength of the correlation, the authors noted that although they were reporting definitive proof that the feeling of helplessness has a major impact on health, we still need to understand the individual, social, and environmental conditions that underlie this feeling and to find the best approach to counteract it.

Their results were recently confirmed by an impressively widescale meta-analysis of 165 studies published in 2008 by psychobiologists at University College London.[35] The authors concluded that psychosocial factors linked to stress are correlated with an increase in the risk of cancer in healthy people and with a reduction of survival rates in people who have cancer. The authors defined "psychosocial stress" as a hybrid category including both stressful events (such as the death of close family members, divorce, exhausting work, etc.) and individual reactions to these events, notably feelings of helplessness. The more long term the study, the clearer the effect on mortality, which implies that psychosocial factors have a slow but cumulative effect on cancer.

The impact of such psychosocial factors on mortality from cancer is, of course, far smaller than that of "heavy-duty" factors like tobacco or obesity. But it is not negligible. In fact, it is roughly comparable to the risk associated with hormone replacement therapy in post-menopausal women. Although the dangers of that treatment have been widely communicated, our medical authorities remain modestly silent with respect to the equally dangerous health consequences of prolonged negative mental states. Perhaps this is because they are not sure how to help those who struggle with such feelings. To address this issue, I will detail later in this chapter some of the practical methods that each of us can learn in order to avoid sinking into such despair.

The Physiology of Helpessness

Is there an identifiable mechanism through which negative mental states influence the way the body functions, facilitate the onset of cancer, or enhance its progress?

It's possible that the physiological effect doesn't stem directly from negative emotions, but from the high-risk behaviors that are often a close companion. For example, a depressed or discouraged person will likely not have the necessary willpower to stop smoking, eat in a more healthy way, or exercise with regularity. His sleep may be poor, he may neglect his weight, drink too much, or even forget to take medication.

However, researchers from University College London observed that the effects of psychosocial factors persist even in people who display none of these behaviors. The logical conclusion is that there exists a direct, physiological mechanism linking body to mind. These days we have a much better understanding of how the biology of stress impacts the development of cancer. It is now known that feelings of helplessness cause the release of hormones that activate the body's "emergency" systems—such as the inflammatory response—which can facilitate the growth and spread of tumors. At the same time, stress slows down all the functions that can be "put on hold," such as digestion, tissue repair, and the immune system.

In the last twenty years, a new scientific field has opened up that explicitly investigates the link between psychological factors and the activity of the immune system. It is referred to as psychoneuroimmunology. Let me briefly break down the three dimensions of this approach; that is, psychology, neurology, and immunology. The psychological aspect refers to the emotional response to difficult life experiences. When people have the feeling that their life is no longer manageable, or that it leads to more suffering than joy (this is the "psychological" part), the neurological response to this stress is the release of stress hormones like adrenalin and cortisol. These hormones in turn activate the nervous system, accelerating heart rate, raising blood pressure, and tensing muscles so they will be prepared to make an effort or stave off attack (this is the "neurological" part). This neurological response is commonly referred to as the fight-or-flight response. But we know today that its effects are felt much more broadly. These same chemical substances that activate the neurological and visceral reflexes of stress also act on immune cells. White blood cells have receptors on their surface that detect the presence of stress hormones and react according to fluctuations in the levels of these hormones in the bloodstream. Some of these cells respond by releasing inflammatory cytokines and chemokines. Natural killer cells are blocked by noradrenaline and cortisol, remaining passively glued to the walls of blood vessels rather than attacking viruses or abnormal precursor cancer cells.

Immune Cells and the Will to Live

We saw in chapter 4 that mice capable of fully mobilizing their immune cells—the descendants of "Mighty Mouse"—are "resistant" to cancer, even when injected with massive doses of extremely aggressive cells. Following along these same lines, at the National Cancer Institute, the laboratory of Ron Herberman, MD (now head of the Cancer Institute of the University of Pittsburgh), studied the NK cells of women recently operated on for breast cancer. He showed that the more active these cells were in the weeks following the operation, the better the women's chances of long-term survival.[36, 37]

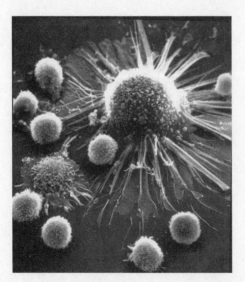

Figure 18. White blood cells of the immune system attack a cancer cell (larger size). They receive signals from the emotional brain, and they respond by sending signals back to the brain. Cells of the immune system are thus part of what Candace Pert, PhD, refers to as the "mobile brain."

Professor Herberman also demonstrated that women with breast cancer who are better able to face the disease psychologically had much *more* active NK cells than those who sank into depression and helplessness.[38] In 2005

Susan Lutgendorf, PhD, of the University of Iowa, confirmed these results in women with ovarian cancer. Those who felt loved and supported and who kept up their morale had more combative NK cells than those who felt alone, helpless, and emotionally distraught.[39]

Everything suggests that the white blood cells of the immune system (the NK cells and the T and B lymphocytes) are particularly sensitive to feelings of helplessness—a conviction that nothing can be done to overcome the disease—and the ensuing loss of the will to live. Martin Seligman's rats—exposed to electric shocks they could not avoid—acted helpless in ways very similar to traumatized humans. Their behavior suggested they had lost all confidence in their abilities. Confronted with competition, they were submissive and passive. They no longer fought back when attacked. And it was exactly in such circumstances that their immune system also gave up. It's as if the emotional state observed from the outside in the individual's behavior is reflected in the internal behavior of immune cells. When the rat—or the person—gives up, feeling that life is no longer worth living, the immune system lays down its arms as well.

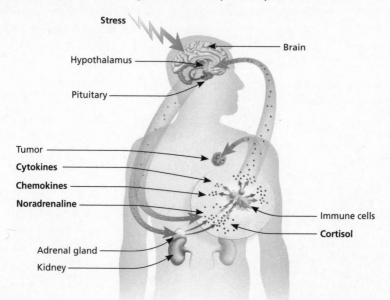

Figure 19. Helplessness and cancer. Psychological stress leads to the release of nonadrenaline and cortisol. They disturb the balance of immune cells, causing overproduction of proinflammatory cytokines and chemokines and inhibition of the normal response to the presence of abnormal cells. In turn, immune cells also release cytokines and chemokines that affect the brain and influence behavior.

In contrast, rediscovering in oneself the will to live often accompanies a decisive turning point in the course of the disease.

Helen was fifty-two when she learned that she suffered from an aggressive lymphoma. The first six rounds of chemotherapy had no effect. Two more treatments only increased the cancer's virulence. Her only hope lay in recourse to a particularly dangerous intervention: an autologous bone marrow transplant. This procedure requires the use of drugs so toxic that they lead to the total destruction of the immune system. After undergoing the transplant, Helen had to spend three weeks in an isolation chamber. Following strict sterilization procedures, her visitors entered her room dressed in outfits that made them look like astronauts; Helen had the unpleasant feeling that she was no longer living on the same planet as these strange visitors and that she might never get back home.

After three weeks, her condition had worsened and she wasn't able to leave the isolation chamber. Her visitors found her so thin and frail that they wondered if they weren't seeing her for the last time. They could neither hug her nor hold her hand. They couldn't even smile, because their faces were hidden behind sterile masks. With hope hanging by a thread, feeling as if her body was giving up, Helen clung to the one thing that had always been there, like a faithful and affectionate companion—the sensation of breath in her chest. Hanging on to one breath at a time, she connected in her deepest being with the will to live. This inner force seemed to link her to everything alive around her: the tree with its foliage visible through the window, the laughs and cries of children going down the corridor, sometimes the stars after nightfall. She experienced a strange feeling of peace. She took comfort in the knowledge that the life flowing through her would continue on in the outer world.

Psychotherapists today who work with people who have cancer understand the importance of nurturing the patient's will to live. There are many ways to cultivate this force, this flame that always flickers deep within us. I have experimented with some that have gained my respect and gratitude, both as a therapist and as a patient. I would like to talk to you about those that seem to me the most important.

PART TWO: RECONNECTING WITH THE LIFE FORCE

Facing the crises of everyday life, its complex schedules and sometimes terrifying events, we often allow ourselves to be submerged by feelings of helplessness and fear. This is understandable and, often, inevitable. However, if these feelings become a constant state of mind, they are accompanied by changes in physiology that may damage our body's defenses against cancer. Avoiding stress at any cost would be impossible. But what can be done is to release tensions regularly. With experience, one can learn to let stress just glide by—like the proverbial water off a duck's back, at least for a period of respite.

In the first minutes after I learned that my tumor had come back, in exactly the same location, I felt overpowered. Soon my body was rebelling in alarm. Anxiety had always had that particular way of gripping me from the inside, making my heart beat faster, putting pressure on my chest, tightening my throat, or making it harder to breathe. My mind was starting to race about all the consequences. I could see the turmoil of going through treatment all over again, and thought I wouldn't have the strength to do it a second time. I had just left my wife, my son, and my home and wouldn't have any support. I pictured myself with my head shaven, emaciated, exhausted, and alone. Staring at the computer screen with the neuroradiologist's report that I had just brought up on the hospital's information system, I thought I might lose control of my body. Perhaps I might even faint. Then I remembered something I once heard the Dalai Lama say. A journalist had asked him if the Chinese invasion of his country, the destruction of temples, the imprisonment and torture endured by so many of his friends, weren't cause enough to disturb his serenity. He answered, "The Chinese took everything from me. I am not going to let them take my soul, too." I recalled some simple relaxation exercises I had learned in a particularly enjoyable yoga class. I had been practicing them at home occasionally and always felt a little better afterward. I thought this might be the time to find out if they worked when you really needed them.

I sat up straight, took some deep breaths, and focused on the smooth sensation of air flowing in my chest. I reassured my mind that I would give this situation all the attention it deserved and would seek all the help I needed, but that, for now, it did not help to envision a movie of all the worst possible outcomes. Gradually, my body calmed down; my mind slowly returned to its normal state. Within about fifteen minutes I could feel my heart rate becoming normal, and see the color returning to my face. I resigned myself to teaching a class to residents, as planned, since I knew they had been really looking forward to it. And it worked. The class was a welcome opportunity to feel useful and think about something else. Helplessness had released its hold on me, at least for that moment.

Focus on the Self in the Present

We can all learn to cultivate our inner strength. Over the past five thousand years, all the great medical and spiritual traditions in the East—such as yoga, meditation, tai chi, and qigong—have taught that any individual may take over the reins of his or her inner being and bodily functioning. This can be achieved simply by concentrating the mind and focusing on the breath. Today we know, thanks to a number of studies, that this mastery is one of the best ways to reduce the impact of stress.* It's also one of the best ways to reestablish harmony in a person's physiology and, as a result, stimulate the body's natural defenses.

The first step in any process of mastering physiology consists of learning to focus one's attention and turn it inward. It's an understatement to say that most of us haven't had much practice at this. Everything in our usual way of life turns us away from our inner being.

Joel and the "Monkey Mind"

When I met Joel, he left me with the impression that I hadn't succeeded in meeting him. He had come to our Center for Integrative Medicine in Pittsburgh for complementary treatment of a metastatic prostate cancer that had spread to his spinal column. Tall, slim, a bit too elegant for a medical consultation, he talked so much that I could hardly get in a question. He had trouble sticking to one subject and jumped around in the conversation at a dizzying pace. His life as a movie producer in Los Angeles seemed marked with the same disorder as our conversation. Instead of talking to me about his cancer, he told me how he used communication technology to reduce his stress. Thanks to his BlackBerry phone (one of the first), he was "hyperconnected" and could "work anywhere." What pleased him most was receiving calls and e-mails and claiming he was at the office when actually he had gone home. He could play chess with his son while reading his messages. And when he had gotten his son into a difficult spot that required time to think, Joel took advantage of the opportunity to answer his messages. I wondered where he was in truth, since he seemed to be neither in his office nor at home. He was neither fully with his phone and e-mail correspondents nor with his son. Since his real attention was with no one, the experience of this effervescent activity must have resembled a no-man's-land without substance. Everyone spends a lot of time in this no-man's-land. Eastern traditions refer to this as the "monkey mind." In this state, one's thoughts hop around in all directions, like agitated monkeys jumping around in a cage.

When I talked to a colleague who knew Joel about the difficulties I'd encountered during the examination, he smiled: "I know. Before we could help him, he'd need to spend two weeks alone sitting on a rock in the desert

---

* I've addressed this topic in much greater detail in my earlier book, *The Instinct to Heal* (also known as *Healing without Freud or Prozac* outside the United States and Canada).[40, 41]

to learn to refocus. At *least* two weeks . . . " He was only half joking. Like Joel, many of us have become strangers to our inner world, gone astray in everything that seems more urgent and more important—e-mails, television programs, telephone calls. Like Joel, many of us need to begin by making contact with ourselves.*

Positive attention is a force that does good to anything it touches. Children, dogs, cats often know more about it than we do. They come to us for no particular purpose, to show us a picture they've made, a bone they've found, or a mouse they've caught in the garden. Or sometimes just for a hug or a scratch under the chin. We know how important this is to them and offer it willingly. But when do we show this benevolent attention to ourselves?

At the Commonweal Center, where I stayed after my relapse, and nowadays in most residential seminars for cancer patients, this is the first thing they learn: for a week, practically no telephone calls, no e-mail, no television. Instead, they participate in two one-hour sessions of yoga or meditation every day. Jon Kabat-Zinn, PhD, a former MIT biologist, has been teaching meditation to medical patients for thirty years. His program is used now in more than 250 hospitals in the United States and Canada (including large university medical centers such as Duke, Stanford, Pittsburgh, the University of California at San Francisco, the University of Washington, Sloan-Kettering, Wisconsin, and Toronto) and also in Europe.†

Kabat-Zinn always insists that spending time every day alone with oneself is "a radical act of love." Like the great tradition of shamans, who always prescribe a ritual of purification to be performed alone, this reflective solitude is the essential precondition to harmonizing the inner healing forces of the body.

The Breath: A Gateway to Biology

In yoga, meditation, qigong, and modern Western methods, the gateway to the inner self is breathing.

Begin by sitting comfortably, with your back straight, in what the Tibetan master Sogyal Rinpoche calls a "dignified" posture.[43] It gives full freedom to the flow of air that slips down through the nostrils toward the throat, then

---

* In his last book—*Coming to Our Senses*—Jon Kabat-Zinn explains that the more connected we are to the outside world (cell phone, e-mail, Internet), the less connected we are to our inner selves.[42]

† Hospitals in Germany, Holland, Sweden, Norway, the United Kingdom, Belgium, and Switzerland offer this program in "mindfulness-based stress reduction."

the bronchi, and finally to the bottom of the lungs, before reversing its route. With your attention focused, take two deep, slow breaths to begin relaxation. A sensation of comfort, lightness, and well-being will settle into your chest and shoulders. As you repeat this exercise, you will learn to let your breathing be led by your attention and to let your attention rest on your breath. As you relax, you may feel your mind become like a leaf floating on water, rising and falling as waves pass underneath. Your attention accompanies the *sensation* of each intake of breath and the long exhalation of air leaving the body gently, slowly, gracefully, all the way to the end, until there is nothing more than a tiny, barely perceptible breath left. Then there is a pause. You learn to sink into this pause, more and more profoundly. It's often while resting briefly in it that you feel in most intimate contact with your body. With practice, you can feel your heart beating, sustaining life, as it has been doing indefatigably for so many years. And then, at the end of the pause, notice a tiny spark light up all by itself and set off a new cycle of breath. What you feel is the spark of life, which is always in us and which, through this process of attention and relaxation, you may discover for the first time.

Inevitably, your mind is distracted from this task after a few minutes and is drawn toward the outside world: the concerns of the past or the obligations of the future. The essential art of this "radical act of love" consists of doing what you would do for a child who needs undivided attention. You recognize the importance of these other thoughts, but while patiently promising to attend to them when the time comes, you push them to the side and come back to the person who really needs you in the present moment, that is, yourself. When this practice is taught, simply and unadorned, to a group of patients, it is not uncommon to see tears streaming down some faces. It is as if these individuals are experiencing benevolence and calm for the first time. They discover an immense sense of simple well-being, which has been absent in their everyday lives. Later, people who meditate learn that at any point in time they can access the mellowness and calm they find during meditation. With a little practice, they will seek it while in line at the supermarket, stuck in a traffic jam, or facing abuse from a colleague at the office. All they need to reconnect with this source of peace is to focus their attention on a long exhalation and the pause that follows.

Breathing is the only visceral function that is totally autonomous with regard to the conscious mind (like digestion or heartbeats, breathing goes on even if we're not thinking about it) and yet easily regulated by the will. The control center for breathing, located at the base of the brain, is sensitive to all the molecules that are constantly exchanged between the emotional brain and the organs of the body, including the immune system. Attention to breathing brings people closer to the pulsations of vital body processes and connects them to conscious thought. Fortunately, it isn't necessary to "believe" in this in order to see it happen and benefit from it. There is a perfectly objective way to measure the relationship between exercises such as yoga and meditation and what is happening in the body.

The Mantra and the Rosary

Over the past fifteen years, Luciano Bernardi, MD, PhD, of the University of Pavia in Italy, has been interested in autonomous body rhythms that form the foundations of physiology: variations in heart rate, blood pressure, respiration, etc. He explored the way these rhythms fluctuate from one moment to the next and at different times of day. He knew that a sound balance between these various biorhythms is perhaps the most accurate indicator of good health; in some studies, measures of this balance can accurately predict survival forty years down the line.[44, 45]

Dr. Bernardi tracked the conditions that could lead to a temporary disorganization of these rhythms and examined the way the body then recovered its equilibrium. To do so, he had his subjects perform exercises such as doing arithmetic in their heads or reading aloud, all the while measuring the microvariations in their heart rate, blood pressure, blood flow to the brain, and breathing patterns. He was thus able to observe that the slightest stressful mental exercise had an immediate effect on these rhythms. They reacted by adapting to the effort, however minimal it might be. But the great surprise came from what is called the "control" condition.

In order to measure the physiological changes set off by the mental exercises, they had to be compared with a so-called neutral condition—a condition in which the subjects talked aloud but without mental effort or stress. In Dr. Bernardi's experiment, the neutral condition consisted of getting the subjects to recite a text they knew by heart, thus requiring no particular attention. As the subjects lived in Lombardy, a deeply Catholic region of Italy, he quite naturally thought of having them recite the rosary.

When Dr. Bernardi's subjects started reciting a stream of Ave Marias in Latin, the laboratory instruments recorded a totally unexpected phenomenon: All the different biological rhythms being measured started to resonate. They all lined up, one after the other, mutually amplifying one another to create a smooth, harmonious pattern. A miracle? Not necessarily. Dr. Bernardi soon realized that the explanation was something much more simple. In Italy the congregation recites the rosary taking turns with the priest. Each recitation occurs in a single exhalation. The inhalation that follows takes place during the priest's turn.* The subjects had quite naturally adopted this rhythm while reciting the prayer during the experiment. In doing so, they had adjusted mechanically—and subconsciously—to a frequency of six breaths a minute, which happens to be the natural rhythm of fluctuations in the other biological functions Dr. Bernardi was measuring (heart rate, blood pressure, blood flow to the brain). The result of this synchronization was that the rhythm of each function resonated with the others, mutually reinforcing each other, just as when one is seated on a swing and the forward thrust of the legs, timed precisely with the upswing, amplifies the movement.

His curiosity aroused, Dr. Bernardi concluded that if the rhythms of the Ave Maria had the capacity to modulate the rhythms of physiology, other religious practices might have a comparable effect. He postulated that the effect would be more intense within those religions that place awareness of the body at the center of spiritual practices, such as in Hinduism or Buddhism. In order to investigate this hypothesis, he had individuals who had never practiced an Eastern discipline learn to recite the best-known mantra in Buddhism: *Om Mani Padme Hum.* As in yoga practice, the subjects learned to let their voices carry each syllable of the mantra, so that they could feel the sounds vibrating in their throats. They would then continue to follow their exhalation until they felt like breathing in again for the next repetition. Bernardi noted exactly the same results as seen with the recitation of Ave Marias. The subjects' breathing automatically adopted a pace of six breaths a minute, a harmonization, or coherence, with the rhythms of other autonomous physiological functions. Intrigued, Bernardi wondered if this surprising similarity between such distant religious practices could have sprung from common roots. In fact, he found a historical source suggesting that the rosary had been introduced in Europe by crusaders who received it from the Arabs, who had in turn adapted it from practices of Tibetan monks and yoga masters in India.[46] Clearly, the discovery of practices that bring forth the harmonization of biological rhythms for well-being and health go back to the most distant past.

In 2006, Julian Thayer and Esther Sternberg, researchers at Ohio State University and at the National Institutes of Health, published, in the *Annals of the New York Academy of Sciences,* a review of all the studies concerning the amplitude and variations of biological rhythms. They concluded that everything that amplifies variations—as happens in the states of resonance or

---

* The Ave Maria in Latin is recited as follows: The priest says, "Ave Maria, gratia plena, Dominus tecum. Benedicta tu en mulieribus, et benedictus fructus ventris tui, Jesus"; then the congregation answers, "Sancta Maria, Mater Dei, ora pro nobis peccatoribus, nunc et in hora mortis nostrae. Amen."

"coherence" described by Bernardi—is associated with a number of health benefits,[47]* in particular:

- better functioning of the immune system,
- reduction of inflammation, and
- better regulation of blood sugar levels.

These are, precisely, three of the principal factors that act against the development of cancer.

Between birth, when the amplitude of biological rhythms is the greatest, and the approach of death, when it is lowest, amplitude of variations (referred to technically as "variability") declines by approximately 3 percent a year.[48] This means that the body progressively loses its adaptability; it has

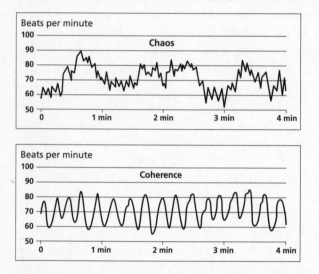

Figure 20. Chaos and coherence. In states of stress, anxiety, depression, or anger, the natural variation in cardiac rhythm becomes weak and irregular or "chaotic." In states of well-being, compassion, or gratitude, or when attention is centered on breathing, this variability is greater and becomes "coherent": Alternation between increases and decreases in cardiac rhythm is regular and aligns itself with other biological rhythms. The same state is induced by reciting the Buddhist mantra *Om Mani Padme Hum* or the rosary in Latin.[49] (This image © HeartMath. ® It comes from the emWave ® PC Stress Relief System developed by Quantum Tech, Inc., in Boulder Creek, California, USA.)

---

* The parameter most commonly used as the index of biological rhythms is "heart rate variability," which is the object of this particular article. It's also the one that is measured by biofeedback methods centered on "cardiac coherence" (see *The Instinct to Heal*). It is important to note that the state of "coherence" is associated with a *greater variability* (amplitude of variations) of heartbeats. What is regular in coherence is not the heartbeat itself, but the pattern of variation.

increasing difficulty maintaining balance when faced with the hazards of our physical and emotional environment. The weakening of this equilibrium in the body's functions is associated with a number of health problems linked to aging: high blood pressure, cardiac insufficiency, complications from diabetes, infarction, sudden death, and, of course, cancer. But it so happens that this balance—which we can easily evaluate by measuring the amplitude of heart rate variations—is also one of the biological functions that responds best to training in breathing and concentration (see figure 20). This is exactly what Dr. Bernardi discovered by showing the impact of practices as ancient as a Buddhist mantra and the rosary.[50]

Like Dr. Bernardi's subjects, everyone can learn to influence the balance of autonomous rhythms, which are central to states of health. Some will do it by reciting a mantra or a prayer. For most people, it can be done simply by directing attention within.

Meditation in the Laboratory

In his laboratory at the University of Wisconsin, Richard Davidson, PhD, studies changes in activity within the brains of people who have practiced meditation for years. Several Tibetan monks have participated in the experiment—among them Matthieu Ricard, PhD, a former cell biologist turned Buddhist monk and philosopher, who helped set up the experiment. During meditation, their cerebral rhythms register a larger amplitude of oscillations than in nonmeditative states. In addition, activity measured within the different brain regions begins to oscillate in harmony. The regions are said to "synchronize." On the scale of the brain, it's a phenomenon comparable to establishing coherence in the body's biological processes. Still better, Davidson and his collaborators have discovered that this synchronization lasts even beyond meditation sessions.[51]

Fortunately, the health benefits of such states can accrue even in beginners. The same laboratory ran an experiment with executives from a large biotechnology firm as the test subjects. Two groups were studied. Members of the first group didn't change anything in their habits, while those in the second group were trained in "mindfulness meditation," as it is taught in the hospital program established by Jon Kabat-Zinn. After a scant eight weeks, among those who had made a short period of meditation part of their everyday habits, significant changes had taken place in the electric activity of their brains as measured by EEG. Regions associated with positive mood and optimism (the left frontal regions) were distinctly more active compared to their earlier state or to that of the control group. And this effect reached further than the brain or the subjects' mood: Their immune systems reacted to the flu vaccine more forcefully than those of the members of the control group. All these changes occurred with only two months of practice.[52]

In Calgary, Canada, the research team of Professor Linda Carlson, PhD, at the university's cancer center studied breast and prostate cancer patients who practiced this same meditation program. After some eight weeks, they reported sleeping better, feeling distinctly less stressed, and sensing that their lives were richer. Meditation benefited their immune systems too. Their white blood cells, including NK cells, recovered a normal profile, far more propitious for fighting cancer.*

Bob, for example, was sixty and worked for the board of education in 1999 when he found he had prostate cancer.

After radiotherapy to the area, he started a mindfulness meditation program at the Calgary Hospital. In the beginning, he would meditate only five to ten minutes a day, but after several weeks he discovered how to make the exercise last easily for thirty minutes. According to Bob, "Meditation gives me a mastery over my own mind and body I never had before. It calms me down enough so that I can put things in perspective and see what's happening, not only around me but also inside myself. It may seem crazy, but to be perfectly honest I must admit I'm grateful to have had cancer, because meditation set me on a different life path. It transformed the way I live with my family, with the people around me. It has given me a sense of direction I didn't have before."

Eight years later, Bob was doing fine. As part of the study, Carlson measured his immune responses before, during, and twelve months after his eight-week initiation into meditation. His responses greatly improved (she noted a reduction in inflammatory cytokines, TNF-alpha, and interferon gamma, and an increase in interleukin-10, which fights inflammation). At the same time, Bob's cortisol level had gone down. Apparently, both his body and his mind had been calmed by his new life path.

A recent study at the University of California at Los Angeles confirmed the positive effect of mindfulness meditation on the immune systems of patients

---

* These results are compatible with other studies in Richard Davidson's laboratory. They show that greater activity in the left hemisphere, such as that observed after practicing meditation, is also associated with greater activity of NK cells and a stronger response to vaccines.[53] At Imperial College in London, Professor John Gruzelier has shown similar results in AIDS patients. Those with greater activity in the left hemisphere (of the kind meditation brings about) have better morale and are more resistant to the spread of disease.[54] At Ohio State University, Professor Janice Kiecolt-Glaser has also demonstrated that elderly patients who practice relaxation exercises for a month show significant increases in their immune cells' activity (NK and T lymphocytes).[55]

with AIDS.[56] For eight weeks, fifty HIV-seropositive men followed a weekly course in this meditation method. They then practiced meditation daily for thirty to forty-five minutes. A control group (with comparable initial characteristics) attended only a one-day training session, following which they did not meditate daily.

Eight weeks later, in the group that did not practice daily meditation, levels of CD4 cells had declined. (These are immune cells whose numbers diminish when the AIDS virus propagates.) However, the CD4 cell count did not drop below its initial level in the men who had meditated daily. And the greater their commitment to the program, as measured by their attendance at training sessions, the higher their CD4 cell count was at the end of the study.

Precisely what mechanism allows meditation to boost the immune system is not yet known. The most probable explanation is that a more serene state of mind is linked to a lower secretion of adrenaline and cortisol, which means that immune cells are better able to fulfill their function of defense.

While the benefits of meditation were clear for Bob, who adopted the practice willingly, for Joel (the patient who introduced us to the concept of "monkey mind"), the undertaking was anything but easy.

Joel Settles Down for the First Time

When we measured Joel's physiological rhythms, they seemed as disorganized as his mind. There was 100 percent chaos and no coherence in the variations of his heart rate. Furthermore, he had a lot of trouble directing his thoughts inward. I doubt he would ever have had the patience to settle down for twenty minutes to concentrate on his breathing without the "excuse" of wanting to measure the state of his inner functions on a computer screen using biofeedback software. While listening to my instructions, he twisted and turned in his chair every two or three minutes. I could tell from his frown that he was making an effort to follow my advice, but as is typical with this type of inward directed exercise, the harder he worked to "get it," the more elusive the quest became. He had to learn how to listen first, to be attentive, patient, well meaning. Jon Kabat-Zinn compares this initial period of suspended action to the situation of a photographer of wild animals. She must station herself discreetly, silently, without moving, until the animal she hopes to see feels safe enough to show itself. If she approaches it nervously, impatiently, there is very little chance that it will allow a glimpse of the beauty of its presence in the midst of nature.

Most of us have learned to mistreat our inner being. Like Joel, over the years we have trained ourselves *not* to listen to our inner selves. Concentrating on our concrete objectives—dealing with the crisis at hand, finding a life partner, taking care of the children, responding to the expectations of parents, friends, a boss, colleagues, etc.—we have chosen to stifle these profound but tenuous movements murmuring deep inside.

If we had listened to these movements, this is what we probably would have heard: "I don't feel very well. I'm deprived of things that really matter to me. I need more integrity, more beauty, generosity, joy, tenderness. . . . There isn't enough. . . . I'm missing something essential. . . . " It's easier to turn a deaf ear and spend time on another phone call, e-mail, film, bottle of wine, cigarette, joint, or some other mind-numbing helper. Anything goes, as long as our attention doesn't fix on this restless inner animal that we're afraid we may never be able to truly satisfy. And when facing the neglected inner self causes unpleasant feelings, as it did when Joel felt extremely uncomfortable after focusing on his breathing, one tends, like him, to get upset: "What on earth am I doing here? There are surely a million more interesting things to be doing!" Obviously, this irritation only serves to further arouse the feeling of inward discomfort, which makes one even more eager to flee toward whatever distraction presents itself.

Joel went away after his first attempt to achieve inner calm feeling frustrated. But his intelligence had registered the message displayed on the screen, that there was something wrong with his physiology. He had also noted that his scatterbrained tendencies and his discomfort when turning inward only served to aggravate the situation.

Even if he didn't really believe in it, Joel was intrigued by everything he had heard, and now seen, about meditation. Without enthusiasm, but with his characteristic curiosity about everything new and his determination not to reject anything without having first experimented with it (two qualities that had made him an accomplished producer), he accepted my proposal: to settle down for ten minutes twice a day to listen to his breathing and learn to tame, slowly, his vital functions.

I gave him the instructions mentioned in Ian Gawler's book—those that had helped its author to deal with his cancer. The only effort required in this exercise was that of finding the time to practice it. The effort of accepting that for ten minutes the exercise will take precedence over all other concerns. As for the rest, it isn't a question so much of effort as of acceptance and benevolence. "Let your eyes gently close, turn your attention inward and remember that it's a moment devoted to the powers of healing."[57] Two ten-minute sessions a day may seem little, but for Joel it was already a huge step forward.

After leaving the center, he went and bought a candle to light during these two breaks in his day, which he was instructed to think of as "sacred." The small flame would remind him that it was a moment outside of regular time and distinct from his ordinary concerns. During these ten minutes, he had the right to cut himself off from the world, to not think about either the past or the future. The past is gone and will never come back, and the future is unknowable. The small flame would also symbolize what he was trying to find within himself: the faint glimmer of life that flickers under the blowing winds of outside events but that stubbornly never goes out.

His first sessions were not as difficult as he'd expected, and he soon learned to make the ten minutes go by quite quickly. During his meditation, he discovered a phenomenon that amused him. When a pressing thought started to distract him ("I absolutely must call Jack back about my new idea for a film"), he only had to let it slide away as he exhaled, saying to himself, "Not now. I can think about it in ten minutes," and it let go. Often another thought of the same type replaced it: "I haven't had any news from the children today." But it slid away just as easily in turn and disappeared after the pause following exhalation. These thoughts were like soap bubbles that rose to the surface of the mind, then burst gently and disappeared. He had never realized that such thoughts—which had often seemed important, imperious, urgent—could be so light that they could fade away if he didn't pay attention to them.

In less than two weeks, he spontaneously went to two fifteen-minute sessions a day. The more progress he made, the better he was at recognizing the discomfort of inner tension. At the same time, he said to himself that since he was aware of it, it didn't represent the totality of his being. He could sense he was anxious, all the while observing, "But I am not my anxiety." And, strangely enough, he observed that this new perspective brought with it a little more calm. Before he left for Los Angeles, we tested his cardiac coherence once more. He had been happy to practice all alone in his hotel room, without the help of biofeedback software. Without the software, after only ten days he had become capable of reducing the chaos in his heart rate variability to 30 percent, achieving 70 percent coherence as measured by the computer.

We kept in contact after he left, and he reported that as he gained more experience with meditation, his mind was no longer the same during the remainder of the day. He felt more easily present, moved, amused by what surrounded him. He felt more alive. He no longer answered e-mails while he played chess with his son. He also decided not to let his BlackBerry warn him every time he received a new message, but checked his mailbox periodically instead. Six months later, he had developed such a taste for that new inner dimension in his life that he got up earlier to practice for thirty minutes every morning. It had become one of the most important periods in his day, a slot he gave to himself to feel who he really was, without distraction or worry or thought. For these thirty minutes, he was free to simply feel.

Two years later, he sent me an e-mail to tell me how pivotal this discovery had been for him. His cancer had stopped spreading, but meanwhile he had experienced one of the great upsets in his life: A film in which he had invested a great deal was a terrible flop. He clung to his morning meditation like a life raft. There he encountered his fears, his anger, his hopes and accepted them all as part of his being. "I don't know what I would have done without these times of inner peace where I made contact with the force deep within," he wrote. "I don't know how I managed before. Thank you for those difficult moments in Pittsburgh."

In the end, Joel didn't need to sit in the desert. He just needed to breathe.

All Meditations Converge

The oldest discipline of inner awareness is yoga. In Sanskrit, the term "yoga" designates a set of practices aiming at the merging of body and mind for the sake of unity and inner peace—a path to each person's innate "superior being." This tradition sets out the principle that there is not one single pathway. On the contrary, every culture and every individual must find the path that suits them best. The central point common to these practices is the temporary diversion of attention from the outside world and the refocusing of that attention on the chosen subject of meditation.

The subject of meditation varies, depending on the school. It may involve the body and its sensations, as in hatha yoga, which works on postures and breathing. The traditions of tai chi, qigong, nidra yoga, and sophrology and the method of cardiac coherence are different versions of this general form of body-centered meditation. Hypnosis, which concentrates the attention in a particularly powerful way, also mobilizes the profound forces of the body. It's possible as well to concentrate on the flame of a candle, a sacred image, a word ("love," "peace," and "shalom" are often used for this purpose), a prayer (the Ave Maria, a Buddhist mantra, the Sufi "dhikr," etc.), or a landscape (the picture of a lake, mountain, or tree).

In the practice taught by Jon Kabat-Zinn—"mindfulness meditation"—attention is focused simply and repetitively on what is in consciousness in the present moment, without dwelling on it at length, simply observing what emerges spontaneously afterward. If a thought appears, it is labeled "thought." Then we look at what comes afterward. If an emotion emerges, it is called "emotion," and our attention moves on. The same is true for a "sensation," a feeling of discomfort, a desire to stop, etc.*

The tradition of yoga also recognizes as higher forms or practices the study of sacred texts, as well as humanitarian work, when practiced with awareness of the present moment. The key in any case is controlling attention. Through the rigorous use of attention, each path provides the opportunity to enter into the same state of inner coherence that promotes the integration and harmonious functioning of the body's biological rhythms.

What matters most is neither one particular technique nor one particular application. There is no secret, no magic password that can cure cancer. There is no position in tantric yoga capable of lining up all the body's energy exactly. What seems essential to the mobilization of the body's forces is to renew contact every day—with sincerity, benevolence, and calm—with the life force that vibrates constantly within our bodies. And to bow to it.

PART THREE: HEALING THE WOUNDS OF THE PAST

For those who have been badly damaged by life, the wounds of the past remain close to the surface. Turning their attention inward may in such cases prove to be too painful or too disturbing. These poorly healed scars drain a significant portion of energy, and they hamper the body's capacity for self-defense. In such cases it may be necessary to find and cure the buried trauma that is the source of emotions so powerful that they have left a persistent mark in the psyche. There are many methods for overcoming such psychological trauma. I have experienced a few, the most effective in my opinion being eye movement desensitization and reprocessing (EMDR).

Mary's Abandonment

When Mary found out that her breast cancer markers were going up, she was not surprised. For several months she had been so desperate and depressed that she sometimes thought of suicide. If her body were to carry out the act instead, that would be just as well. At fifty-five, she had just experienced the greatest love story of her life with a man twenty years younger. He told her time and again that she was the love of his life, that he couldn't imagine himself for a single instant with anyone else, and that she had transformed and

---

* The clear and simple phrase that Kabat-Zinn teaches to recall what we must do with our attention so as to approach full awareness is "Aim your attention and sustain it. Aim and sustain. Aim and sustain."

fulfilled him, opened him up to life. Mary had believed in the sincerity of this unusual but unfaltering passion. For the first time in her life, she abandoned herself to this gentle, protective love. During the six years the relationship lasted, she cut herself off from the world. Then one day, he left. While thanking her for everything she had helped him to understand about himself, he told her that he wanted children and he had found another woman with whom he could pursue this new dream. Shattered, Mary felt totally impotent. When she was a child, her father had abandoned his family and never again paid any attention to her. Later, her young husband had found a mistress and their marriage ended in divorce. Like Marty Seligman's rats exposed to unavoidable electric shocks, Mary had "learned" in the course of these experiences that it was useless to try to protect herself. Her feeling of helplessness, of inevitability, led her to thoughts of suicide. Perhaps these feelings contributed, also, to the rise in her cancer markers.

At the University of Helsinki in Finland, Kirsi Lillberg, MD, PhD, has shown in a study of more than ten thousand women that the loss of an important emotional relationship doubles the risk of breast cancer. Breakups and painful divorces may even be more directly correlated with cancer than is the death of a spouse.[58] The loss of love causes intense feelings of helplessness in many people, perhaps by tapping into psychological wounds received in childhood through experiences of rejection or criticism.

The feeling of helplessness can transform a painful event into a full-fledged trauma. This is familiar to soldiers who have experienced war. The most terrible memories are not those of battles in which they fought and were caught up in the action. The worst are those in which they couldn't do anything to save a wounded comrade or when they were trapped, powerless to defend or fight, under an interminable bombardment.

When the trauma is particularly serious and, as in Mary's case, when there was no one to help her get over it because she had let her network of friends dwindle, the risk of developing a disease rises. One study suggests that the risk of developing breast cancer may be nine times greater in people who feel alone when dealing with this sort of emotional and psychological challenge.[59] In the effort to ward off cancer, it is thus essential to combat the psychology of helplessness.*

---

* Generally, states of mourning and post-traumatic stress are clearly associated with a deterioration of the immune system and a decline in the activity of white blood cells and NK cells.[60-62] Still more significantly, psychological traumas are associated with a wide variety of medical problems,[63, 64] with a major reduction in survival time after a heart transplant,[65] and specifically with a greater frequency of cancers.[66] Fortunately, traumas can be treated with brief therapies such as cognitive behavior therapy or EMDR (see below).[67-69]

Helplessness Is Traumatic

"Trauma" is the term for a shock (or a series of shocks) that leaves a painful and profound mark on a patient's brain. Small challenges or setbacks that occur in the normal course of life may disturb someone for several days, but the brain is capable of "healing." Just as a small cut will quickly be repaired and will leave no scar, the brain also possesses a natural mechanism for healing emotional wounds. These wounds leave no lasting scar and are often the impetus for maturation and personal growth.

In other instances, certain events are so painful that they tear deeply into the image people have of themselves or the trust they have in the world around them. This is true with particularly disturbing events such as rape, frightening or life-threatening accidents, and even some romantic breakups. It is also the case with the absence or loss of love or repeated humiliations experienced in childhood, as this is the age when people are the most emotionally and psychologically vulnerable. Such wounds tend to form a sort of psychological abscess. The brain tries to isolate and skirt around them as much as possible; the individual's consciousness may even "deny" the event. But just as pressure on an abscess will show that it is still sensitive, life may brutally remind a person of his traumatic past, causing him to become aware of the still-tender psychological wound.

When reactivated, the traumas of the past may take over the individual's entire mental and physical functioning. For Mary, at the time when Paul leaves her, the traumatic memories of her father's departure fifty years earlier and of her husband's twenty years earlier once again become the stark reality of the moment. She believes that she doesn't deserve to be loved, that she's useless, destined to fail. She feels the same sadness and weeps the same tears, her body produces the same stomach cramps and goes so far as to assume the same position—that of a little girl hunched over, her arms around her knees.

Inwardly, the emotional wound also affects deep vital processes. Just as a lesion on the skin activates repair mechanisms, a psychological wound sets off mechanisms of the stress response: release of cortisol, adrenaline, and inflammatory factors, as well as a slowdown in the immune system. As publications in *Nature Cancer Reviews* and *The Lancet* have shown, these physiological stress mechanisms can contribute to the growth and spread of cancer.[70, 71]

However, what unhealed traumas lead the person back to is a *false* sense of helplessness. Although this impotence may have been real in the past, it is not a true reflection of the present. Allowing a patient to realize this illusion is the key to therapy.

In Mary's case, her doctor found a simple and direct way to rekindle her inner strength. Since she was a journalist and a published author, he encouraged her to write down the story of her passion and its devastating failure. Despite her despondency, she found this idea engaging. As the story flowed through her fingers on the keyboard, she felt gradually restored to life. After her new book was published, she returned to see her doctor. Not only had she left behind her ideas of suicide, but her cancer markers had returned to a perfectly normal level. Having a focused, attainable goal had empowered Mary to let go of the illusion of helplessness and recover her desire to live. Her body responded as well, returning to health and gaining control over her potential cancer.* For Mary, devoting herself to writing provided her with a vital source of energy, a sort of life force. For others, it might be planning a long-wished-for trip, building a dream house, or simply being more involved in the lives of family and friends. The key is for the activity to be rich in meaning for the individuals and capable of bringing them into closer contact with their own life force.

Some people, like Mish, whom I described in chapter 5, manage to endure life's trials thanks to the love of a close family member. A husband, wife, daughter, or son who holds your hand through every stage, and who allows you to lay your tired head on his or her shoulder, can help keep you from feeling helpless. But recent studies show that a network of friends can sometimes play a role that is just as important, whether in a cure or in survival long beyond statistical life expectancy.

In a book published in 2009, Jeffrey Zaslow tells the story of a group of eleven childhood friends who scattered across the United States after leaving high school.[73] Their friendships survived almost forty years and all the ups and downs of life—success and failure at university, marriages, divorces, and difficulties with children. In September 2007, one of them—Kelly—was told that she had breast cancer and that she would need family support. Instead of turning to her family, however, she confided the news by e-mail to her far-flung high-school girlfriends, and it was as if she had sparked an "instant shower of love." She was deluged with e-mails, phone calls, letters, cards, packages. When her chemotherapy caused painful mouth ulcers, one of her girlfriends sent a machine to make milk shakes to soften her mucous membranes. Another, whose daughter had died from leukemia, knitted her a woolen hat so she wouldn't catch cold after losing her hair. A third made

---

* Similarly, at the University of Auckland in New Zealand, Dr. Keith Petrie and his colleagues have shown that the simple fact of writing down the most difficult events of one's life over four consecutive days increases the capacity of the immune system to make antibodies in reaction to a hepatitis vaccine.[72]

Anticancer
Action

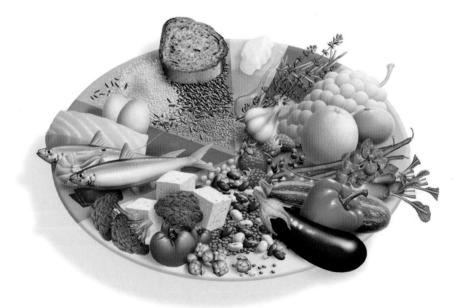

Little Changes That Make a Big Difference

Protecting Yourself

Avoid products containing industrial chemicals whenever possible:

- Air out your dry-cleaned clothing
- Avoid pesticides and insecticides
- Avoid chemical cleaning products
- Avoid skin contact with aluminum
- Avoid parabens and phthalates in cosmetic products
- Avoid skin-care products that contain estrogens or placental by-products
- Avoid foods and liquids that have been in contact with hot plastics (microwave plastic bowls, plastic mugs, plastic kettles, many canned foods)
- Avoid inorganic phosphate additives (in many commercial sodas, commercial baked goods, processed meats)

Diet

- **Eat grass-fed organic animal products:**
  – meat, milk, cheese, yogurt, omega-3 eggs (the organic label is preferable but less important in choice of vegetables, fruits, and grains)
- **Balance your diet**
  – reduce your intake of sugar, white flour, products containing omega-6s—sunflower oil, corn oil, soybean oil, safflower oil, margarine, hydrogenated (trans) fat, nonorganic animal fat (meat, eggs, dairy products)
  – increase your omega-3 intake (found in fish, grass- or flaxseed-fed animal products, flaxseeds and oil)
  – increase your intake of anticancer products (turmeric, green tea, soy, specific anticancer vegetables and fruits)
- **Filter tap water:**
  – use a carbon filter or an inverse osmosis filter or drink mineral water or spring water

Activity

- **Spend 20 to 30 minutes of physical activity per day**
- **Expose yourself to sunlight for 20 minutes each day (creates vitamin D)**

Meditation

- **Practice a method of relaxation and self-centering** (such as yoga, cardiac coherence, qigong, tai chi, etc.)

Free Yourself of Your Feelings of Powerlessness

- **Resolve past traumas**
- **Learn to accept your emotions, including fear, sadness, despair, and anger**
- **Find someone with whom you can share your emotions**

What Inhibits and What Activates Immune Cell Production

Inhibits	Activates
traditional Western diet (proinflammatory)	Mediterranean diet, Indian cuisine, Asian cuisine (antiinflammatory)
persistent anger or despair	facing one's difficulties
social isolation	support from family and friends
denial of your true identity (for example, your sexuality)	acceptance of self with one's values and past history
sedentary life-style	regular physical activity

Various studies prove that white cells react to food intake, the environment, physical activity, and emotional state. (See chapters 4 and 9.)

Principal Influencing Factors on Inflammation

Aggravates		Reduces	
	traditional Western diet	Mediterranean diet, Indian cuisine, Asian cuisine	
	unmanaged stress, anger, and depression	laughter, lightheartedness, serenity	
	less than 20 minutes of physical activity a day	a 30-minute walk 6 times a week	
	cigarette smoke, atmospheric pollution, domestic pollutants	clean environment	

Inflammation plays a key role in the development of cancer. We can reduce inflammation using natural methods available to all. (See chapters 4 and 6.)

Anticancer Plate

Animal proteins (optional)
fish, organic meat, omega-3 eggs, organic dairy products

Grains
multigrain bread, whole-grain rice, quinoa, bulgur . . .

Fats
olive, canola, or flaxseed oil, omega-3 butter

Herbs and spices
turmeric, mint, thyme, rosemary, garlic . . .

Vegetables, fruits, and vegetable proteins
lentils, peas, beans, tofu . . .

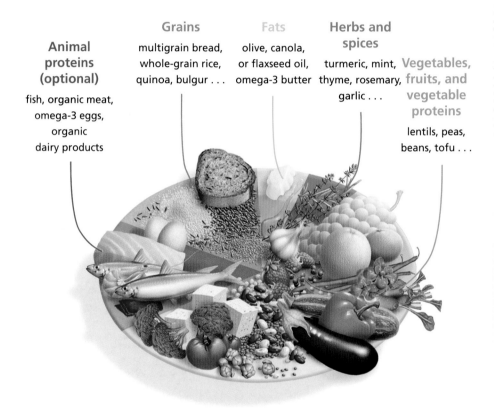

The anticancer diet is made up primarily of vegetables and legumes prepared with olive, canola, or flaxseed oil, or omega-3 butter, herbs, and spices. Unlike the traditional Western diet, meat and eggs are much less prominent; they are served as accompaniments in small amounts.

Choosing Foods Based on Their Glycemic Index

High Glycemic Index (avoid)	Low Glycemic Index (use liberally)
sugar: white or brown, honey, syrups: maple, fructose, dextrose	natural sweeteners: agave nectar, stevia, acacia honey, coco flower sugar, xylitol, dark chocolate (>70% cocoa)
white bleached flours: white bread, white rice, overcooked white pasta, muffins, bagels, croissants, rice cakes	mixed whole-grain cereals: multigrain bread (not just wheat) or leavened (sourdough) bread, rice—whole-grain or basmati or Thai—pasta and noodles cooked al dente (preferably multigrain), quinoa, oats, millet, buckwheat
potatoes (except for the rare Nicola variety), especially mashed potatoes	lentils, peas, beans, sweet potatoes, yams
cornflakes, Rice Krispies (and most of the other bleached or sweetened breakfast cereals)	oatmeal (porridge), muesli, All-Bran, Special K
jams and jellies, fruit cooked in sugar, fruit in syrup	fruit in its natural state: particularly blueberries, cherries, raspberries, which help to regulate blood sugar levels (if necessary, use agave nectar for sweetening)
sweetened drinks: commercial fruit juices, sodas	water flavored with lemon, thyme, or sage
	green tea (without sugar, or use agave nectar), which combats cancer directly
alcohol (except during meals)	1 glass of red wine a day with a meal
	garlic, onions, shallots: when mixed with other food, help lower insulin peaks

Many studies have shown that an overconsumption of refined sugar increases the insulin and IGF levels in our system, thereby contributing to cancer growth.

The Most and Least Contaminated Fruits and Vegetables

Most Contaminated (prefer organic)

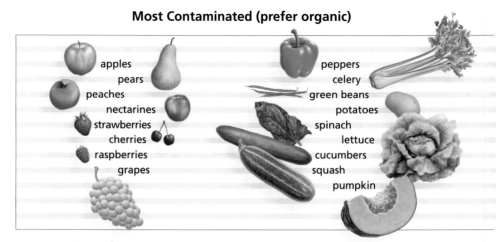

apples
pears
peaches
nectarines
strawberries
cherries
raspberries
grapes

peppers
celery
green beans
potatoes
spinach
lettuce
cucumbers
squash
pumpkin

Everyday Household Products to Avoid

Avoid as Much as Possible

perchloroethylene/tetrachloroethylene in dry cleaning
deodorants and antiperspirants containing aluminum (especially for women who shave their armpits, which facilitates penetration of aluminum)
cosmetics, shampoo, lotions, gels, hair dye, nail polish, sunscreen containing estrogens or placental products (common in hair products for Afro hairstyles), or with parabens or phthalates. Phthalates to avoid include: BBP and DEHP.* Parabens to avoid include: methylparaben, polyparaben, isoparaben, butylparaben
perfumes containing phthalates (nearly all of them do)
chemical household pesticides and insecticides
heating foods or liquids (coffee, tea, baby formula) in plastic containers made with PVCs (which are liberated into the food when heated), polystyrene, or Styrofoam
preparing food in scratched Teflon pans
common cleaning products such as liquid detergents, disinfectants, toilet bowl sanitizers with alkylphenols (nonoxynol, octoxynol, nonylphenol, octylphenol, etc.)
excessive exposure to electromagnetic fields of cell phone

Everyday cancerogenous products that are either proven or suspected of contributing to the development of cancer and their substitutions.

* BBP=benzyl butyl phthalate; DEHP=di (2-ethylhexyl) phthalate.

Least Contaminated (growing methods less important)

bananas	
oranges	broccoli
tangerines	cauliflower
pineapple	cabbage
grapefruit	mushrooms
melons	asparagus
watermelons	tomatoes
plums	onions
kiwi	eggplant
blueberries	peas
mangoes	radishes
papaya	avocados

Replace With

air out dry-cleaned garments in fresh air for several hours before wearing or employ wet cleaning, liquid CO_2 or silicone
natural deodorants without aluminum
natural and organic products free of parabens, phthalates, and estrogens. Many "organic" cosmetics are free of parabens and phthalates. Some companies, such as Body Shop or Aveda, make products without phthalates.
no perfume, or wear only toilet water (which contains fewer phthalates)
use insecticides made from essential oils or boric acid, or diatomaceous earth. See complete list of alternative remedies to most suspect pesticides and insecticides on www.panna.org
use glass or ceramic containers (including when using a microwave oven)
flawless Teflon, or else non-Teflon pans, such as stainless steel 18/10
green or European Ecolabel products. Or replace with white vinegar (for counters and floors), baking soda, or white soap
reduce use of cell phones with an air-tube headset

Omega-3 Content in Fish and Seafood

Type of Fish	Amount Required to Provide the Recommended Daily 1 g of EPA + DHA* (ounce fish or g capsule)
Tuna	
• light, in water, drained	12.0
• white, in water, drained	4.0
• fresh	2.5–12.0
Sardines	2.0–3.0
Salmon	
• chum	4.5
• sockeye	4.5
• pink	2.5
• chinook	2.0
• Atlantic, farmed†	1.5–2.5
• Atlantic, wild†	2.0–3.5
Mackerel	2.0–8.5
Herring	
• Pacific	1.5
• Atlantic	2.0
Trout, rainbow	
• farmed	3.0
• wild	3.5
Halibut	3.0–7.5
Cod	
• Pacific	23.0
• Atlantic	12.5
Haddock	15.0
Catfish	
• farmed	20.0
• wild	15.0
Flounder/Sole	7.0
Oyster	
• Pacific	2.5
• Eastern	6.5
• farmed	8.0
Lobster	7.5–42.5
Crab, Alaskan king	8.5
Shrimp, mixed species	11.0
Clams	12.5
Scallops	17.5
Capsules	
• cod-liver oil	5.0
• standard fish body oil	3.0
• omega-3 fatty acid concentrate	1.0–2.0

Fish and seafood represent a principal source of long-chain omega-3 (EPA and DHA). The levels vary depending on the type, the source, the raising, and the season in which they are fished.

Classification of the Effects of Certain Foods on Several Specific Cancers

Colon Cancer

Inhibition of Cancer Cell Growth

20 0 20 -40 -60 -80 -100

garlic
leeks
scallions
brussels sprouts
savoy cabbage
cabbage
beets
spinach
kale
asparagus
cauliflower
fiddlehead fern
onions
broccoli
red chicory
turnips
eggplant
red cabbage
Boston lettuce
green beans
celery
potatoes
bok choy
fennel
romaine lettuce
squash
carrots
endive
red peppers
cucumbers
control

Some foods specifically inhibit cell growth in certain cancers. Dr. Béliveau's laboratory was able to test crude extracts from different foods on the cells of several different cancers. Based on the results, they drew up a list of foods especially recommended in a diet targeting a particular cancer. Note that garlic, onions, and leeks (of the alliaceous family) rank high among the most effective foods for all the cancers listed below. The last line of each graph is the control line that shows cancer cell growth without the exposure to any particular vegetable.

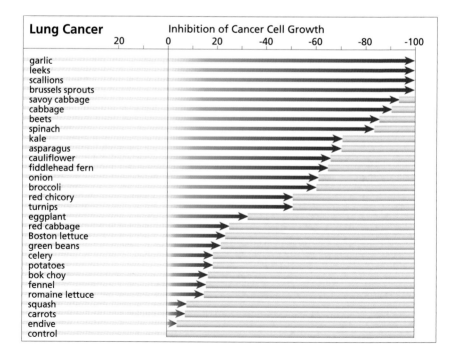

Brain Cancer — Inhibition of Cancer Cell Growth

20 · 0 · 20 · -40 · -60 · -80 · -100

garlic
leeks
brussels sprouts
beets
cabbage
scallions
kale
broccoli
cauliflower
spinach
savoy cabbage
onion
green beans
red cabbage
asparagus
celery
turnips
fiddlehead fern
squash
jalapeño peppers
cucumbers
tomatoes
red chicory
fennel
carrots
bok choy
potatoes
endive
romaine lettuce
Boston lettuce
orange peppes
eggplant
control

Lung Cancer — Inhibition of Cancer Cell Growth

20 · 0 · 20 · -40 · -60 · -80 · -100

garlic
leeks
scallions
brussels sprouts
savoy cabbage
cabbage
beets
spinach
kale
asparagus
cauliflower
fiddlehead fern
onion
broccoli
red chicory
turnips
eggplant
red cabbage
Boston lettuce
green beans
celery
potatoes
bok choy
fennel
romaine lettuce
squash
carrots
endive
control

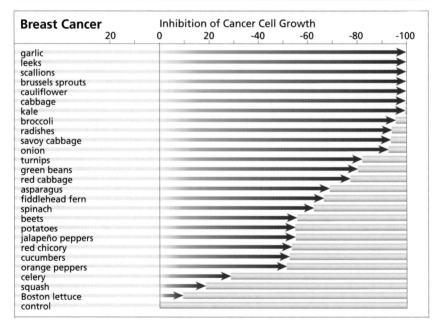

Prostate Cancer   Inhibition of Cancer Cell Growth

	20	0	20	-40	-60	-80	-100

garlic
brussels sprouts
scallions
leeks
broccoli
cauliflower
savoy cabbage
onion
cabbage
kale
beets
fiddlehead fern
jalapeño peppers
red cabbage
celery
turnips
orange peppers
spinach
cucumbers
red chicory
asparagus
squash
fennel
radishes
eggplant
potatoes
tomatoes
bok choy
endive
Boston lettuce
green beans
romaine lettuce
carrots
control

Breast Cancer   Inhibition of Cancer Cell Growth

	20	0	20	-40	-60	-80	-100

garlic
leeks
scallions
brussels sprouts
cauliflower
cabbage
kale
broccoli
radishes
savoy cabbage
onion
turnips
green beans
red cabbage
asparagus
fiddlehead fern
spinach
beets
potatoes
jalapeño peppers
red chicory
cucumbers
orange peppers
celery
squash
Boston lettuce
control

The Competition of Omega-3 and Omega-6 Fatty Acids in Our Organism

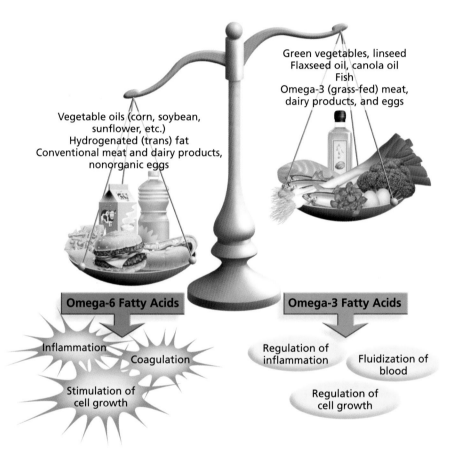

The imbalance between omega-6 and omega-3 fatty acids in our diets increases inflammation, coagulation, and the growth of adipose and cancer cells.

Energy Spent in Different Activities Measured in MET*

Activity	MET	Category
Sitting, watching television	1.0	**Daily Activities**
Sitting, sewing	1.5	
Walking from house to car or bus	2.5	
Loading/unloading car	3.0	
Taking out trash	3.0	
Walking the dog	3.0	
Household tasks, moderate effort	3.5	
Vacuuming/Lifting items continually	3.5	
Raking lawn	4.0	
Gardening (no lifting)	4.4	
Mowing lawn (power mower)	4.5	
Playing the piano	2.3	**Mild Activities** (fewer than 3 MET per hour)
Canoeing (leisurely)	2.5	
Golf (with cart)	2.5	
Walking (2 mph, 3km/h)	2.5	
Dancing (ballroom)	3.0	
Walking (3 mph, 5km/h)	3.3	**Moderate Activities** (3 to 7 MET per hour)
Cycling (leisurely)	3.5	
Calisthenics (no weights)	4.0	
Golf (no cart)	4.4	
Swimming (slow)	4.5	
Walking (4 mph, 6.5 km/h)	4.5	
Chopping wood	4.9	
Tennis (doubles)	5.0	**Vigorous Activities** (5 to 12 MET per hour)
Dancing (ballroom, fast or square)	5.5	
Cycling (moderately)	5.7	
Aerobics	6.0	
Rollerblading	6.5	
Skiing (cross-country or downhill)	6.8	
Climbing hills (no load)	6.9	
Swimming	7.0	
Walking (5 mph, 8 km/h)	8.0	
Martial arts training adapted for cancer patients	8.0	
Jogging (6 mph, 10 km/h)	10.2	
Jumping rope	12.0	
Sustained martial arts training	12.0	
Squash	12.1	

Studies show that physical exercise helps the body fight cancer, but the required dose isn't the same for all cancers. Doses are calculated in units called MET (metabolic equivalent). One MET is defined as the energy it takes to sit quietly.* For breast cancer, there seems to be a measurable effect after three to five hours a week of walking at normal speed (9 MET a week). For cancer of the colon and rectum, twice as much (18 MET a week) is needed to have a comparable effect. This means either walking twice as long or twice as fast, or finding activities requiring more effort to replace walking (for example, bicycling at a speed that requires effort adds up to twice as many MET as walking). Two weekly sessions of karate practiced by Dr. Bouillet's patients corresponded to a dose of 18 MET a week. Finally, to have an effect on prostate cancer, 30 MET a week are required, the equivalent of three hours of jogging spread out over the week. (They can be done in six sessions of 30 minutes each.) Weight training depends on the amount of weight, so it is not possible to give a generic estimate.

Anticancer Shopping List

Anticancer Foods

Proteins

• fish and shellfish *(selenium, vitamin D, and long-chain omega-3)*, especially salmon, mackerel, whole anchovies, sardines (even canned sardines, but only those conserved in olive oil and not sunflower oil), eel, cod liver, and occasionally white albacore tuna canned in water or olive oil

• organic meat and poultry (in moderation)

• omega-3 eggs (in moderation)

• vegetable proteins (lentils, peas, beans, chickpeas, mung beans)

• organic soy: tofu, tempeh, miso, soy steak, soy sprouts, soybeans, soy milk, soy yogurt *(isoflavones and genistein)*

Grains and Carbohydrates

• multigrain or sourdough bread

• whole-grain rice (or basmatic or Thai rice)

• quinoa

• bulgur

• oatmeal (porridge), muesli, All-Bran, Special K, or combination of oats, bran, flaxseed, rye, barley, spelt

• Nicola potatoes

• sweet potatoes, yams

• vegetable proteins (see above)

Fats

• olive oil

• flaxseed oil *(vegetal omega-3s and lignans)*

• omega-3 butter

• cod-liver oil *(vitamin D)*

• canola oil

• omega-3 margarines

Vegetables

• cabbages: brussels sprouts, bok choy, Chinese cabbage, broccoli, cauliflower, etc. *(sulforaphane and indo-3-carbinols/i3c)*

• beta-carotene–rich vegetables: carrots, sweet potatoes, yams, squash, pumpkins, certain varieties of potimarron squash (also known as Hokkaido squash), tomatoes, beets, etc. *(vitamin A and lycopene)*

• spinach *(magnesium)*

Mushrooms

• shiitake, maitake, enoki, crimini, portobello, oyster, thistle oyster, or turkey-tail *(polysaccharides and lentinian)*

Herbs and Spices

• turmeric *(curcumin)* mixed with black pepper and olive oil

• curry

• labiates: mint, thyme, marjoram, oregano, basil and rosemary *(terpene)*

• parsley and celery *(apigenine)*

• alliums: garlic, onion, leek, shallots, chives *(diallyl disulfide)*

• cinnamon *(proanthocyanidins)*

• ginger *(gingerol)*

Probiotics and Prebiotics

- organic yogurt and kefir, soy yogurts enriched with *Lactobacillus acidophilus* and *Bifidobacterium bifidum*
- sauerkraut, kimchee
- garlic, onions, tomatoes, asparagus, bananas, wheat

Seaweed

- nori, kombu, wakame, arame, and dulse *(fucoidan)*

Fruits

- berries: strawberries, raspberries, blueberries, blackberries, and cranberries *(ellagic acid and polyphenols)*
- cherries *(glucaric acid)*
- citrus fruit: oranges, tangerines (even with the peel if they are organic), lemons, and grapefruit *(flavonoids)*
- persimmons and apricots *(vitamin A and lycopene)*
- pomegranate juice

Dried Fruits

- walnuts and hazelnuts *(vegetal omega-3 and magnesium)*
- pecans *(ellagic acid)*
- almonds *(magnesium)*

Desserts

- dark chocolate—more than 70% cocoa *(proanthocyanidines)*
- all fruits
- sweeten with agave nectar, stevia, acacia honey, coco flower sugar, xylitol

Drinks

- red wine *(resveratrol)* in moderation (1 glass per day)
- filtered water, mineral water, spring water (as long as the plastic bottles haven't sat in the sun and the water doesn't smell like plastic, which indicates the presence of PVCs)
- lemon-flavored water (or flavored with thyme, sage, tangerine, or orange rind)
- all green tea *(EGCG)*, especially Japanese green tea (sencha, gyokuro, matcha, etc.)
- gingerroot infusion *(gingerol)*

Anticancer Products

- natural deodorants without aluminum
- natural and organic cosmetics free of parabens and phthalates
- pesticides made from essential oils or boric acid
- white vinegar or natural cleaning products (without pesticides) or the European Ecolabel
- use glass or ceramic containers for use in a microwave
- flawless Teflon, or else non-Teflon pans, such as stainless steel 18/10

Summary Detoxified Diet

Reduce	Replace With
foods with a high glycemic index (sugar, white flour, etc.)	fruit, flour, and starches with a low glycemic index
hydrogenated or partially hydrogenated (trans) oils sunflower, soy, and corn oil conventional dairy products (too rich in omega-6) fried food, chips, fried appetizers	olive, canola, or flaxseed oils organic grass-fed dairy products (balanced in omega-6/omega-3, free of rGBH), or soy milk, soy yogurts hummus, olives cherry tomatoes, sliced fennel
nonorganic red meat, poultry skin	vegetables, legumes (peas, beans, lentils), tofu, miso organic poultry and omega-3 eggs organic grass-fed red meat (max 300 g/ 12 ounces a week) fish (mackerel, sardines, salmon, even farmed)
skins of nonorganic fruits and vegetables (pesticides cling to their skins)	fruits and vegetables peeled or washed, or else labeled "organic"
tap water in areas of intensive farming because of the presence of nitrates and pesticides liquids exposed to polycarbonate ("hard") plastics, especially if heated	tap water filtered through carbon filter or reverse osmosis mineral or spring water in plastic bottles, provided the bottles are from a reputable brand and made of PET (number "1" plastic), not PVC (number "7" plastic)

Summary of major steps to take to protect our everyday diets. (See chapters 6 and 8.)

pajamas from special cloth to make night sweats less unpleasant. Kelly often found it easier to talk about what she was going through with her girlfriends than with her doctors. "We've known each other so long, we can tell each other anything," she said joyfully.[74]

Research confirms the importance of a network of friends. In the *Nurses' Health Study,* a large-scale study of nurses in the United States, women with breast cancer who could name ten friends had a four times better chance of surviving their illness than women who could not. The geographical proximity of these friendships was not significant; the protective effect seemed to stem from the simple fact of feeling connected.[75] Friendship also plays a major role for men: A Swedish study of 736 men found that friendships had as strong an effect on health as the fact of being married.[76] On the other hand, the study found that only smoking affected health as negatively as feelings of loneliness and isolation.

Michael's Smile

For me it started with a friend's gaze. After my relapse and the subsequent long year of chemotherapy, I too had begun to lose my footing in life. I'd had to stop working, since I no longer had the physical strength to run my division of psychiatry and the Center for Integrative Medicine at the university, nor even to continue seeing patients. As for my personal life, Anna and I no longer agreed on anything concerning our son's upbringing. The tension generated by this dissension was so great that she eventually agreed to undertake couples therapy. We were not succeeding in our efforts to save the marriage, perhaps in part because of the stress of my illness, which made give-and-take difficult. I was losing my wife, my family, my work, and my health all at once. I could feel my life slipping through my hands. I feared that any benefits of treatment were being compromised by the stress of my shattering life. This is when I met Michael Lerner.

Michael is not a physician. He is a sociologist and a psychotherapist. He also runs several NGOs. A former professor of sociology at Yale University, founder of the Commonweal Center in California, and the author of a key work on different approaches to the treatment of cancer, he has become one of the great American thinkers, examining the connection between medicine and the individual in the modern world.[77] He has met hundreds of patients at his retreats and has gained considerable wisdom from his experiences.

When I met him, he asked me a few key questions. Rather than focusing on what was going wrong in my life, he got me to talk about what gave me the most satisfaction. For instance, what was the "music of life" I would like to dance to? What was the "song"—unique, personal—I wanted to be sure to have sung at least once in my life? On hearing these questions, which were both direct and full of tact, I felt my heart beat a little faster. I answered with some hesitation and talked of a project I was thinking about—and also of the fear that it might only be a presumptuous dream. I sometimes saw myself writing a book about what I had learned as a neuroscientist using natural methods to treat depression and anxiety. But I had never written a book, and this ambition seemed beyond reach, especially in my current state of fatigue. Raising my eyes, I saw his gaze fixed on me. He looked happy. He had found what he was looking for. "David," he said, "I don't know what else you should do in your life, but I know that you have to write that book." A short time later, with Michael's words and smile in my heart, I started to write.* And like Mary, I found my way back. Like a shaman, Michael had succeeded in kindling the small flame of life in me that, a few months earlier, had started to waver.

Healing Helplessness

Like all psychiatrists, I was familiar with the problem of post-traumatic stress syndromes and dreaded them, since most treatments have little effect. Even drugs, which must be prescribed over the long term if they are to be of any use, usually reduce symptoms by only a third or a half.[78–81] I was therefore extremely skeptical when I heard of nonpharmacological treatment methods that promised to free a majority of patients from symptoms related to some of the most painful experiences of their lives, and often only in a few weeks. Some studies even report a positive response rate of 80 percent (which is comparable to results of antibiotics in the treatment of pneumonia in hospitalized patients).[82–85]

Shortly after finishing my training in treating psychological trauma,[†] I started to offer this almost systematically to cancer patients. I asked them to make a list of the ten most painful events of their lives. I saw these events as screws fastening down a large metal plate crushing their desire to live. If these screws were "unscrewed" one by one, patients were often awakened to a totally different way of living. Once relieved of the weight they had been carrying around, they were able to look at everything differently. Although relieving patients of the pain of trauma is not a treatment for cancer, it often enables natural defenses to recover their strength, which can aid in the fight against disease.

---

* *The Instinct to Heal: Curing Depression, Anxiety, and Stress Without Drugs and Without Talk Therapy* (Emmaus, PA: Rodale, 2006).

† The therapy I have found most helpful and readily acceptable to patients is EMDR, which uses eye movements comparable to those taking place spontaneously during REM sleep.[86]

Lilian Overcomes Her Fear

Lilian was an actress who taught in a well-regarded university program. She had acted on stages all over the world. Fear was a familiar feeling to her, and she knew everything there was to know about self-control. Yet she was now sitting in my office because her old enemy—fear—had her in its grip. A few years earlier, she had been operated on for an extremely dangerous myosarcoma (cancer of the muscles), and she had made a sound recovery. But she had just found out that the tumor was back and that she probably had only a few months to live. She was so frightened when she talked about her disease that her halting breath prevented her from finishing her sentences. I tried to help her recover her calm, but nothing worked. She repeated over and over while she sobbed: "In any case, you can't understand. Nobody can understand. I'm going to die and nobody can do anything." I had just started a year of chemotherapy myself, following my relapse. Lilian's words echoed the fear I too had experienced. Although I had adopted a rule to never talk about my disease with my patients, that day was the one and only time I broke the rule. Our session was being filmed on video to serve as instruction for students and residents. I unfastened the microphone and got up to speak into her ear, and I whispered, "You know, Lilian, I never talk about it, but I too have cancer, and I'm frightened. The only thing I can say is that it's possible to find peace and strength inside oneself. It's essential, so as to give yourself your best chances of recovering. That's what I'd like to help you do." Her sobs stopped almost immediately. She turned toward me with relief. She was no longer alone. We hugged for a few moments, and then we were able to begin our work.*

I learned that she had been raped several times by her father. The helplessness she now felt facing this disease probably echoed the impotence she had experienced as a child. She remembered every detail of the day when, as a six-year-old, she cut the inside of her thigh on a garden gate. Her father had taken her to the doctor and sat by while she had stitches put in, all the way up to her pubis, without anesthesia. Back home, her father had laid her flat on her stomach and, holding her down with his hand on the nape of her neck, raped her for the first time.

Lilian had begun by telling me that, in the course of several years of conventional therapy, she had talked at length about incest and her relationship with her father. She didn't think it would be useful to go back over these old memories. "I'm really over that," she said. But the connection between

---

* I've already written about Lilian's case in my earlier book, *The Instinct to Heal,* without mentioning the scene concerning me.

that childhood scene—combining the themes of illness, total impotence, and fear—and the anxiety she was now experiencing over her cancer seemed, to me, too powerful to set aside. She finally concurred and agreed to evoke these memories again and work on them with me.

When she brought back the memory of what had happened, she reexperienced in her body the childhood terror. An idea came back to her, an idea she'd had at the time: "What if it was my fault? Wasn't it my fall in the garden and the fact that my father saw my genitals at the doctor's that led him to do that to me?" Like almost all victims of sexual abuse, Lilian felt partly responsible for the atrocious acts. As we continued our work, at one point, she suddenly realized that it hadn't been her fault. She had only been a very small child, and her father should have looked after her and protected her. That was now self-evident to her; she had done nothing that could justify such an act of aggression. She had simply fallen. What could be more ordinary for an active, adventurous little girl? The connection between the adult standpoint and the old, childish distortion preserved in the scar from the trauma was taking shape as I looked on.

Progressively, her emotion changed. Fear turned into justified anger: "How could he do such a thing to me? How could my mother let him do it for years?" The physical sensations, which seemed to have as much to say as her words, changed as well. After experiencing anew the pressure on her neck and the fear in her belly, she felt a strong tension in her chest and jaw, such as anger can bring on. Several schools of psychotherapy consider that the objective in treating rape victims is precisely to bring them to the exact point where fear and impotence change into legitimate anger. However, in my view, the treatment should really go on in the same mode as long as the patients notice changes taking place inwardly, and they should not be left with negative feelings, be they anger or sadness, if they can move beyond them.

As our work went on, Lilian saw herself as a lonely little girl, emotionally abandoned and physically assaulted. She then reexperienced a profound sadness, together with great compassion for this poor child. As in the stages of mourning described by Elisabeth Kübler-Ross,[87] anger had turned into sadness. Then she realized that the competent adult she had become could take care of this child. After all, hadn't she ferociously protected her own children—as she said, "like a lioness"? Finally, she came round to telling her father's story. An early member of the Resistance in Holland during the Second World War, he had been arrested and tortured. She had always heard her mother and her grandparents say that he had never been the same again. When evoking these memories, she felt a wave of pity welling up in her. She now saw him as a man with a great need for love and compassion that his wife, who was hard and cold, had never given him. Nor had his parents, trapped in a cultural tradition that attached no importance to emotions. A confused, lost soul who had lived through such harsh experiences that "it was enough to make anyone go mad," she said. And she saw him as he now was: "A pitiful old man, so weak that he has trouble walking. His life is so difficult. I'm sad for him."

During her short therapy, she went from the terror of a little girl who had been raped to acceptance and even compassion for her aggressor—the most adult point of view conceivable. None of the usual stages of mourning, as described in conventional therapy, had been omitted. It was as if months or years of conventional psychotherapy had been condensed into a short time. She had woven the necessary strands between the events of the past and her perspective as an adult woman. Once these links were established, the traumatic memory was digested—"metabolized," as biologists say—and had lost its capacity to set off overwhelming and debilitating emotions. Lilian even became capable of referring to the memory of the first rape and looking at it without the slightest trouble: "It's as if I were a simple observer. I look at it from afar. It's only a memory, an image."

Stripped of its emotional charge, the traumatic memory loses its virulence and its grip weakens. This is a big first step. But the resolution of traumas is not confined to neutralizing old memories. It opens those who experience it to a new way of life. Once Lilian's terrible childhood traumas were resolved, she discovered an inner strength she had never suspected. She was then able to confront her disease, as well as the prospect of death, with much greater serenity. Through her healing experiences, she rediscovered the vital energy within her and acquired a kind of radiance that impressed all those who approached her.*

Neither shamans nor therapy for trauma can cure cancer. But shamans sometimes cure feelings of helplessness, and good therapy nearly always does.†

We can no longer hide behind the argument that there is insufficient proof that mind-body methods have an impact or are effective. Studies, and in particular the recent studies that I've listed in this chapter, indicate that in fact the

---

* I received the sad news of Lilian's death just as I was finishing this book. I had spoken to her a few months earlier. Seven years after the news of her relapse, she was continuing to make the most of life.

† The effectiveness of EMDR as a brief therapy for trauma is largely established, at the time of my writing, by eighteen controlled studies, six meta-analyses, and an authoritative Cochrane Review.[88] On the other hand, the mechanism leading to the rapid healing of traumatic memories through the stimulation of attention with eye movements (or other techniques used in EMDR) has not yet been fully elucidated, though several hypotheses are being actively pursued in neuroscience research.[89, 90]

opposite is true. Here is one last study, published two years after *Anticancer* first appeared, and perhaps the most impressive of all.

Barbara Andersen, a professor of psychology at Ohio State University, directed a particularly illuminating prospective, long-term study of survival after cancer treatment. In this study, she observed over eleven years 227 women who had received every conventional treatment after breast cancer that had spread to the lymph nodes (stage II or III). Following treatment, some of these women undertook a year-long practical program aimed at acquiring lifestyle techniques and information similar to what is described in this book. The program included information about nutrition and the importance of physical exercise and had a strong emphasis on learning stress management techniques, such as a very simple method for "progressive muscle relaxation" inspired by yoga. A control group received only conventional treatment and follow-up meetings for psychological evaluation. The results were remarkable. The group that received practical advice about lifestyle changes had a 56 percent lower mortality risk over the eleven-year period. They had learned to practice this basic relaxation method for twenty minutes three times a week while listening to an audio recording. After the first few months, they were able to reach that relaxed state after only two minutes. The data from the study showed that the more they had practiced, the better they were at reducing the feeling of helplessness in their lives. And the more they did that, the more the immune system was strengthened.[91-93]

If results like these were ever achieved with a new drug, every oncologist in the world would feel obligated to prescribe it.

Whether it's learning to relax and better control our minds, or better nourishing ourselves, or practicing regular physical exercise, there's really only one secret. We need to give ourselves a way in which we can steer the course of our own lives instead of being subjected to them in helplessness and distress.

CHAPTER 10

Defusing Fear

Pronounce the word "cancer" and it's enough to arouse the fear of death. Fear paralyzes. That's its nature. When an antelope senses a lion's presence, its nervous system sends out a signal, and it freezes. Evolution has programmed the antelope to preserve a tiny chance of survival in extreme circumstances: By remaining completely still, the animal has a better chance of evading detection. Perhaps the lion will pass nearby without noticing the antelope.

When we find out our lives are seriously endangered, we often experience this strange paralysis of body and mind. But the disease won't pass us by. Fear blocks our life force at the time when we need it most.

Learning to fight cancer consists of learning to nourish the life in us. But it's not necessarily a fight against death. To carry through this apprenticeship is to touch the essence of life, to find a completeness and peace that make it more beautiful. Death may be part of that success. Some people live their life without appreciating its true value. Others live their death with such richness, such dignity, that it seems like an exceptional accomplishment and gives meaning to everything they have experienced. And in preparing for death in this way, we sometimes release the energy needed to live.

The Train to Omaha

In the weeks after the discovery of my cancer, I dashed from one appointment to another. At the end of a rainy afternoon, I was awaiting my turn in a fifteenth-floor waiting room. I stood in front of a plate glass window and watched the small figures in the street below scampering around like ants. I was no longer part of their world. They were alive; they had errands to run, plans for the future. As for me, my future was death. I had left the ant heap, and I was frightened. I remembered the poem "Limited" quoted by the psychiatrist Scott Peck.[1]

The poem's narrator writes about a train barreling at top speed across the endless expanse of the Great Plains. He knows the final destination of these steel coaches—the scrap heap; and the fate of the men and women laughing in the compartments—dust. He asks a fellow passenger where he's going. The man answers: "Omaha."

In the end, even if the other ants didn't know it, we were all going to the same place. Not to Omaha, but to dust. The last stop was going to be the same for everyone. The only difference was that the others weren't thinking about it, whereas I was.

Like birth, death is part of life. Of mine too. I was no exception. So why was I afraid? Over the months and years that have followed, my patients have taught me how to recognize and come to grips with that fear. Through their experience, I've come to understand that the fear of death isn't just one fear but many fears. And once they are examined one by one, they are much less overwhelming.

The Fear of Suffering—The Fear of Nothingness

When I met Denis, he was preparing to die at the age of thirty-two. We were almost the same age, and like me, he was a physician. A lymphoma had been consuming him for several months, and the treatments no longer worked. Without knowing what I was going through myself, he must have sensed that I was moved by his anxiety, and he asked to see me regularly. He said he wanted to understand, to remain fully conscious, despite his fear, even face to face with emptiness. He did most of the talking, and I listened. To be honest, he seemed to understand a lot more than I did.

"What helped me at first was to realize one morning that I wasn't the only one who has to die. Even if I'm going to die young, I suddenly saw that we're all in the same boat. All those people in the street, the TV anchor, the president, and even you," he said as he averted his eyes. "You're going to die too. It sounds crazy, but thinking about that reassured me. This fate we have in common means I'm fully human and linked to all of you and all our ancestors and all our descendants. I haven't lost my membership card."

In his dreams Denis was often chased by vampires—a transparent symbol of death's hunting him down. He always woke up before they got to him. But one day his dream had a different ending. The vampires caught him and sank their teeth and nails into his flesh. Denis yelled out in his sleep and woke up in a sweat. Up to now he had never thought about what he had just grasped: "Not only am I afraid of dying, but now I realize I'm terrified that it will be painful."

As young doctors, we both realized that we didn't know much about dying. We didn't even know if it really was painful. No one had considered it useful to teach us about that in medical school. So we read books together that described clearly how the body and mind go through the transition to death.[2, 3] With relief we found out that death isn't painful in itself. In the final days, the dying no longer feel like eating or drinking. The body dehydrates progressively. No more secretions, no more urine or stools, less phlegm in the lungs. Thus less pain in the abdomen, less nausea. There is no more vomiting, no more coughing. The whole body slows down. The mouth is often dry, but it's easy to relieve the dryness by sucking on small ice cubes or a damp cloth. Fatigue sets in, and the mind grows more distant, usually with a feeling of well-being, sometimes even mild euphoria. The dying are less interested in talking, simply holding a hand or looking through the window at the sunlight or listening to birdsong or particularly beautiful music instead. In the final hours, one some-times hears a different kind of breathing called the "death rattle." And then there are usually several final incomplete breaths (the "last breath") and invol-untary contractions of the body and face, which seem to be resisting the loss of the life force. These do not betray suffering but are simply a sign of the lack of oxygen in the tissues. Then the muscles let go and everything is over.

But Denis was afraid that his various tumors wouldn't allow him to experi-ence such a peaceful end. Already on one occasion his nerves had been com-pressed and the pain had been terrible. He was only reassured when we drew up a detailed plan with his oncologist. If necessary, he wanted to be given sufficient doses of painkillers to block all pain. He understood that high doses could lead to such a feeling of peace that he might stop breathing. But the risk of shorten-ing his life a little was less important than the certitude that he wouldn't suffer.

Then Denis had another dream he described vividly. "It was the end of the world. I was enclosed in a covered stadium. My old school friends were there, and we were in the midst of a huge crowd. We knew that there were only a few hours left, perhaps a night. People were milling around and shout-ing wildly. Some of them were making love with anyone and everyone; others were committing suicide or killing each other. The anxiety was unbearable. I woke up with the impression that my head was going to explode. I could hardly breathe. I have never been so frightened. And yet that dream changed everything. Because that scene was much worse than the idea of my own death. Yes, I'm going to die, but . . . it's not the end of the world!"

Denis was profoundly atheistic, and this relief baffled him. He had always imagined that with the extinction of his consciousness the world was going to disappear with him. "What does it matter if the world goes on after me?" he asked. "Why this unexpected comfort?"

Together we read Viktor Frankl, a Viennese psychiatrist and a student of Freud and Adler. He had been deported to Auschwitz and Dachau. After his liberation, he developed a new form of psychotherapy, "logotherapy" ("logo" for "meaning"), which relieves anxiety by helping people find more meaning in their lives, even at the point of death.[4] I remember a passage in his book in which he speaks of a dying woman in a bunkhouse who looks out through a tiny window onto a branch swaying against the sky. She says to her companions, "See that leaf? Nothing is serious because life goes on." Just a leaf, not even a human existence. The feeling of connection to life discussed by Frankl can go very far, beyond humanity, to all of nature. Many people encountering their imminent death discover, as Denis did, the universal dimension of existence, which is profoundly reassuring. Even if they had never looked at the world from that angle before.

Denis discovered what he later called his "soul"—how each of his choices, each of his actions in the course of his life, had been imprinted forever on the fate of the world through its infinite repercussions. Like the proverbial butterfly of chaos theory, whose fluttering wings in China influence the hurricanes of America, Denis became aware of the importance of each thought, of each one of his words. And even more of demonstrations of love to others or even to the earth. He now saw them like seeds for an eternal harvest. He had the feeling, for the first time, of living in the moment. Of blessing the sun that caressed his skin, like the water that refreshed his throat. This same sun had already given life to the dinosaurs. This same water had quenched their thirst. The water had been part of their cells before once again becoming clouds, then oceans. "Where does this gratitude come from—in me, a dying man?" he asked. And the wind too, the wind on his face. "Soon I'll be the wind and the water and the sun. And, above all, the sparkle in the eyes of a man whose mother I took care of or whose child I saved. You see, that's my soul. What I've made of myself, which already lives everywhere and will always live on."

When he began to get really weak, he took to his bed, aided by home hospice care. His sister and a few friends visited him regularly. Together, they made sure he was comfortable. They smoothed his sheets, kept him clean, brought him flowers for his room and the music he loved. I went up to that room as one prepares to enter a shrine. A smile from him felt like a blessing.

In the final days, he wanted to talk about what happens after death. Neither of us was a believer. But we had both been struck by the experiences described by certain patients of ours who had been "clinically dead" and had come back to life. Nobody really knows how to interpret these so-called NDEs ("near-death experiences"). We found out that the principal features of such experiences are found in antique paintings as well as medieval frescoes. We also learned there is an astonishing similarity in descriptions of NDEs, whatever the cultural differences, the religious or the historical background. And clinical studies, as well as a famous article in *The Lancet,* suggest that they are very common (found in nearly one person in five whose heart had stopped beating for some length of time before being medically "resuscitated").[5, 6] In

The Tibetan Book of Living and Dying, by Lama Sogyal Rinpoche, we found an "instruction manual" for a person preparing to die. He speaks of a welcoming white light and suggests simply turning toward it. Everything else takes care of itself.[7]

Denis found these accounts comforting. Keeping his distance from a theoretical "hereafter," he never became a believer. But he no longer saw death solely as a confirmation of the nihilists' great nothingness. To him it became "a mystery." Something much more open, like a return to the enigma of what had been, before he was an embryo in his mother's womb.

In the last days, he almost stopped talking. He died late one evening. One of his friends was massaging his feet. The next morning on my desk I found a note from my assistant: "Denis M.: C.T.B." A common euphemism in the hospital for "ceased to breathe." And I wondered if he hadn't just begun.

The Fear of Being Alone

Along with the fear of suffering and the fear of nothingness can often be found the anxiety of facing alone what in *The Death of Ivan Illych* Tolstoy called "the formidable and solemn act of one's own death." We are afraid there will be no one there to console us at the end, facing such a terrifying circumstance. This loneliness often causes more suffering than physical pain.

One day I was asked to speak to a patient's wife because she was "upset" and was disturbing the smooth running of the department. She harassed the nurses and interns with questions and instructions on what should or shouldn't be done for her husband. She raised her voice in the corridors in a manner that disturbed the other patients. Deborah and her husband were both forty-two. They had been brilliant students at one of the best business schools and then had become high-flying traders. But for the past year, Paul had been suffering from very serious hepatitis. They were "fighters." They had explored all the existing treatments and followed the toughest protocols. Nothing worked, and the doctors had told Deborah there was no hope left. She was resolutely opposed to telling Paul. Pale and brusque in her gestures, she explained to me that it was still possible for the latest treatment to have an effect, that he should maintain a positive outlook. He mustn't in any case imagine that he might be dying.

When I entered his room, Paul was pitiful to look at. Jaundice had further heightened the frailty of his sunken cheeks. As we introduced ourselves, his hands nervously wrinkled and smoothed the sheets. While respecting Deborah's directives, I asked him what he thought of his condition and how in his opinion it might evolve. He thought he could recover. He thought he ought to remain optimistic. Hope, right up to the end, is important to us all.

But wasn't he sometimes afraid that things might not turn out as well as he hoped? For a long time he remained silent. Then he said that he often thought of it but never spoke about it because his wife wouldn't be able to bear it.

I felt a deep sadness for Paul and Deborah. They protected each other so well that they wound up preventing each other from discussing what frightened them most. What a terrible solitude they were both experiencing! We talked about their first meeting, their happiest memories together, their intention to have a child after much hesitation. At the end of the conversation, I asked Paul what he would think if their roles had been reversed. What would he say if Deborah was in his place, if she said to herself that perhaps she was going to die and she chose not to talk to him about it? If she slipped quietly away one morning without giving him a chance to tell her everything he had shared with her? He promised to think about it.

When I returned several days later, Deborah had changed. She greeted me in the corridor more graciously; she had better color in her face; she looked like she had slept. She told me that Paul had spoken to her. He had told her he was afraid that there might not be any remaining hope. He said he felt terribly guilty about letting her down because he was so sick. That he held it against himself not to be able to share the future they had planned together. She told him that in her whole life nothing had counted as much as her relationship with him. In the following days, they reminisced; he told her everything that had mattered most to him—often details that she had not noticed herself at the time. She told him how frightened she was and how much she would miss him if he had to go. And then she gathered her courage and said to him: "I want you to know that if ever you feel it is time, you can leave." It was terribly sad. They wept. But they were once again *together*. Paul died a few days later, holding her hand. Although he almost had, he didn't die alone.

Dr. David Spiegel, who for thirty years has been conducting support groups for people who are seriously ill, believes firmly in the importance of humor and optimism to stimulate the body's natural defenses. But he often reminds his patients not to let themselves be locked in what he calls "the prison of positive thinking." There is every reason to believe that the solitude the seriously ill impose on themselves when they don't talk about their fear of dying contributes to making their condition worse.

In fact, studies show that the connection between social isolation and the risk of death is as great as the link between cholesterol or tobacco and the risk of death.[8–12] Anything that prevents us from having a genuine connection to others is in itself a step toward death.

The mantra that David Spiegel likes to repeat to his patients has always seemed more sensible and useful to me than the naive commandments of "positive thinking." It's the realist's credo: What's most important is to always hope for the best but be prepared for the worst.

The Fear of Being a Burden

We are often more accustomed to looking after others than to being looked after. And we set great store by our autonomy. The idea of a slow decline toward death also terrifies us because it condemns us to being terribly dependent on others precisely at a time when we no longer have anything to give them.

However, in the course of the last days of our existence, we will have to accomplish one of the greatest tasks of transmission in our lives. For each of us, the idea we have of our own death usually comes from the examples we have witnessed through the deaths of our grandparents, our parents, our brothers or sisters, or a close friend. These scenes will be our guides when our own turn comes. If they have shown us how to prepare, how to say goodbye, how to nurture a certain calm, we will feel ready for this ultimate stage in our lives. When we approach our own death, rather than be "useless," we in turn become pioneers and masters for everyone close to us.

At Harvard Medical School this teaching goes beyond the family circle. Patients on the threshold of death are now invited to meet with first-year students to speak to them about what they are experiencing. A retired secondary-school teacher dying of a virulent leukemia had agreed to meet with several of them. When her husband joined her, she turned toward him, her eyes still tear-filled from her conversation with her young visitors, and said: "Honey, I have one last teaching gig."[13]

I too had the good fortune of having a grand master—my grandmother. She was a reserved woman and revealed little about herself, and yet she was a constant presence in all the passages of childhood that seemed difficult to me. When I was a young adult, I went to see her on what we both knew was her deathbed. Inspired by her beauty and her calm in her impeccable white nightdress, I held her hands and told her how much she had mattered to the child who had now grown up. Of course I cried and didn't know what to do with my tears. She took one of those tears on her finger and showed it to me, smiling gently: "You know, for me, your words and your tears, they're pearls of gold, and I'll take them with me." I have carried with me the image of her final days. Although she had lost her autonomy and her body had abandoned her, she gave her children and grandchildren the gift of love that remains when there is nothing else left to give.

The Fear of Abandoning Your Children

Of all the fears, I've often felt that the most terrible is that of a mother (or father) who won't be there to help her children grow up. Leslie was forty-five and had two adolescent children of twelve and thirteen. Her ovarian cancer was already metastatic, and after a second chemotherapy, which hadn't worked, she had been given six months to live. Her greatest anxiety was over abandoning her children. We tried to deal with that fear during a therapy session in which she visualized what she imagined would be the worst that could happen after her death. First she saw herself as a phantom spirit who could see her children as they went about their lives but who could neither touch nor speak to them. They were sad and lost, and the impotence she felt at her inability to help them was heartrending. Leslie's chest was so oppressed that on seeing these images she had trouble breathing. I suggested stopping the session, but she wanted to go on. Then she saw her daughter getting ready for one of her cello concerts, where Leslie used to accompany her. Little Sophie felt totally lost at having to go alone. Once on the podium, she sat with shoulders slumped and empty eyes. Imagining that scene, Leslie's face was still more contorted, and I began to wonder if the session might do more harm than good. But at the very moment when I was preparing to interrupt it, she saw her daughter smile. She seemed to hear her thoughts: "Mom isn't here, but the memory of all the times she accompanied me here is still so strong. . . . I hear her words and her encouragements in my head. I feel her strength in my backbone. I feel her love in my heart. It's as if she was everywhere with me now. . . ." And Leslie saw her start to play as never before, with depth and maturity. Now the tears running down Leslie's cheeks were tears of confidence. Some part of herself had authorized her to leave in peace by reminding her, in her deepest being, of what she had already passed on to her children. Two years later, I received a letter from Leslie. She was still alive. Still undergoing treatment. She remembered that session as one of the most difficult moments she had experienced. But letting go of her fear and gaining confidence had enabled her to go on fighting the disease.

The Fear of Unfinished Stories

Death is the final departure. To leave in peace, we have to bid farewell. The fact is that it's very difficult to turn the page on unrealized ambitions, dreams of travel, or relationships that once mattered but were broken off too soon. Often the best way to say farewell is to make one last try. Writing the poems we have always wanted to write, making the trip we have dreamed of all our lives—while it is still possible. As these are the final attempts, even if everything doesn't work out, we forgive their imperfections. But what is often hardest of all is letting go of a painful relationship that has marked our lives.

At thirty-six, Jennifer was dying of a particularly aggressive breast cancer that no longer responded to treatment. Her father had abandoned her family when she was six and her brother eleven. He lived in Mexico and had never tried to see them again. She had long hesitated before writing to him. How would he react? After thirty years' absence, would he be too ashamed to respond? Would he be indifferent and not even answer? If that was the case, would she be devastated? But the solemn moment of death often opens a door to the most hardened hearts. Jennifer's father came. He was frightened, he was ashamed, but he came. In the one and only conversation of their adult lives, she was able to tell him she would have liked to have known him, she would have liked him to protect her, to teach her what he knew of life. She showed him photos of herself—still radiant before she had fallen ill—and of her son. Facing this emaciated body and face, he didn't have the heart to defend or justify himself. He listened. He ended up saying that he was sorry too. That he had done what he could under the circumstances of that earlier time, with the anxieties he had experienced at that age, that he probably wouldn't act the same way today but it was too late. He begged her forgiveness. She died a short while afterward a little more at peace.

HOW TO START A DISCUSSION ON THE POSSIBILITY OF DEATH

Never impose a discussion on the possibility of death with a person who isn't prepared to talk about it. It's important to recognize that the person isn't ready and come back to the subject diplomatically later.

With someone who has not been told how serious their illness is, you can explore what they might want to talk about by simply asking, "What do you understand from everything your doctors tell you? Do you sometimes wonder whether they might have overlooked something?" If the answer is "no" the first time, the question still gives the person a chance to come back to the subject with you later.

With someone who is familiar with their diagnosis but doesn't talk about what might happen, you can begin by gently asking an open question, such as "I wonder if you sometimes think of what might happen if your present treatments didn't work?" If the person answers, "Why are you asking me that?" you can answer, "Because I sometimes think about it, and it occurred to me that you may wonder about it too." This is usually enough to start a conversation that becomes increasingly frank, during which it's important to *listen* rather than speak.

Being Alive

We often hear it said of people struck down by an unexpected heart attack that "it was a good way to go." Nevertheless, it's an end that leaves us without any chances for preparation, exchange, or transmission, or any occasion to seek closure in an incomplete relationship. This is not what I wish for myself.

Today the word "cancer" is no longer synonymous with death. But it suggests its shadow. To many patients, as it was to me, this shadow is an occasion to think about our life, about what we want to do with it. It's the occasion to begin living in such a way that the day we die, we can look back with dignity, with integrity. That on that day we can say farewell with a feeling of peace. I've found that realistic attitude in almost all the people who have survived their cancer well beyond the statistics they were given. "Yes, I may die earlier than foreseen. But it is also possible that I'll live longer. Whatever happens, I'm going to live my life as well as I can from now on. It's the best way to prepare for whatever happens."

CHAPTER 11

The Anticancer Body

Touch as a Mother Would Touch Her Child

When Linda arrived at the Commonweal Center in California for a seven-day retreat, she was at the end of her rope. After several operations, then chemotherapy and radiotherapy, she felt that she had been spared nothing. "I was slashed, poisoned, and burned," she said, reducing to their most brutal expression the treatments whose marks were printed in her flesh. She never looked at herself in the mirror anymore. With scars for breasts, her limbs all skin and bones, a grayish complexion, this frightful vision had driven her to despondency.

Massage was part of the treatment, but when the time came, Linda had trouble disrobing. Wasn't she sickening to look at? Who could possibly want to touch her? But under the filtered light, with the scent of purity given off by the essential oils, and calmed by Michelle's sweet smile and attentive expression, Linda agreed to lie down on the massage table, covered with a light sheet and showing only her back. First Michelle put her hands on Linda's head and lightly massaged her temples and scalp. Linda relaxed. Little by little she recovered enough confidence to turn over and show her torso. Michelle then placed one hand—gentle, strong, and reassuring—over her heart on the scar where once her left breast had been. She left it there several minutes without moving, centered and present. Linda felt that soothing hand, and something in her was moved. Imperceptibly, then more and more powerfully, a tremendous sob rose out of her. Linda then grasped Michelle's hand like a child who doesn't want her mother to leave.

Overwhelmed by the loneliness of the long months of treatment, Linda was again aware of the fear she'd had to keep in for so long. But now the fear was mixed with immense affection for her skinny, bruised body that had courageously held on. Michelle had neither moved nor spoken. And as mysteriously as they had come, the sobs died down. In their place, Linda now felt great calm and warmth in her chest, and she welcomed it like the sun after a storm. Michelle barely spoke. She only said, "Your face has more color. Now your cheeks are rosy." At the end of the session, the two women hugged for a minute before saying goodbye.

Michael Lerner and Dr. Rachel Naomi Remen, who codirect the Commonweal Center, attach great importance to massage, which they have fully integrated into their program. "Touching," Dr. Remen explains, "is a very old way of healing. Touch as a mother would touch a child, because what a mother is saying through her touch is 'live.' Something in touching strengthens the will to live in us. Healing is evoking the will to live in another person. It comes about not by doing something but by letting another person know that their pain and their suffering and their fear matter. They really matter."

In intensive care units for premature infants, the importance of touch in encouraging life became clear in the eighties.[1] Despite ideal physical conditions—controlled temperature, ultraviolet light, perfect humidity and oxygen supply, diet calculated to the milligram, a sterile environment—these frail little beings often wouldn't grow. Human, physical contact was not part of the regimen, in large part because of instructions advising nurses and parents not to touch the infants. A single night nurse changed everything. Incapable of resisting their lonely cries, she had discovered that she could get her tiny patients to calm down by gently stroking their backs. And, although no one understood why at first, those infants exposed to her touch set about growing.

At Duke University, Saul Schanberg, MD, PhD, and his team demonstrated the biological basis of this phenomenon with a series of experiments on baby rats isolated from their mothers at birth. They proved that in the absence of physical contact, the body's cells literally refused to divide and grow. In each cell, the part of the genome responsible for producing the enzymes needed for growth was no longer expressed; thus, the whole organism went into a form of hibernation. On the other hand, stroking a baby rat's back with a wet brush, to imitate the way a mother rat responds to her babies' cries, immediately triggers enzyme production and, with it, growth.[2] From this experiment we may conclude that very probably, attentive physical contact—such as massage practiced with benevolent intention—stimulates the life force in human adults, not just on an emotional level, but on a biological level inside their very cells.

As with Linda, touch also fosters acceptance of one's body, bruised as it may be. The body responds in its own way to the implicit physical message, the message that it "matters," is accepted, and still has its place among humans. At the medical school of the University of Miami, Tiffany Field, PhD, runs a research institute on massage. Working with Dr. Saul Schanberg's laboratory, her team has shown that three weekly thirty-minute sessions of massage slowed down the production of stress hormones and increased the number of NK cells in women with breast cancer.[3, 4] These women were also more serene and felt less physical pain after just the very first session—a well-known effect of massage.[5]

The Body in Motion

There are many different ways to tell our body it matters, that it is loved and respected, and to get it to sense its own desire to live. The best way is to let it practice what it was designed for: movement and physical activity. Several studies have demonstrated that the regulation and defense mechanisms that contribute to fighting cancer can be directly stimulated by exercise.

Jacqueline was fifty-four when she found out she had a rare cancer of the fallopian tube. Several members of her immediate family had died of cancer, and she had always thought that her turn would come someday. Her physician told her frankly that her chances for survival were slim, but that they would try every possible treatment. After surgery she started six months of chemotherapy to limit the risk of metastases. But her oncologist, who had some original ideas, didn't stop there.

Medical director of the Institute of Radiotherapy at the Avicenne Medical Center of the University of Paris, Thierry Bouillet, MD, was also a black belt in karate. He had once been the physician for the French karate team. An expert in sports medicine, he was naturally intrigued by the many recent studies showing fewer cases of cancer among the most physically active patients, as well as distinctly fewer relapses in active subjects compared to other cancer patients.[6–20]

Dr. Bouillet himself had treated patients whose regular exercise seemed to play a major role in their healing. He particularly remembered a thirty-nine-year-old airline pilot who was a former marathon runner and developed metastatic cancer of the lung. Despite a prognosis for survival of two years at most, he wanted to keep his body in shape up to the end. After his right lung was removed and he underwent harsh chemotherapy, he began to run again as soon as he was able. He started by running two hundred meters as best he could, and eventually he succeeded in increasing the respiratory capacity of his remaining lung to the point where he was again able to run in semimarathons. But even more impressive, he was still alive seven years later.

As Dr. Bouillet also knew, there are numerous mechanisms by which exercise improves overall physiology. First, it reduces the quantity of adipose tissue, the principal storage site of carcinogenic toxins (in humans, as well as in polar bears, see chapter 6). At the University of Pittsburgh, Devra Lee Davis refers to excess fat as the "toxic waste site" of the human body. According to her, any form of physical activity capable of reducing fat, taking with it its stockpile of contaminants, is a prime method for "detoxifying" the body.

Moreover, physical exercise modifies our hormonal balance. It reduces the excess estrogens and testosterone that stimulate the growth of cancers (in particular, cancer of the breast, prostate, ovary, uterus, and testicles).[21] Exercise also reduces blood sugar levels and, as a result, the secretion of insulin and IGF (see chapter 6), which contribute so dramatically to tissue inflammation and to the growth and spread of tumors.[22-24] Physical exercise even acts directly on the cytokines responsible for inflammation by lowering their level in the blood.[25] Finally, physical activity, like meditation, has a direct effect on the immune system, seemingly protecting it against the stress of bad news.

At the University of Miami, Arthur LaPerrière, PhD, examined the protective effect of exercise against stress. He chose a particularly painful experience to study: when a person is informed he is HIV positive. At the time the study was carried out, long before the development of antiretroviral tritherapy, this diagnosis was equivalent to a death sentence. It was up to each patient to deal with it psychologically as best he could. In most patients, upon learning of their fate, the level of NK cells dropped rapidly. This reaction was not seen in those patients who had been randomly assigned to exercise for a month prior to the diagnosis (forty-five minutes of cycling in a gym three times a week).[26] In another study from the same group, the effect of exercise on improving the immune system (measured by the increase in CD4 count) was comparable in magnitude to that of the AIDS drug AZT.[27]

Incorporating this data into his approach to Jacqueline's treatment, Dr. Bouillet knew that his advice would startle his patient. He also knew some of his colleagues didn't fully "believe" in it. But the scientific data seemed compelling to him. "Jacqueline," he said, "this may be a little hard, but when you begin chemotherapy, you'll also have to exercise." He recommended a karate club that specialized in looking after cancer patients.* The idea seemed strange to Jacqueline. She had done gymnastics in the past but had never imagined herself practicing a martial art, and she didn't particularly want to participate in a group made up exclusively of cancer patients. In fact, it was the last thing she would have liked to do with her free time.

---

* The association CAMI—Cancer, Martial Arts, and Information—located in the suburbs of Paris, is organized by patients who are coached by former European karate champion Jean-Marc Descotes.

A Martial Energy

Arriving at the dojo on the outskirts of Paris, Jacqueline was struck at first by the youth of the people in white kimonos who greeted her with smiles. Several of them were barely forty. Aside from one, whose shaved head betrayed her courses of chemotherapy, nothing in their look or attitude suggested illness. She realized suddenly that nothing in *her* appearance suggested it either. That was already reassuring. Before beginning the physical exercises, in accordance with Japanese ritual, all the students lined up on their knees facing the instructor. Then, as he did, with a bow from the waist, they saluted what they were about to do together—undertake an act of respect for their own bodies, in contact with their individual life force. Sensing the serene determination of these people, who had all suffered as she had, who had chosen to fight as she had, who were full of hope as she was, Jacqueline was moved. She knew, at that very instant, that she had been right to come.

When she stood up, the young master—a former European champion—pointed out that she was standing bent over, looking down at the floor. Jacqueline examined herself in the mirror and saw that it was true. Since her two operations, she had taken on the look of a "little old woman." Inwardly, as well, she felt she had aged. Standing at her side, the master then demonstrated the striking motions. She watched him as he moved, slowly at first, then at full speed. The movements were brisk, intense, and powerful, and he accompanied them with the traditional shout, "kaï," rising from the inner reaches of his body. Jacqueline smiled. This wasn't for her. She had never fought in her life, not even to say "no" to her family or friends, who had long taken advantage of her. She was definitely not a karateka. But since the beginning of her treatment, Dr. Bouillet's voice had been there to support her. He'd said, "You'll see. It's terrific." As everything he'd predicted had actually proved true, she decided to mobilize her body and strike the imaginary blow with a small, timid shout. Though barely audible, it was already a giant step for her.

At the end of the first session, she was soaked in perspiration. She had pushed and pulled on her body in ways she hadn't known were possible. She had struck the air with her hands and her feet. She had shouted. She had sensed her . . . strength. Jacqueline was thoroughly astonished at what had happened, at the energy she had discovered deep inside her body and whose existence she had never suspected. Thanks to this physically grueling session, she felt herself perk up.

Throughout the six cycles of chemotherapy she was to undergo, she attended classes religiously, twice a week. Still, her exhaustion was sometimes so great that she had visions of death. On the way to the club, in the subway, she was often nauseated. Or she would have trouble standing up straight. During those times, she wondered how she was going to make it. But she didn't give up. Today she realizes the friends she made at the club helped her keep up her courage. Even when she was assailed by doubts, seeing people who she knew were also burdened by disease and yet were so vigorously active reminded her that she was still alive. Moving her body, shouting out from the depth of her being—against her disease, against everything she was undergoing—restored her physical strength. In her karate sessions she felt herself fighting her enemies again and again, all the invisible enemies who had tried to steal her life. In the end, after each session she was less tired than before it began.

Many patients remember extreme fatigue at certain periods of their chemotherapy. They recall dragging themselves from bed to couch during the two weeks following injection of liquid chemicals that both heal and poison. Fatigue from cancer, added to exhaustion from treatments, is one of the most discouraging sides to the disease. It affects as many as nine out of ten patients, and it sometimes goes on for years after the treatments are over. Rest has no effect, nor does sleep. The whole body feels sheathed in lead.

Forty years ago, cardiac patients were still being told after an infarction that their fatigue came from the weakness of their heart. From this they learned that they were "cardiac cripples." Full-time rest was prescribed, but it did nothing to relieve their exhaustion and still less to improve their morale. Today cardiac patients are told to start exercising as soon as possible. Oncology is still at the very beginning of this same revolution in thinking, and very few patients receive this advice. Still, as Amit Sood, MD, of the Mayo Clinic, says, today we know that physical exercise is one of the most proven methods to relieve fatigue resulting from disease or from its treatment.[28]

CAUTION: CERTAIN EXERCISES MAY BE DANGEROUS

Some cancers may affect parts of the body that make certain exercises dangerous (arm movements after surgery in the armpit, jogging for individuals who have bone metastases, etc.). It is imperative for patients to consult their oncologists before choosing a kind of physical activity, in order to adapt it to their condition.

As for Jacqueline, she has never stopped karate. Four and a half years after her initial diagnosis, her oncologist told her she was free of disease.

Surviving her type of cancer was extremely rare and meant that the disease had been vanquished. But she had developed a taste for this new relationship with her body and with her life, for rediscovering her body at each session, sensing that she could act on it and seek energy deep in her inner being. To her, it's become a way of keeping the disease at bay. Twice a week, in her white kimono, she takes up the posture of combat. She stands straight, her gaze steady. She hears herself saying firmly to the ghost of her cancer, in case it should have the vaguest thought of returning, "Let's have it out."

Jacqueline is right to go on. Today there is every reason to believe that regular practice of physical exercise substantially reduces the risk of a relapse. As concerns breast cancer, in an editorial in the greatest international journal of oncology, the *Journal of Clinical Oncology,* Wendy Demark-Wahnefried, PhD, of Duke University, evokes a drop in relapse rate of 50 percent to 60 percent with exercise. This is such an impressive effect that she doesn't hesitate to compare it to the powerful effects of chemotherapy with Herceptin (for HER2-positive breast tumors), a revolutionary drug qualified in 2005 as a "major turning point in the eradication of suffering and death from cancer."*

Two studies, one by the Mayo Clinic, the other by the University of North Carolina, show comparable effects of exercise on estrogen-negative breast cancers.[30, 31] Moreover, still better than Herceptin, physical exercise provides benefits to patients with a broad variety of cancers. A comparable level of protection has been shown against recurrence or aggravation of cancer of the prostate (as much as a 70 percent drop in the risk of death in men over sixty-five), of the colon, and of the rectum. A protective effect has also been documented against cancer of the ovaries, the uterus, the testicles, and the lung.[†32–45]

A Morale Booster

"I'll never manage. . . . Anyhow, it's useless to try. . . . It won't work. . . . I'm never lucky. . . . It's my fault. . . . I'm letting everyone down by getting sick. . . . Other people may get over this, but I don't have enough energy, strength, courage, willpower, etc." Cancer is often associated with dark, pessimistic thoughts, which demean the self and even others. These ideas take on such an

---

* This quote is from Andrew C. von Eschenbach, MD, director of the National Cancer Institute of the United States.[29]

† On the other hand, the amount of physical exercise required to reduce relapse rates for colon cancer is higher (at least one hour of sustained walking five to six times a week), and greater still for prostate cancer (studies suggest three to five hours a week of "sustained exercise" such as jogging, singles tennis, bicycling, swimming, etc.).

automatic character that it is difficult to determine to what extent they express the disease rather than an objective truth.

Since the sixties and the remarkable work of a Philadelphia psychiatrist, Aaron Beck, MD, the founder of cognitive therapy, we have learned that the simple fact of repeating these statements maintains depression. Conversely, Beck has also shown that the act of voluntarily ceasing to say—or think— them sets patients on the path to better psychological balance.[46] One of the benefits of prolonged physical effort is that it can help eliminate the unceasing flow of ruminations, at least temporarily. Pessimistic thoughts rarely surface spontaneously in the course of exercising. If they do, they are chased away in the flow of physical movement, simply by focusing attention on breathing, on contact of the feet with the ground, or on the sensation of standing up straight.

Joggers attest, for example, that after twenty or thirty minutes of sustained effort, they enter a state where spontaneously positive, even creative, thoughts spring forth. Less aware of themselves, they get caught up in the rhythm of the effort that sustains and carries them forward. This is what is commonly called the "runner's high." It may be reached after several weeks of persever-ance. Even if it's subtle, this state may become addictive. Some can no longer do without their twenty minutes of running, even for a single day. According to a number of studies, the runner's high is an example of the mood-enhancing effect of physical exercise. This effect is so striking that physical activity is now recommended by the Ministry of Health of the United Kingdom on par with chemical antidepressants as a first intervention for depression.[47]

Keys to Success

A few very simple secrets ease the transition toward this new relationship with our bodies.

Begin slowly, gently

When beginners come back from the sporting goods store with their new Pumas, the major mistake they make is to want to run too fast and too far. There is no "magic" speed or distance valid for everyone. As Mikhail Csik-szentmihalyi, PhD, who researched "states of flow," has brilliantly shown, what enables us to enter the optimal mental and physical state of "flow" is persevering in an effort that keeps us at the limit of our capacities.[48] *At the limit,* not beyond. For someone just starting to run, this inevitably means for a short distance and with small strides. Later, it will mean running faster and longer to reach and maintain "flow," but this progression takes time. When jogging, it is usually recommended not to go beyond a speed at which you can still talk, but no longer sing. Make sure that you feel less tired after exercising than before, not the contrary.

Exercise everywhere and anywhere. The first step is recognizing we needn't do a lot, and after that, what's important is getting in the habit. Studies on breast cancer show that two to five hours a week of walking at a normal speed has a powerful effect on preventing relapse. There is no need to wear sweatpants. Walking in the subway, on the way to the office, or on daily errands counts as well. It's much better to include a little regular physical exercise than to exhaust yourself in a fitness center once and never go back. Some patients I know traded their car in for a bicycle, which is what I've done, too. Getting around by bicycle takes me the same amount of time as using public transportation, but I spend that time outdoors and sensing that my body is alive. At the end of the day, instead of having spent minutes of my life in a subway car, I've had fifty minutes of physical exercise, all with the feeling of being on vacation.

Try easy activities

Exercises such as yoga or tai chi, which stimulate the body gently, can be practiced by almost all cancer patients, whatever their condition. There is no study indicating that they are as effective as more vigorous activities, but they maintain attentive contact with the body and its energies. They are also a precious help in deepening and harmonizing breathing, and thus cardiac coherence. Several studies note that they also improve morale.[49-54]

Join a group

Encouragement and the support of others, or simply emulation in a group devoted to the same exercise, make a great difference in our capacity to stick to a program. Social activity helps to provide motivation on rainy days, or when you're behind schedule or there's a good movie on TV. Those who exercise in groups are more mindful of the need for regular attendance, which is so crucial to success.

Have fun

It's essential to choose a kind of exercise you enjoy. The more entertaining the exercise, the easier it is to keep up. In the United States, for example, there are informal basketball or softball teams organized at a good many companies. Just getting together three times a week for an hour after work can make a huge impact. This works just as well with volleyball or soccer, provided that the sessions are regular (and that you don't end up as the goalkeeper every time!). If you love swimming and hate running, don't force yourself to jog. You won't stick with it.

Get in the picture

This advice has turned out to be useful for several of my patients, and I've benefited from it as well. You can turn the use of a stationary bike, treadmill, or elliptical trainer into entertainment thanks to a DVD player. All you need to do is exercise while watching an action film, and only allow yourself to watch it as long as you go on. This method has several advantages: First, action films, like dance music, tend to be physiologically activating. They make you want to move. Second, a good film has a hypnotic effect that gets you to forget the passing time. The standard twenty-minute session goes by before you have a chance to think about checking your watch. Finally, if you follow the rule and don't watch the movie after you've stopped exercising, suspense makes you want to go on the next day, if only to find out what happens next.

Figure out the dose

Studies show that physical exercise helps the body fight cancer. But the required dose isn't the same for all cancers. Doses are calculated in units called MET.* For breast cancer, there seems to be a measurable effect after three to five hours a week of walking at normal speed (9 MET a week). For cancer of the colon and rectum, twice as much (18 MET a week) is needed to have a comparable effect. This means either walking twice as long or twice as fast, or finding activities requiring more effort to replace walking (for example, bicycling at a speed that requires effort adds up to twice as many MET as walking). Two weekly sessions of karate practiced by Dr. Bouillet's patients correspond to a dose of 18 MET a week. Finally, to have an effect on prostate cancer, 30 MET a week are required, the equivalent of three hours of jogging spread out over the week. (They can be done in six sessions of thirty minutes.)

The Energy of Life

My chemotherapy was spread out over thirteen months. Every four weeks, I had to ingest a daily dose of medicine for five days. Luckily for me, the drug probably wasn't as harsh as others may be. Also, perhaps because of all I was doing in parallel to the treatments I received, I was able to go on working almost up to the end. Generously, my colleagues organized our work so that I didn't have to come in before noon, and while I usually stayed at the hospital until 8 P.M., my days were nevertheless much lighter. At night I slept in a

---

* One MET is defined as the energy it takes to sit quietly. For the average adult, this is about one calorie per kilogram (2.2 pounds) of body weight per hour. Someone who weighs 160 pounds would burn approximately 70 calories an hour while sitting or sleeping. An activity level of 5 MET burns five times this basal level of energy expenditure.

separate room in the house, with our dog Mishka, a white German shepherd with hazel eyes. When I woke up with nausea, and sometimes with fear in my gut, he came and put his head on my knees. I patted him gently until I felt better. In the morning, he meditated with me. (Aren't dogs always in the process of meditating, effortlessly connected to the here and now?) Then he would stretch with half-closed eyes, as if yoga came naturally to him. He would look at me, tilting his head to the side toward the street. That meant that it was time to go running together.

We ran every morning that year, I think, and always for twenty minutes. In the snow, wrapped up in several layers of fleece and with earmuffs, in the rain with a slicker, in spring sunshine in a T-shirt, in the humid heat of East Coast summer days with a headband on my forehead to keep the sweat out of my eyes. When I didn't do it for myself, I did it for him. We kept up the same pace, but he pulled me on. I sensed the drug's ferocity in my body, increasing my heart rate and dragging my energy down. But every step forward, every gulp of air, gave me the feeling of getting the upper hand over the disease. I believed I could feel the drug's healing power circulating throughout my cells, eliminating its toxicity. I had the feeling we were working together—the drug, my body, and I.

I was very lucky to have a dog. Not everyone so easily finds their way to the kind of exercise that suits them best. Even for those completely won over to the principle, nothing is more difficult than including regular exercise in their daily lives. All the more so when they are worn down by disease or by treatments. But there is no doubt it is one of the most important things we can do to help ourselves. In the end, it comes down to deciding whether to give in to disease or to sustain the energy of life.

TABLE 9: ENERGY SPENT IN DIFFERENT ACTIVITIES MEASURED IN MET[55]

Activities of Daily Living	
Lying quietly	1.0
Sitting, watching television	1.0
Sitting, sewing	1.5
Walking from house to car or bus	2.5
Loading/unloading car	3.0

Activities of Daily Living	
Taking out trash	3.0
Walking dog	3.0
Household tasks, moderate effort	3.5
Vacuuming	3.5
Lifting items continuously	4.0
Raking lawn	4.0
Gardening (no lifting)	4.4
Mowing lawn (power mower)	4.5

Exercise	
Mild (less than 3 MET an hour)	
Playing the piano	2.3
Canoeing (leisurely)	2.5
Golf (with cart)	2.5
Walking (2 mph, 3 km/h)	2.5
Dancing (ballroom)	2.9
Moderate (3 to 5 MET an hour)	
Walking (3 mph, 5 km/h)	3.3
Cycling (leisurely)	3.5
Calisthenics (no weights)	4.0
Golf (no cart)	4.4
Swimming (slowly)	4.5
Walking (4 mph, 6.5 km/h)	4.5
Chopping wood	4.9

Vigorous (5 to 12 MET an hour)	
Dancing (fast or square dancing)	5.5
Cycling (moderately)	5.7
Aerobics	6.0
Roller skating	6.5
Skiing (cross-country or downhill)	6.8
Climbing hills (no load)	6.9
Swimming	7.0
Walking fast (5 mph, 8 km/h)	8.0
Martial arts training adapted for cancer patients	8.0
Jogging (6 mph, 10 km/h)	10.2
Jumping rope	12.0
Sustained martial arts training	12.0
Squash	12.1

CHAPTER 12

Learning to Change

As we have seen, while cancer can be triggered by any number of factors, it can only develop and spread if the terrain is favorable. There is no way to prevent cancer or slow down its growth (once it has already taken root) without changing this terrain in depth. Basically, seeing our response to cancer as a war or even a combat may not be the right metaphor. Rather than fighting insurgents, we may be better off changing mentalities. Our guiding principle, above all, should be to bring more awareness into our lives in order to change our attitude and that of our cells. But to what extent can we really *change*? One of the world's greatest cancer surgeons, William Fair, MD, experienced this inner revolution against his will.

Dr. Fair's Transformation

A specialist in prostate and kidney cancer, Bill Fair was head of the prestigious Department of Urology at Memorial Sloan-Kettering Hospital in New York when he learned he had colon cancer at a very advanced stage. After two operations and a year of intravenous chemotherapy (which didn't prevent him from operating several times a day), his tumor returned. This time it was even more aggressive, so aggressive that his doctors, chosen from among his hospital colleagues, told him sadly that his cancer was now "incurable." In their opinion, he had only a few months to live. Bill Fair was too "emotionally shattered" to react, as he later recounted. His wife, a former nurse in the armed forces, took things in hand. She told him the time had come for him to look after his "terrain." Spurred on by his wife, this workaholic, who was on deck seven days a week and often worked thirty-six hours at a stretch, took up meditation and yoga. Instead of grabbing a bite to eat at a fast-food counter in the hospital cafeteria, he was initiated to the benefits of a vegetarian diet. As a prominent member of the Western medical elite, he had never taken an interest in what the world's other medical traditions had to offer. Now he asked to meet researchers who had started a program investigating traditional Chinese medicine at the National Institutes of Health in Washington. This transformation was anything but easy. With his sharp mind, his biting tongue, and his characteristic surgeon's arrogance, Bill Fair had long cultivated a profound contempt for all these "alternative" approaches. His son remembered his former references to "touchy-feely West Coast nonsense."[1] Summoning up her courage and a great deal of patient kindness, Fair's wife finally convinced him he had nothing to lose. He could approach these other ways of looking at life with the mind of a researcher. He could keep what worked for him and leave the rest. He could preserve his critical mind and at the same time listen to his explorer's instinct. Bill Fair went along with it. Very haltingly. For example, after a training program in California on relaxation, he jumped on the red-eye to New York the same night because he wanted to be back at work early the next morning. But little by little, with yoga, meditation, a careful diet, Bill Fair changed. From the overbearing surgeon, from the authoritarian researcher and self-assured author of more than three hundred articles published in international cancer journals, he calmed down. He became a gentler, friendlier man. He learned to carefully choose the people he would spend time with, and in turn he would give them all his attention. Impressed by what he found out about himself, about his new relationship with his body, his mind, and the people around him, in a few years Bill Fair became the person he basically would have always liked to be. He was asked three years later what he thought of the benefits of this approach focused on improving the "terrain." Benevolently, he answered, "I've already lived three years beyond my colleagues' prognoses. As a scientist, I know that doesn't prove anything; it may just be luck. But there is one thing I'm sure about: I don't know if I extended my life, but I certainly expanded it."

His whole life Bill had been under pressure to be the best among the brightest, and to hold on to his hard-won place at the top of one of the greatest medical and research institutions. He had loved his work, but, at heart, he hadn't liked that brutal, intense style of practicing it so common among surgeons of his rank. He had girded himself with a sort of armor so as to function in an environment where categorical judgments are tossed around like so many blows and where you learn to give as good as you get.

His disease had given him the opportunity to discover approaches he had long despised. They had brought him peace and well-being. These mattered a lot to him now. He felt as if he were unloading himself of whole facets of his former personality. He learned, like many other patients, to pay more attention to what really mattered to him, independently of others' judgment. He no longer had to play the role of "brightest in the class." Bill Fair never renounced his passion as a physician or his scientific rigor. He continued to underscore the importance of conventional cancer treatments. He insisted that complementary approaches had to undergo strict evaluation. But, month after month, he became more genuine, more patient, and gentler. More receptive to the mystery and the richness of life.

Little by little, Bill Fair became a defender of these new approaches. He wanted them to be integrated into teaching and treatment programs. He organized a dinner for several deans and some of the principal oncologists of New York medical schools, so that they could meet one of the most respected American activists, Ralph W. Moss, a science journalist and an ardent promoter of complementary methods in oncology. In the course of the dinner, Fair leaned over to Moss and said: "I imagine ten years ago you would never have dreamed you would one day find yourself at dinner with these people." The activist answered: "Ten years ago, I would never have dreamed of finding myself at dinner with *you,* Bill."[2] Bill Fair had indeed changed a great deal.*

The path Dr. Fair followed is open to whoever may decide to take it. Hemmed in as he was in a culture that systematically denigrated that personal quest, this change was more difficult for him than for anyone else. If Bill Fair was able to transform his attitude toward life so radically, we must all be able to follow his example.

Changing Personalities?

At the University of Toronto, the psychologist Alastair Cunningham, PhD, has been looking after groups of cancer patients for thirty years; he teaches relaxation, visualization, meditation, and yoga. He helps his patients find the strength to become themselves, to draw as close as possible to their deepest values. He often works with patients considered "incurable," who have been given only a few months to live. By following them systematically, he has identified the attitudes that help predict which patients will have a chance of living far beyond their prognoses.[4, 5] Some of the patients he has followed from this group have outlived their prognosis by more than seven years. His studies suggest that these are people who, perfectly calmly, have asked the fundamental questions "Who am I really?" and "Where do I want to go?" Then they have drawn the consequences. One of his patients put it this way:

> Cancer sort of shifted the way I was developing in life and the goals I was pursuing. . . . I was totally focused on building a "bigger me." . . . I was

---

* Bill Fair's ideas and his transformation have been discussed in several publications. One of the most noteworthy was a piece in the *New Yorker* by Jerome Groopman, MD, a professor of medicine at Harvard Medical School and a writer.[3] I met Bill Fair myself in Washington in October 2001, three months before he finally succumbed to cancer. He had survived four years longer than his doctors' prognoses.

sort of following what our culture says is the approved path and then when I faced the fact that I might not live very long, I realized that all of that would die . . . and I started to question who I was really, if all that went. . . . It seemed like the whole focus of my life then shifted. [And now] I think I would be able to experience life today more fully [and] . . . to accept life as it comes to me and be part of that and just enjoy."[6, 7]

The closer Alastair Cunningham's patients got to their true values, the less constrained they felt to act only for the sake of propriety, or out of obligation, or for fear of causing disappointment and losing the affection of others. Another patient says:

I was one to follow the rules quite a bit and please everybody; I think I feel more comfortable with my place in the world now than I did before I was diagnosed. Definitely.

Most of them then discovered a real pleasure in making choices they hadn't allowed themselves up until then, and even in saying no. A third patient whose survival was exceptionally long:

Now I even say no, but before I would've been paranoid to say no. Now I can say, "No, not today, that doesn't suit me." . . . And there was no guilt when I made the decision not to go back to work next year. . . . It's not what I want to do. . . . I'm very happy with what I do now, and it's much easier to make a decision on the spur of the moment, and go to see a movie because you feel like going to see a movie, or sitting down and trying to sketch even though you know you're not good at it but it's so peaceful and pleasant. That's all.

What these patients have succeeded in doing in their lives, Cunningham comments, is ridding themselves of their "type C personality," of always trying to avoid making waves (see chapter 9). Rather than going through life passive and submissive, little by little they have learned to appropriate their freedom, their authenticity, and their autonomy. Cunningham calls that "de-type-C'ing" themselves.

This change is also visible in the way these patients approach their treatments, including their way of stimulating their natural defenses. I asked Dr. David Spiegel what was different about the three women in the support groups who had survived their metastatic cancer for more than ten years at a time when available treatments had little effectiveness. He described them this way:

They didn't stand out; they often remained calm and silent. But they had very specific ideas about what they would or wouldn't do to help themselves. They accepted certain treatments and refused others. They seemed imbued with a quiet strength.

This attitude of awareness and freedom of choice applies to natural methods too. Whether it's a question of diet, or yoga, or psychological support. These approaches are not all equally valid for everyone or at all times. On one day the most beneficial method will be meditation; on another, keeping a diary; the day after that, exercise. What we recognize in these exceptional survivors is their clear-eyed capacity to say "This is what I need now" and, firm but flexible, to move forward in their lives.

This change often amounts to more than learning to say no and asserting personal choices. Patients who have managed to survive for a substantial length of time have a strength buttressed by another attitude that is also often new to them—gratitude. They have become capable of perceiving another dimension to life that had escaped them earlier. As if a sort of x-ray enabled them to see the essential through the fog of the ordinary. One of them explained, for example, that one evening at dinner his wife and children started to quarrel. It was a familiar scene that never failed to exasperate him. But on that particular evening, instead of feeling angry, he saw all the love that was flowing around the table. If their feelings flared up, it was basically because they each cared so much about what the others thought. The affection that sustained this family suddenly seemed so palpable that tears came to his eyes and he was overcome with gratitude.

I experienced some of this same gratitude years after my separation from Anna. We had settled our painful divorce, after the legal process had dragged on for three very difficult years. We were sitting, again, at the kitchen table in the small blue wooden farmhouse we had lived in together in Pittsburgh. The crackles of a fire in the cast-iron stove filled the silences when we could not find words or even really look at each other. Sacha, now eleven, was playing by himself upstairs. I had loved this kitchen, this fire, the garden outside where I planted almost all the trees with Sacha looking on. And I had loved this woman. Then the words came. I was able to say that if that divorce had been so difficult, it was perhaps because a big part of me still loved her and loved what we had created together. That behind what I may have done in anger there was mostly my pain. As I could imagine hers too. And that now I was grateful for this love that remained between us, a love that would help our son grow. She did not say much, only wiped a few tears that had started to roll down her face. As I left the house—again—she put her hands on my arms, smiled shyly, and said, "I love you too." We had parted.

In the end, the best protection against cancer is a change in attitude arising from the process of growth valued by all the great psychological and spiritual traditions. To describe the very foundation of the life force, Aristotle speaks about "entelechy" (the need for self-fulfillment that starts with the seed and comes to full fruition in the tree). Jung describes a "process of individuation," transforming the person into a human being different from all others, capable of fully expressing his or her unique potential. Abraham Maslow, the founder of the human potential movement, refers to "self-actualization."[8-10] The spiritual traditions encourage "awakening" by developing the unique—in other words, the sacred—in the self.[11] It is very important that we define our most authentic values and put them to work in our conduct and in our relationships with others. From that approach springs a feeling of gratitude for life as it is—and our body, and its biology, basks in its grace.

CHAPTER 13

Conclusion

We have now finished touring some of the mysteries of cancer and of our natural defenses. What essentials should we keep in mind to prevent or fight the disease? To help people who may be threatened by cancer? To help rescue our wounded planet, no longer capable of providing us an environment that sustains our health? The key ideas that I have presented in this book, and that I use every day for my own protection, can be summed up in three points:

- the importance of our "terrain"
- the effects of awareness
- the synergy of natural forces

Let us review them one by one.

The Importance of Our "Terrain"

My Tibetan colleagues willingly admit that Western medicine treating a specific disease with a specific drug or intervention is marvelously effective in a crisis. Every day it saves lives, thanks to an operation for appendicitis, to penicillin for pneumonia, to epinephrine for an acute allergic reaction.

But it rapidly reveals its limits when dealing with a chronic illness. A myocardial infarction is probably the most striking example. A patient arrives in the emergency room on the point of death—pale, suffocating, with a crushing pain in her chest. The medical team, guided by years of cutting-edge research on tens of thousands of patients, knows exactly what to do: In a few minutes, oxygen is flowing through nasal prongs; nitroglycerin is dilating her veins; a beta-blocker is slowing down her heart rate; a dose of aspirin is preventing the creation of additional clots; and morphine is relieving her pain. In less than ten minutes, this woman's life has been saved. She breathes normally, she speaks to her family, and she even smiles. This is the miracle of medicine in what it has most spectacularly and also most admirably to offer.

And yet beyond this stunning success, the disease itself—the progressive obstruction, by cholesterol plaques, of the coronary arteries in a state of chronic inflammation—has not been affected by the emergency room intervention. Even the use of a stent, an act of technical prowess that consists of inserting a small tube inside the obstructed coronary artery to restore blood flow, is not adequate protection from relapses. In order to avoid them over the long term, the terrain must be changed: diet corrected, mental attitude altered, and body strengthened by exercise.*

Recent discoveries concerning the mechanisms of cancerous growth lead us to a similar conclusion. Cancer is the quintessential chronic disease. It is unlikely that we can stamp it out by focusing all our efforts on new techniques for screening and targeting tumors. Here again, we must look after the terrain. As emphasized by the 2007 report of the World Cancer Research Fund, approaches reinforcing the body's defense mechanisms—such as nutrition and exercise—are at the same time truly *preventive* and essential contributions to *treatment*. Because they rely on natural processes, they dissolve the frontier between prevention and treatment. On one hand, they prevent the microtumors we all carry in us from developing (prevention). On the other, they enhance the benefits of surgery, chemotherapy, and radiotherapy in the prevention of relapse (treatment).

Everyone knows people who have had cancer—sometimes a very serious one—but whose tumor has regressed thanks to treatment, and who have lived normally ever since. Sometimes their scan detects a tumor that has decreased in size. One way or another, their natural defenses now keep the disease at bay and prevent it from interfering with their health. As Judah Folkman, who discovered angiogenesis, writes in *Nature,* these people are carrying "cancer without disease."[2]

René Dubos, who spent his whole career at Rockefeller University in New York, is considered one of the great twentieth-century thinkers in biology. He discovered the first antibiotic put to medical use.† He became an ardent defender of ecology because of the interdependence he observed between living organisms and their environment. The quotation heading this book, which opened the journey we have just taken together, was written at the end of his career: *"I have always felt that the only trouble with scientific medicine is that*

---

* A major study recently published in the *Journal of the American Association of Cardiology* even shows that physical exercise is *more effective* than a high-tech intervention such as angioplasty with a stent in terms of preventing relapse.[1]

† It was gramicidin, which was used for several years before penicillin.

it is not scientific enough. Modern medicine will become really scientific only when physicians and their patients have learned to manage the forces of the body and the mind that operate via vis medicatrix naturae [*the healing power of nature*].*"*

From this point of view, we are, paradoxically, unwitting victims of the formidable achievements of Western medicine. Surgery, antibiotics, radiotherapy are extraordinary steps forward. But they have led us to overlook the body's own healing power. However, it's possible, as I hope I have convinced you, to enjoy the benefits of medical progress and the body's natural defenses at the same time.

The Effects of Awareness

Every one of us can make the most of this revolution in our knowledge of cancer to protect as well as to take care of ourselves. But this first calls for a revolution in our *awareness*. Above all, we must be conscious of the value and beauty of the life in us. We must pay attention to it and look after it as we would care for a child entrusted to us. This awareness helps us avoid damaging our physiology and encouraging cancer. It enables us to make the most of everything that nourishes and sustains our vital force.

We don't need to have cancer to start to really take our life seriously and to perceive its beauty. To the contrary. The closer we are to our own values and the more sensitive we are to the vibrant beauty of existence, the more chances we have of being protected against disease and also benefiting fully from our passage on earth.

By choosing a lifestyle that is more aware, we are not just doing what's good for ourselves. When we demand food from animals raised with respect for their biological needs, we gradually set off a chain reaction whose effects will be magnified down the line. Thus, our awakening will have an impact on rivers and streams. We will be contributing to reducing their pollution (with pesticides from cornfields and waste from feedlot-raised animals). Our choice will have an impact on the equilibrium and the renewal of land left fallow for the sake of regeneration. It will even have an effect on animals that give us their milk, eggs, and flesh, since they will be in better health when they are fed naturally. Globally, our awareness will have repercussions that extend to our planet's equilibrium: As we saw in chapter 6, consuming fewer animal products and demanding healthier food for animals contribute to considerably reducing the greenhouse effect responsible for global warming. Awareness, as the Buddha (whom I finally read!) insisted, truly has universal effects.

The eclipse of awareness weighs on us all, and even more so on the most destitute among us. Restoring the global balance of our environment would reduce one of the most terrible social injustices. For the most disadvantaged members of our Western societies are also those who have the highest cancer rates.[3] They are the most vulnerable to economic forces. They must content themselves with the cheapest food products, which are also the unhealthiest (with the most sugar and the largest quantities of omega-6 fatty acids and trans fats) and the most tainted by pesticides. Professionally, the disadvantaged are the most exposed to products known for contributing to cancer (wall and floor coverings, paint, cleaning products, etc.). As for their housing, which is concentrated in the most polluted areas (near incinerators, toxic waste dumps, factory smoke, etc.), they are exposed to industrial wastes that burden the body's anticancer defenses.[4] The disadvantaged are the most glaring victims in our affluent world, those who most need to make use of the natural means of resisting such aggressions but who have the least access to them.

The Synergy of Natural Forces

Fortunately, we can begin to protect ourselves against the biological mechanisms of cancer without adopting to the letter *all* the methods that have a positive effect. The body is a huge system in equilibrium, where each function interacts with all the others. Alter just one of these functions and the whole is inevitably affected. Thus, each of us can choose where we want to start: with diet, physical exercise, psychological work, or any other approach that brings more meaning and awareness into our lives. Every situation, every person, is unique; each person's way forward will be too. What matters above all is nourishing the desire to live. Some will do it by participating in a choir or by watching comedies, others by writing poetry or keeping a diary or getting more involved in the lives of their grandchildren.

We discover that increasing awareness in one domain almost automatically leads to progress in others. At Cornell, the researcher T. Colin Campbell observed, for example, that rats on a diet of vegetable rather than animal proteins started to exercise more, as if the balance in their diet made physical exercise easier.[5] In the same way, the practice of meditation or yoga links awareness to the body. Little by little, we lose a taste for an unbalanced diet—whose "heaviness" on the stomach and overall impact begin to weigh on the body. We lose the taste for tobacco—whose effect on breathing and on an accelerating heartbeat becomes more tangible, as is its odor on hair and fingers. We also lose our attraction to alcohol, whose influence on clear thinking and fluid movement is more easily detected. Health is a whole. Every step taken toward greater equilibrium makes the next ones easier.

"If It Were That Simple . . . "

When this book was first published, a professor of oncology—who had not yet taken the time to read it—was questioned about it by a reporter. His answer: "If it were that simple, you do realize we'd all know about it."

It is indeed difficult to imagine that effective approaches to cancer treatment and prevention could exist and yet not be widely put into practice. Sadly, when it comes to medical progress, this is more the norm than the exception. For example, in the early 1980s Dr. Barry Marshall discovered that a specific bacteria was the principal cause of ulcers in the stomach and duodenum. Nobody wanted to believe him. It wasn't until after he deliberately gave himself an ulcer by swallowing large quantities of the bacteria that he began to be taken seriously. And yet, despite the remarkable efficacy of the new ulcer treatment, which produced a definitive cure after a few weeks on a very cheap and well-tolerated antibiotic, it took almost ten years for his discovery to begin to influence the manner in which ulcers are treated. It was another ten years before Marshall was awarded the Nobel Prize for medicine.[6]

What could possibly explain this reluctance to embrace new medical strategies? I decided to discuss this issue with one of the biggest names in European oncology, Professor Lucien Israel, whom I met after *Anticancer* was first published.* In the 1950s, while he was working in a pulmonary ward specializing in the treatment of tuberculosis, young Israel saw an ever increasing number of cases of lung cancer. These patients were in fact among the first casualties of the growing epidemic linked to tobacco use. At the time, there were only three chemotherapy agents available for treatment of lung cancer. The protocol was to deploy one at a time, moving on when one of the agents was shown not to work, as was very often the case. Israel knew that doctors had only managed to cure tuberculosis when they realized that they had to use the various antituberculosis agents *at the same time*. So he asked a world-renowned chemotherapy specialist, who was presenting his protocols at a medical conference, "Why don't you use the three drugs together, instead of sequentially?" The response was curt: "Your mind is completely twisted, young man! Even if it worked, we would never know which agent was effective!"

Israel was less than impressed by the man's logic, which clearly valued academic knowledge over the beneficial treatment of patients. He became

---

* I conducted an interview at his house on May 20, 2009.

one of the first doctors to use polychemotherapy—deploying several agents at once—and to combine it with radiotherapy too.*

Today Professor Israel is retired and is writing his memoirs. An eternal combatant (he is a second-dan black-belt judo master) he continues to be appalled by the lack of willpower and imagination shown by academic medicine in the fight against cancer. "Given all the mechanisms that cancer cells employ to survive and develop, we need to go much further in what we're doing and multiply the means at our disposal, if we're going to win," he told me. "We have to use all the known nontoxic approaches *at the same time,* as complements to conventional treatments." He insisted on the importance of reinforcing the immune system, reducing inflammation, angiogenesis, and IGF, and exploiting the arsenal of nutrients known to be capable of contributing to the death of cancer cells. (He cited vitamin D, resveratrol, omega-3 fatty acids, and melatonin—secreted during sleep.) He emphasized, "I've observed it all through my career: When we help patients in this way, we considerably increase the rate of cure."

Listening to Professor Israel, I wondered how it was possible that a cancer specialist of his stature, who had published in international journals and obtained such remarkable results, should today be ignored. Is it possible that it really is that simple, and yet we don't all know about it?

It is, alas, possible. Professor Israel discussed the obstacles that he encountered when pushing the boundaries of cancer treatment. "It's very difficult to do studies on these combined approaches. Biostaticians are reluctant to evaluate several treatments administered at the same time, for fear we'll never know what is really effective. And in addition, there isn't much motivation to set up expensive research protocols for treatments that aren't patentable and won't bring in money. My publications didn't convince the medical world to invest in such studies. The doctors I trained do continue to practice these methods, but they aren't making inroads among the more conventional oncologists. To be frank, this unwillingness to go beyond standard protocols has always shocked me."

Today, the studies that Professor Israel dreamed of are beginning to appear. In this book, I've described two: the study from the University of California at San Francisco (chapter 2) with lifestyle interventions in prostate cancer[7] and the very recent Ohio State University study looking at nutrition, physical

---

* Several years later, Professor Israel was the first to use ambulatory chemotherapy, which avoids long and difficult periods of hospitalization without sacrificing the efficacy of treatment. Today, this method is used by millions of people around the world.

activity, and stress management in breast cancer patients (chapter 9).[8] Their conclusions converge: There is a dose-effect relationship between patients' adoption of anticancer lifestyle changes and the slower progression of their cancer. The *more* these patients are involved in a program to modify their "terrain," the *greater* the benefits. Similarly, researchers at the University of San Diego and Stanford University have shown that women who have had breast cancer and who begin *both* to eat a healthier diet *and* to walk for thirty minutes six days a week reduce their risk of relapse by almost half.[9, 10] It is, indeed, the *combination* of approaches—whether they are purely medical or involve lifestyle—that allows us to slow down cancer, or eliminate it.

False Hope?

At the end of this book, I must confess I'm concerned about the reactions of my fellow physicians and scientists. One of a physician's—and in particular an oncologist's—greatest worries is "not to give false hope." We have all learned that nothing is more painful for a patient than the feeling of having been betrayed by ill-considered promises. There is also a danger that certain patients will naively believe that, thanks to natural approaches, they can go on smoking, neglect screening mammograms, or refuse difficult treatments such as chemotherapy. Because of these concerns—all legitimate—my colleagues are sometimes tempted to refuse out of hand all approaches outside the confines of existing conventional practices. But this comes down to restricting ourselves to a conception of medicine that withholds the power every one of us has to take charge of ourselves. As if we couldn't do anything to protect ourselves actively against cancer—before *and* after the disease. Encouraging this passivity creates a culture of *hopelessness*.

What's more, it's a *false* hopelessness, since all the scientific evidence shows that we can have a substantial impact on our body's capacity to defuse the mechanisms of cancer. This is exactly what the resounding report of the World Cancer Research Fund emphasized when it stated that "in principle, most cancer is preventable."[11] I personally have refused to resign myself to the passivity of this false hopelessness, by putting into practice all the approaches described here. In writing this book I have not sought to impose recommendations to change their lifestyle on people who may not be ready to do so. Every one of us can decide for him- or herself what best fits his or her situation. However, I have chosen to share my experience and what I learned from the scientific literature with everyone who would like to explore how to become more active in his or her own health. I would like to believe that the majority of my colleagues can understand and identify with this reasoning.

Basking in the Light

The last time I saw my neurooncologist for the customary checkup, he made a surprising comment. "I don't know whether I should tell you this," he started out with a slightly embarrassed frown, "but I'm always very happy to see you. You are one of my rare patients who is doing well." I shivered inside. Despite his kindness, he had reminded me of the shadow hanging over my head—a shadow that nowadays I often forget. By talking about my case in this book, I'm exposing myself to receiving this kind of reminder more often than I would wish.

I'm aware that my personal history risks arousing two sorts of reactions—common in people who don't readily admit whatever ventures off the beaten track. Some of them may well say, "If he's doing well today, it's because his cancer wasn't that serious." How I wish—despite a relapse, a second operation, and thirteen months of chemotherapy—that were true. . . . My neuro-oncologist also said, "It's strange. Our genetic analyses show that your tumor has an aggressive biology, but its behavior with you is quite civilized." Perhaps it's just a matter of luck. Or perhaps it's because of what I do every day to live differently, as I've laid out here. In any event, my case is not a scientific experiment. It cannot serve to settle this debate. Only ongoing studies can transform our collective methods of preventing and treating cancer.*

But there is another "typical" reaction to the story of my case that could conceivably come up—a reaction that in a sense would amount to a wager against life. Some skeptics might say, "Before following his advice, wait and see if he's still alive next year." In other words, rather than examine their preconceived ideas, they might prefer to see no one escape the norm. To those I would answer that I don't know if I'll still be here in a year or in two or in

---

* Since the publication of *Anticancer: A New Way of Life,* I've been asked a lot of questions about the nature of my tumor and my state of health. I understand this need for information, but although I've gone public with my illness, I prefer to keep the details confidential, so people don't start placing bets on how long I'll be around. I can say that I'm not suffering from exactly the same cancer as Senator Ted Kennedy (a grade IV glioblastoma). However, my tumor's aggressive biology led to a relapse, despite very early detection followed by immediate treatment, which could in other circumstances have proved fatal. It has already required two craniotomies, thirteen months of chemotherapy, and five weeks of radiotherapy. Despite this, part of the tumor is still visible on scans. However, I am otherwise healthy and even relatively athletic. I bicycle every day, in Pittsburgh or Paris, I play squash regularly, and in 2008 I began kite surfing. Since commencing treatment I have lost quality of sleep and capacity to work, but I am happier and more balanced today, and I can say with confidence that I have been "living healthy with cancer" for eighteen years.

sixty. They would be right. I am not invulnerable. But there is one thing I'm certain of. I will never regret living as I live today, because the health and the greater awareness that this personal transformation has brought into my life give it a much greater value. Indeed, I have only one wish for every one of my readers as I finish this book. Whether you are well or ill, I hope that you too will choose to open yourself fully to that awareness—it is your birthright—and that your life will long bask in its light.

Follow Dr. David Servan-Schreiber's blog and sign up for his free weekly newsletter at www.anticancerbook.com.

Acknowledgments

Writing this book wasn't my idea. It took shape one May evening in a little Italian restaurant where my brother Franklin and I were dining. We were talking about our future plans. He thought mine lacked passion. "When will you finally make up your mind to talk about what happened to you and everything you discovered when you looked for ways to stay healthy?" he asked. Then he added, with all the powerful persuasion of his tender, penetrating gaze, "You don't have the right to keep that to yourself." I didn't think that I had enough material for a book—in any case, not enough for a book that would be truly useful to others. He set about questioning me about what had changed me the most. By the end of the evening, we had laughed and cried and agreed on the concepts we both thought essential to this book. And in the days that followed, I couldn't get the book project out of my mind. As he had done with so many other people who have had the good fortune to know him, Franklin had lit a flame within me that is still burning today.

Very quickly I sought the advice of three women whose names I never pronounce without immediately adding: "She's amazing." I knew them well but had never before discussed the story of my illness with them.

I spoke to Nicole Lattès, who was the publisher of my preceding book and whose intelligence gives off a kind of warm radiance. To my confused, hesitant, and modest proposal of working together again, she responded with sensitivity, kindness, and wisdom. She knew exactly what to do to channel it all into a book. Nicole is amazing.

I spoke to Susanna Lea, my agent, whose simple charm and innate knowledge of what is coherent and fair gave me a deep sense of confidence and encouragement. We quickly drew up the broad outlines for what this book needed to say, as well as a timetable that would give me a chance to devote myself entirely to writing for almost a year. Along the way, our long talks and our *not* eating the pastries in the best patisserie in Paris together were a delight. Susanna, I can't tell you too many times how amazing you are.

Finally, I met with Ursula Gauthier, a French journalist I admire greatly, on the sunlit terrace of a Paris café. I asked her if she would agree to work with me for a whole week, to help gather the memories of my experience with cancer. I also asked if she would help to edit the manuscript while it was being written. This subject was too sensitive for me to write about without the security of her intelligence and good judgment. That day, we talked about my project for three hours. At first she said she was too busy to take on a new task, but the next day she called to say she'd put everything else on hold in order to have the pleasure of working on this subject with me. My joy upon hearing this news was immense—Ursula, this book would never have come about without you. I've said it to you many times, let me write it now: You're amazing!

I was also rewarded with the encouragement of my former editor, Abel Gerschenfeld. When I explained the book idea to him he was visibly stirred. This reaction—rather unusual from him—was exactly what I needed to convince me the project was valid. Abel, even if we did not work together on this one, I often heard your voice in my head ringing with your benevolent advice.

In Logan, Utah, on the slopes of the Rockies, lives a woman who devotes her energy to treating cancer with nutritional approaches. With her PhD in nutrition, Jeanne Wallace is not a physician. But her encyclopedic knowledge of the biochemical mechanisms that can feed or, to the contrary, greatly limit the spread of cancer impressed me when I heard her present her results at a conference organized by the National Institutes of Health in 2001. As observed by researchers of the NIH, many of the patients Jeanne looked after—while they were receiving conventional medical treatment—survived far longer than originally predicted. I have been following her advice myself since that time. I am in her debt for many of the key ideas in this book—especially her scientific analysis of the different factors constituting the "terrain" and how to influence them with natural interventions. I also owe her, to a large extent, the good health that has enabled me to write, and to enjoy doing it.

Among the intellectual guides whose ideas and friendship have most inspired me, I wish to particularly thank Francine Shapiro, the founder of EMDR therapy, with her exceptional combination of sensitivity, intelligence, and humanism; Michael Lerner (surely an older brother in a previous life), with his quasiclairvoyant vision of the individual and society; and Jon Kabat-Zinn, who has introduced mindfulness meditation to a number of hospitals all over the world and made an enormous contribution to medicine and the well-being of so many people.

In Pittsburgh, the people who have inspired and helped me the most since I began to explore integrative medicine (the integration of conventional medicine with scientifically grounded natural approaches) are Emily Dorrance, who died at twenty-four with the serenity of a saint, from a sudden cancer, and Emily's parents, Susanne and Roy Dorrance. Amid the pain of their loss, they opened their hearts to me. They shared with me their spiritual strength in total respect for my own initial lack of—and on occasion my insensitivity to—religious conviction. I have kept a smiling photograph of Emily with me ever since. It has sustained me when my turn came to endure the anxieties and pains of illness.

My gratitude also goes to Michele Klein-Fedyshin, the librarian of the UPMC Shadyside hospital in Pittsburgh. We've been in contact several times a week, dealing with the 375 scientific references in this book. Michele also generously shared with me the beautiful letter written by her husband, Peter J. Fedyshin, to give her heart and strength during her treatment for breast cancer. The Mish letter is my favorite passage of this book.

Tohra Chalandon has provided constant friendly support and intellectual stimulation, for which I wish to express my great appreciation. The time she has given unsparingly to searching the Web for complex data (sometimes deliberately buried) has made it possible to document certain key passages. Our long summer swims in the sea were moments of simple and pure happiness.

I wish to thank the actor Bernard Giraudeau for talking about his cancer so honestly and courageously. He is an example for many who follow this path of empowerment, myself included.

My gratitude also goes to Marie-France Gizard. She was quite right in her kindly insistence that I follow through on my ideas regarding the mind-body link in relation to cancer. She also knew how to convince me to go much further than I had initially contemplated in the description of my own psychological development. I don't know if that will be as helpful to readers as she claimed, but the effort was certainly useful to me.

I would like to cite the key figures in medicine and research who, despite their heavy schedules, found time to see me and answer my questions, or to comment on the initial versions of the manuscript. I wish in particular to stress the kindness of Annie Sasco, David Spiegel, Devra Lee Davis, Richard Béliveau, Denis Gingras, Bharat Aggarwal, Zheng Cui, Luciano Bernardi, Linda Carlson, Susan Lutgendorf, Alastair Cunningham, Pierre Weill, Jean-Claude Lefeuvre, and Claude Aubert, as well as the French oncologists with whom I had fruitful discussions: Jean-Marie Andrieu, Bernard Asselain, Thierry Bouillet, Yvan Coscas, and Jean-Marc Cosset. My great appreciation is due to all of them for everything this book may contain that's right. As for the ideas they may not necessarily agree with, I willingly take sole responsibility.

My own oncologists and surgeons saved my life, and I salute their passion for a profession that is often trying. I also wish to pay tribute to the open-mindedness with which they accepted my ideas about my own treatment, though these did not always coincide with their own. Some of them even encouraged me to venture off the beaten track, and their support has mattered a great deal to me. My gratitude goes to Richard Fraser, L. Dade Lunsford, David Schiff, Cliff Schold, Frank Lieberman, and Hideho Okada.

The story I tell is mine, but it is also that of the mother of my son. We loved each other very much, before the mutual misunderstanding that took hold between us and caused us both a great deal of suffering. Whatever happened after that, I remain grateful to her for anchoring me to life at a time when I was afraid of the future, and infinitely grateful to her for bringing into the world our son Sacha, and giving him so much love.

Finally, I would like to mention the affection of those around me today who have supported me all along the way, putting up with my prolonged absences graciously: my mother, Sabine, with her generosity, her constancy, and her flashes of brilliance; my two brothers Emile (who picked the photograph for the jacket of the European editions) and Edouard (the first to tell me about the battle of Stalingrad); my son Sacha; sweet and patient Gwenaëlle for the energy we found in each other and for the laughter; my uncle Jean-Louis and my aunt Perla, pillars of wisdom and serenity; my cousin Florence, for the charm and vitality she radiates; my cousin Catherine, for her strength, courage, humor, and sustaining advice; my cousin Pascaline, for making me want to be a doctor when we were five; my cousin Simon, for his integrity and our unending laughter in Oxford or Montreal; Aunt Bernadette, the unconditional protector; the remarkable Liliane, who has been managing our family life nimbly and confidently for forty-five years; my assistant Delphine, who knew how to spare me almost all outside obligations while I was writing and without whom nothing I undertake would be done so efficiently; my friend Daniele Stern, my guardian angel in Pittsburgh and almost a second mother; and then Madeleine Chapsal, at whose home I wrote almost the entire book from summer to winter and then to summer, for the simple pleasure of living side by side with her in her house on the Island of Ré. Her enlightened encouragement, support, and warmth inspired the desire to write and to surpass my own limits.

Certain friends were so good as to read the earliest versions of these chapters and share their comments with me. I made the most of their kindness. I owe my appreciation to Guy Sautai, Pauline Guillerd, Claudia and Anna Sénik, Randa Chahal, Pascal Berti, Christian Regouby, Francis Lambert, Christophe Béguin. And also to Denis Lazat, my friend since we were eleven, an honorary brother, and the first vegetarian I knew (and made so much fun of!).

Thank you also to Anne Schofield-Guy, who shared with me her vast knowledge of English and her keen sense of what sounds and *is* right, for the English translation.

My father died while I was doing this work. He will never read it. Still, I owe my exploration of these virgin paths to his encouragement, from childhood onward, to always look beyond appearances and turn toward whatever restores individual power. I still sometimes sense his presence in me during my morning meditation, especially in difficult moments. I'm certain he will be there when I need strength to further these ideas.

—DSS
Island of Ré

Notes

INTRODUCTION TO THE SECOND EDITION

1. World Cancer Research Fund, *Food, Nutrition and the Prevention of Cancer: A Global Perspective* (London: World Cancer Research Fund and American Institute for Research on Cancer, 2007).

2. Institut National du Cancer, *Nutrition et prevéntion des cancers: des connaissances scientifiques aux recommandations* (Paris: Ministere de la Santé et des Sports, 2009).

3. Knoops, K. T. B., et al., "Mediterranean Diet, Lifestyle Factors, and 10-Year Mortality in Elderly European Men and Women—The HALE Project," *JAMA* 292 (2004): 1433–39.

4. Khaw, K.-T., et al., "Combined Impact of Health Behaviours and Mortality in Men and Women: The EPIC-Norfolk Prospective Population Study," *PLoS Medicine 5*, no. 1 (2008), e12.

INTRODUCTION

1. Harach, H. R., K. O. Franssila, and V. M. Wasenius, "Occult Papillary Carcinoma of the Thyroid: A 'Normal' Finding in Finland: A Systematic Autopsy Study," *Cancer 56*, no. 3 (1985): 531–38.

2. Black, W. C., and H. G. Welch, "Advances in Diagnostic Imaging and Overestimations of Disease Prevalence and the Benefits of Therapy," *New England Journal of Medicine* 328, no. 17 (1993): 1237–43.

3. Stewart, B. W., and P. Kleihues, eds., *World Cancer Report* (Lyon, France: W.H.O. IARC Press, 2003).

4. Yatani, R., T. Shiraishi, K. Nakakuki, et al., "Trends in Frequency of Latent Prostate Carcinoma in Japan from 1965–1979 to 1982–1986," *Journal of the National Cancer Institute* 80, no. 9 (1988): 683–87.

5. Stewart and Kleihues, *World Cancer Report*.

6. Sorensen, T. I. A., G. G. Nielsen, P. K. Andersen, et al., "Genetic and Environmental Influences on Premature Death in Adult Adoptees," *New England Journal of Medicine* 318 (1988): 727–32.

7. Lichtenstein, P., N. V. Holm, P. K. Verkasalo, et al. "Environmental and Heritable Factors in the Causation of Cancer—Analyses of Cohorts of Twins from Sweden, Denmark, and Finland," *New England Journal of Medicine* 343, no. 2 (2000): 78–85.

CHAPTER 2: ESCAPING STATISTICS

1. Spiegel, D., "A 43-Year-Old Woman Coping with Cancer," *JAMA* 282, no. 4 (1999): 371–78.

2. Van Baalen, D. C., M. J. deVries, and M. T. Gondrie, "Psycho-social Correlates of 'Spontaneous' Regression in Cancer," monograph, Department of General Pathology, Medical Faculty, Erasmus University, Rotterdam, The Netherlands, 1987.

3. Lerner, M., oral communication, Smith Farm Retreat, 2001.

4. Ornish, D., G. Weidner, W. R. Fair, et al., "Intensive Lifestyle Changes May Affect the Progression of Prostate Cancer," *Journal of Urology* 174, no. 3 (2005): 1065–69, discussion 9–70.

5. Ornish, D., M. J. Magbanua, G. Weidner, et al., "Changes in Prostate Gene Expression in Men Undergoing an Intensive Nutrition and Lifestyle Intervention," Proceedings of the National Academy of Sciences 105 (on press): 8369–74.

6. Ghadirian, P., S. Narod, E. Fafard, M. Costa, A. Robidoux, and A. Nkondjock, "Breast Cancer Risk in Relation to the Joint Effect of BRCA Mutations and Diet Diversity," *Breast Cancer Research & Treatment* (2009).

7. Fradet, V., I. Cheng, G. Casey, and J. S. Witte, "Dietary Omega-3 Fatty Acids, Cyclooxygenase-2 Genetic Variation, and Aggressive Prostate Cancer Risk," *Clinical Cancer Research* 15 (2009): 2559–66.

8. King, M.-C., J. H. Marks, J. B. Mandell, New York Breast Cancer Study Group, "Breast and Ovarian Cancer Risks Due to Inherited Mutations in BRCA1 and BRCA2," *Science* 302 (2003): 643–46.

CHAPTER 3: DANGER AND OPPORTUNITY

1. Yalom, I., *Existenial Psychotherapy* (New York: Basic Books, 1977).

2. Ibid.

CHAPTER 4: CANCER'S WEAKNESSES

1. Westcott, R., "Can Miracles Happen?" *British Medical Journal* 325, no. 7363 (2002): 553.

2. Everson, T. C., "Spontaneous Regression of Cancer," *Progress in Clinical Cancer* 3 (1967): 79–95.

3. Cole, W. H., "Efforts to Explain Spontaneous Regression of Cancer," *Journal of Surgical Oncology* 17, no. 3 (1981): 201–9.

4. Challis, G. B., H. J. Stam, G. B. Challis, et al., "The Spontaneous Regression of Cancer: A Review of Cases from 1900 to 1987," *Acta Oncologica* 29, no. 5 (1990): 545–50.

5. Bodey, B., B. Bodey, Jr., S. E. Siegel, et al., "The Spontaneous Regression of Neoplasms in Mammals: Possible Mechanisms and Their Application in Immunotherapy," *In Vivo* 12, no. 1 (1998): 107–22.

6. Papac, R. J., "Spontaneous Regression of Cancer: Possible Mechanisms," *In Vivo* 12, no. 6 (1998): 571–78.

7. Van Baalen, D. C., M. J. deVries, and M. T. Gondrie, "Psycho-social Correlates of 'Spontaneous' Regression in Cancer," monograph, Department of General Pathology, Medical Faculty, Erasmus University, Rotterdam, The Netherlands, 1987.

8. Cui, Z., M. C. Willingham, M. A. Alexander-Miller, et al., "Spontaneous Regression of Advanced Cancer: Identification of a Unique Genetically Determined, Age-Dependent Trait in Mice," *Proceedings of the National Academy of Sciences of the United States of America* 100 (2003): 6682–87.

9. Hicks, A. M., G. Riedlinger, M. C. Willingham, et al., "Transferable Anticancer Innate Immunity in Spontaneous Regression/Complete Resistance Mice," *Proceedings of the National Academy of Sciences of the United States of America* 103, no. 20 (2006): 7753–58.

10. Trapani, J. A., and M. J. Smyth, "Functional Significance of the Perforin/Granzyme Cell Death Pathway," *Nature Reviews Immunology* 2 (2005): 735–47.

11. Voskoboinik, I., and J. A. Trapani, "Addressing the Mysteries of Perforin Function," *Immunology and Cell Biology* 84 (2006): 66–71.

12. Whiteside, T., and R. B. Herberman, "Characteristics of Natural Killer Cells and Lymphocyte-Activated Killer Cells," *Immunology and Allergy Clinics of North America* 10 (1990): 663–704.

13. Head, J. F., F. Wang, R. L. Elliott, et al., "Assessment of Immunologic Competence and Host Reactivity Against Tumor Antigens in Breast Cancer Patients: Prognostic Value and Rationale of Immunotherapy Development," *Annals of the New York Academy of Sciences* 690 (1993): 340–42.

14. Levy, S. M., R. B. Herberman, M. Lippman, et al., "Immunological and Psychosocial Predictors of Disease Recurrence in Patients with Early-Stage Breast Cancer," *Behavioral Medicine* 17, no. 2 (1991): 67–75.

15. Imai, K., S. Matsuyama, S. Miyake, et al., "Natural Cytotoxic Activity of Peripheral-Blood Lymphocytes and Cancer Incidence: An 11–Year Follow-Up Study of a General Population," *Lancet* 356, no. 9244 (2000): 1795–99.

16. Schantz, S. P., B. W. Brown, E. Lira, et al., "Evidence for the Role of Natural Immunity in the Control of Metastatic Spread of Head and Neck Cancer," *Cancer Immunology, Immunotherapy* 25, no. 2 (1987): 141–48.

17. Herberman, R. B., "Immunotherapy," in *Clinical Oncology*, ed. R. J. Lenhard, R. Osteen, and T. Gansler (Atlanta, GA: American Cancer Society, 2001), 215–23.

18. MacKie, R. M., R. Reid, and B. Junor, "Fatal Melanoma Transferred in a Donated Kidney 16 Years after Melanoma Surgery," *New England Journal of Medicine* 348, no. 6 (2003): 567–68.

19. Cui, Z., "The Winding Road to the Discovery of the SR/CR Mice," *Cancer Immunity* 3 (2003): 14.

20. Koebel, C. M., Vermi, W., Swann, J. B., et al., "Adaptive Immunity Maintains Occult Cancer in an Equilibrium State," *Nature* 159 (2008): 363–76.

21. Imai, Matsuyama, Miyake, et al., "Natural Cytotoxic Activity of Peripheral-Blood Lymphocytes and Cancer Incidence."

22. Herberman, "Immunotherapy."
23. Levy, S. M., R. B. Herberman, A. M. Maluish, et al., "Prognostic Risk Assessment in Primary Breast Cancer by Behavioral and Immunological Parameters," *Health Psychology* 4, no. 2 (1985): 99–113.
24. Lutgendorf, S. K., A. K. Sood, B. Anderson, et al., "Social Support, Psychological Distress, and Natural Killer Cell Activity in Ovarian Cancer," *Journal of Clinical Oncology* 23, no. 28 (2005): 7105–13.
25. Schantz, Brown, Lira, et al., "Evidence for the Role of Natural Immunity in the Control of Metastatic Spread of Head and Neck Cancer."
26. Dvorak, H. F., "Tumors: Wounds That Do Not Heal: Similarities Between Tumor Stroma Generation and Wound Healing," *New England Journal of Medicine* 315, no. 26 (1986): 1650–59.
27. Balkwill, F., and A. Mantovani, "Inflammation and Cancer: Back to Virchow?" *Lancet* 357, no. 9255 (2001): 539–45.
28. Peek, R. M., Jr., S. Mohla, and R. N. DuBois, "Inflammation in the Genesis and Perpetuation of Cancer: Summary and Recommendations from a National Cancer Institute-Sponsored Meeting," *Cancer Research* 65, no. 19 (2005): 8583–86.
29. Huang, M., M. Stolina, S. Sharma, et al., "Non–Small Cell Lung Cancer Cyclooxygenase-2-Dependent Regulation of Cytokine Balance in Lymphocytes and Macrophages: Up-Regulation of Interleukin 10 and Down-Regulation of Interleukin 12 Production," *Cancer Research* 58, no. 6 (1998): 1208–16.
30. Mantovani, A., B. Bottazzi, F. Colotta, et al., "The Origin and Function of Tumor-Associated Macrophages," *Immunology Today* 13, no. 7 (1992): 265–70.
31. Baxevanis, C. N., G. J. Reclos, A. D. Gritzapis, et al., "Elevated Prostaglandin E2 Production by Monocytes Is Responsible for the Depressed Levels of Natural Killer and Lymphokine-Activated Killer Cell Function in Patients with Breast Cancer," *Cancer* 72, no. 2 (1993): 491–501.
32. Marx, J., "Cancer Research: Inflammation and Cancer: The Link Grows Stronger," *Science* 306 (2004): 5698–966.
33. Wallace, J., "Nutritional and Botanical Modulation of the Inflammatory Cascade—Eicosanoids, Cyclooxygenases, and Lipoxygenases—as an Adjunct in Cancer Therapy," *Integrative Cancer Therapies* 1, no. 1 (2002): 7–37.
34. Crumley, A. B. C., D. C. McMillan, M. McKernan, et al., "Evaluation of an Inflammation-Based Prognostic Score in Patients with Inoperable Gastro-oesophageal Cancer," *British Journal of Cancer* 94, no. 5 (2006): 637–41.
35. Al Murri, A. M., J. M. S. Bartlett, P. A. Canney, et al., "Evaluation of an Inflammation-Based Prognostic Score (GPS) in Patients with Metastatic Breast Cancer," *British Journal of Cancer* 94, no. 2 (2006): 227–30.
36. Forrest, L. M., D. C. McMillan, C. S. McArdle, et al., "Comparison of an Inflammation-Based Prognostic Score (GPS) with Performance Status (ECOG) in Patients Receiving Platinum-Based Chemotherapy for Inoperable Non-Small-Cell Lung Cancer," *British Journal of Cancer* 90, no. 9 (2004): 1704–6.

37. Harris, R. E., S. Kasbari, and W. B. Farrar, "Prospective Study of Nonsteroidal Anti-inflammatory Drugs and Breast Cancer," *Oncology Reports* 6, no. 1 (1999): 71–73.

38. Nelson, J. E., and R. E. Harris, "Inverse Association of Prostate Cancer and Non-steroidal Anti-Inflammatory Drugs (NSAIDs): Results of a Case-Control Study," *Oncology Reports* 7, no. 1 (2000): 169–70.

39. Thun, M. J., "NSAID Use and Decreased Risk of Gastrointestinal Cancers," *Gastroenterology Clinics of North America* 25, no. 2 (1996): 333–48.

40. Karin, M., and F. R. Greten, "NF-kappaB: Linking Inflammation and Immunity to Cancer Development and Progression," *Nature Reviews Immunology* 5, no. 10 (2005): 749–59.

41. Marx, "Cancer Research."

42. Ibid.

43. Calcagni, E., and I. Elenkov, "Stress System Activity, Innate and T Helper Cytokines, and Susceptibility to Immune-Related Diseases," *Annals of the New York Academy of Sciences* 1069 (2006): 62–76.

44. Glaser, R., "Stress-Associated Immune Dysregulation and Its Importance for Human Health: A Personal History of Psychoneuroimmunology," *Brain, Behavior, & Immunity* 19, no. 1 (2005): 3–11.

45. Beevor, A., *Stalingrad: The Fateful Siege: 1942–1943* (New York: Penguin Group, 1998).

46. Folkman, J., "Fighting Cancer by Attacking Its Blood Supply," *Scientific American*, September 1996, 150–54.

47. Folkman, J., "Tumor Angiogenesis: Therapeutic Implications," *New England Journal of Medicine* 285, no. 21 (1971): 1182–86.

48. Ibid.

49. "Cancer Warrior," *NOVA* Online, 2001. (Accessed November 2, 2006, at http://www.pbs.org/wgbh/nova/cancer/program.html.)

50. O'Reilly, M. S., L. Holmgren, Y. Shing, et al., "Angiostatin: A Novel Angiogenesis Inhibitor That Mediates the Suppression of Metastases by a Lewis Lung Carcinoma," *Cell* 79, no. 2 (1994): 315–28.

51. O'Reilly, M. S., L. Holmgren, C. Chen, et al., "Angiostatin Induces and Sustains Dormancy of Human Primary Tumors in Mice," *Nature Medicine* 2, no. 6 (1996): 689–92.

52. Rose, D. P., and J. M. Connolly, "Regulation of Tumor Angiogenesis by Dietary Fatty Acids and Eicosanoids," *Nutrition and Cancer* 37, no. 2 (2000): 119–27.

53. Béliveau, R., and D. Gingras, *Foods That Fight Cancer* (New York: McClelland & Stewart Ltd., 2006).

54. Béliveau, R., and D. Gingras, "Green Tea: Prevention and Treatment of Cancer by Nutraceuticals," *Lancet* 364, no. 9439 (2004): 1021–22.

55. Rose and Connolly, "Regulation of Tumor Angiogenesis by Dietary Fatty Acids and Eicosanoids."

56. Ziche, M., J. Jones, and P. M. Gullino, "Role of Prostaglandin E1 and Copper in Angiogenesis," *Journal of the National Cancer Institute* 69, no. 2 (1982): 475–82.

CHAPTER 6: THE ANTICANCER ENVIRONMENT

1. Dinse, G. E., D. M. Umbach, A. J. Sasco, et al., "Unexplained Increases in Cancer Incidence in the United States from 1975 to 1994: Possible Sentinel Health Indicators?" *Annual Review of Public Health* 20 (1999): 173–209.

2. Institut de Veille Sanitaire, "Estimations Nationales: Tendances de l'Incidence et de la Mortalité par Cancer en France entre 1978 et 2000," Ministère de la Santé, de la Famille et des Personnes Handicapées, 2002.

3. Surveillance Epidemiology and End Results (SEER). Cancer incidence public use database, 2006; see http://seer.cancer.gov/.

4. McGrath, K. G., "An Earlier Age of Breast Cancer Diagnosis Related to More Frequent Use of Antiperspirants/Deodorants and Underarm Shaving," *European Journal of Cancer Prevention* 12, no. 6 (2003): 479–85.

5. Steliarova-Foucher, E., C. Stiller, P. Kaatsch, et al., "Geographical Patterns and Time Trends of Cancer Incidence and Survival Among Children and Adolescents in Europe Since the 1970s (the ACCIS Project): An Epidemiological Study," *Lancet* 364, no. 9451 (2004): 2097–2105.

6. Post, P. N., D. Stockton, T. W. Davies, et al., "Striking Increase in Incidence of Prostate Cancer in Men Aged <60 Years Without Improvement in Prognosis," *British Journal of Cancer* 79, no. 1 (1999): 13–17.

7. Institut de Veille Sanitaire, "Estimations Nationales."

8. Ries, L. A. G., M. P. Eisner, C. L. Kosary, et al., "SEER Cancer Statistics Review 1975–2001," National Cancer Institute, Bethesda, MD, 2004.

9. Institut de Veille Sanitaire, "Estimations Nationales."

10. Ries, Eisner, Kosary, et al., "SEER Cancer Statistics Review 1975–2001."

11. Ferlay, J., F. Bray, P. Piesci, et al., eds., WHO International Agency for Research on Cancer (IARC), IARC Cancer Epidemiology Database, Globocan 2000, *Cancer Incidence, Mortality and Prevalence Worldwide* (Lyon, France: IARC Press, 2000).

12. King, M-C., J. H. Marks, J. B. Mandell, et al., "Breast and Ovarian Cancer Risks Due to Inherited Mutations in BRCA1 and BRCA2," *Science* 302, no. 5645 (2003): 643–46.

13. Institut de Veille Sanitaire, "Estimations Nationales."

14. Rosenberg, C. E., *The Cholera Years: The United States in 1832, 1849, and 1866* (Chicago, IL: University of Chicago Press, 1962).

15. Steingraber, S., *Living Downstream: A Scientist's Personal Investigation of Cancer and the Environment* (New York: Vintage Books, 1998).

16. Davis, D., *The Secret History of the War on Cancer* (New York: Basic Books, 2007).

17. Waterhouse, J., C. Muir, K. Shamnugaratnam, et al., eds., *Cancer Incidence in Five Continents*, vol. IV (Lyon, France: IARC-W.H.O., 1982).

18. Sasco, A. J., "Migration and Cancer," *Revue de Médecine Interne* 10, no. 4 (1989): 341–48.
19. Davis, *The Secret History of the War on Cancer.*
20. Waterhouse and Shamnugaratnam, *Cancer Incidence in Five Continents.*
21. Stewart, B. W., and P. Kleihues, eds., *World Cancer Report* (Lyon, France: W.H.O. IARC Press, 2003).
22. National Cancer Institute, *Executive Summary of Cancer Etiology Think Tank* (Bethesda, MD: National Cancer Institute, 2004).
23. Eaton, S. B., and M. Konner, "Paleolithic Nutrition: A Consideration of Its Nature and Current Implications," *New England Journal of Medicine* 312, no. 5 (1985): 283–89.
24. Cordain, L., S. Eaton, A. Sebastian, et al., "Origins and Evolution of the Western Diet: Health Implications for the 21st Century," *American Journal of Clinical Nutrition* 81, no. 2 (2005): 341–54.
25. Ibid.
26. Grothey, A., W. Voigt, C. Schober, et al., "The Role of Insulin-Like Growth Factor I and Its Receptor in Cell Growth, Transformation, Apoptosis, and Chemoresistance in Solid Tumors," *Journal of Cancer Research & Clinical Oncology* 125, no. 3–4 (1999): 166–73.
27. Long, L., R. Navab, and P. Brodt, "Regulation of the Mr 72,000 Type IV Collagenase by the Type I Insulin-Like Growth Factor Receptor," *Cancer Research* 58m, no. 15 (1998): 3243–47.
28. Dunn, S. E., R. A. Hardman, F. W. Kari, et al., "Insulin-Like Growth Factor 1 (IGF-1) Alters Drug Sensitivity of HBL 100 Human Breast Cancer Cells by Inhibition of Apoptosis Induced by Diverse Anticancer Drugs," *Cancer Research* 57, no. 13 (1997): 2687–93.
29. Cordain, L., S. Lindeberg, M. Hurtado, et al., "Acne Vulgaris: A Disease of Western Civilization," *Archives of Dermatology* 138, no. 12 (2002): 1584–90.
30. Smith, R., N. Mann, A. Braue, et al., "The Effect of a Low Glycemic Load, High Protein Diet on Hormonal Markers of Acne," *Asia Pacific Journal of Clinical Nutrition* 14 (supp.) (2005): S43.
31. Smith, R., N. Mann, A. Braue, et al., "Low Glycemic Load, High Protein Diet Lessens Facial Acne Severity," *Asia Pacific Journal of Clinical Nutrition* 14 (supp.) (2005): S97.
32. Santisteban, G. A., J. T. Ely, E. E. Hamel, et al., "Glycemic Modulation of Tumor Tolerance in a Mouse Model of Breast Cancer," *Biochemical & Biophysical Research Communications* 132, no. 3 (1985): 1174–79.
33. Parkin, D., F. Bay, J. Ferlay, et al., "Global Cancer Statistics, 2002," *CA: A Cancer Journal for Clinicians* 55 (2005): 74–108.
34. Weiderpass, E., G. Gridley, I. Persson, et al., "Risk of Endometrial and Breast Cancer in Patients with Diabetes Mellitus," *International Journal of Cancer* 71, no. 3 (1997): 360–63.
35. Hankinson, S. E., W. C. Willett, G. A. Colditz, et al., "Circulating Concentrations

of Insulin-Like Growth Factor-I and Risk of Breast Cancer," *Lancet* 351, no. 9113 (1998): 1393–96.

36. Chan, J. M., M. J. Stampfer, E. Giovannucci, et al., "Plasma Insulin-Like Growth Factor-I and Prostate Cancer Risk: A Prospective Study," *Science* 279, no. 5350 (1998): 563–66.

37. Chan, J. M., M. J. Stampfer, J. Ma, et al., "Insulin-Like Growth Factor-I (IGF-I) and IGF Binding Protein-3 as Predictors of Advanced-Stage Prostate Cancer," *Journal of the National Cancer Institute* 94, no. 14 (2002): 1099–1106.

38. Michaud, D. S., S. Liu, E. Giovannucci, et al., "Dietary Sugar, Glycemic Load, and Pancreatic Cancer Risk in a Prospective Study," *Journal of the National Cancer Institute* 94, no. 17 (2002): 1293–1300.

39. Michaud, D. S., C. S. Fuchs, S. Liu, et al., "Dietary Glycemic Load, Carbohydrate, Sugar, and Colorectal Cancer Risk in Men and Women," *Cancer Epidemiology, Biomarkers & Prevention* 14, no. 1 (2005): 138–47.

40. Franceschi, S., L. Dal Maso, L. Augustin, et al., "Dietary Glycemic Load and Colorectal Cancer Risk," *Annals of Oncology* 12, no. 2 (2001): 173–78.

41. Augustin, L. S. A., J. Polesel, C. Bosetti, et al., "Dietary Glycemic Index, Glycemic Load and Ovarian Cancer Risk: A Case-Control Study in Italy," *Annals of Oncology* 14, no. 1 (2003): 78–84.

42. Gunter, M. J., et al., "Insulin, Insulin-Like Growth Factor-I, and Risk of Breast Cancer in Postmenopausal Women," *Journal of the National Cancer Institute* 101 (2009): 48–60.

43. McMillan-Price, J., et al., "Comparison of 4 Diets of Varying Glycemic Load on Weight Loss and Cardiovascular Risk Reduction in Overweight and Obese Young Adults: A Randomized Controlled Trial," *Archives of Internal Medicine* 166, no. 14 (2006): 1466–75.

44. Collectif LaNutrition.fr., *Le Régime IG Minceur: comment perdre du poids en maîtrisant son sucre sanguin* (Vergèze, France: Thierry Souccar Editions, 2007).

45. Heini, A. F., and R. L. Weinsier, "Divergent Trends in Obesity and Fat Intake Patterns: The American Paradox," *American Journal of Medicine* 102, no. 3 (1997): 259–64.

46. Willett, W.C., "Dieary Fat Plays a Major Role in Obesity: No," *Obesity Reviews* 3, no. 2 (2002): 59–68.

47. Weill, P., *Tous Gros Demain?* (Paris, France: Plon, 2007).

48. Ibid.

49. Ailhaud, G., and P. Guesnet, "Fatty Acid Composition of Fats Is an Early Determinant of Childhood Obesity: A Short Review and an Opinion," *Obesity Reviews* 5, no. 1 (2004): 21–26.

50. Ailhaud, G., F. Massiera, P. Weill, et al., "Temporal Changes in Dietary Fats: Role of n-6 Polyunsaturated Fatty Acids in Excessive Adipose Tissue Development and Relationship to Obesity," *Progress in Lipid Research* 45, no. 3 (2006): 203–36.

51. Weill, P., B. Schmitt, G. Chesneau, et al., "Effects of Introducing Linseed in Livestock Diet on Blood Fatty Acid Composition of Consumers of Animal Products," *Annals of Nutrition & Metabolism* 46, no. 5 (2002): 182–91.

52. Ailhaud and Guesnet, "Fatty Acid Composition of Fats Is an Early Determinant of Childhood Obesity."

53. Simopoulos, A. P., "The Importance of the Ratio of Omega-6/Omega-3 Essential Fatty Acids," *Biomedicine Pharmacotherapy* 56, no. 8 (2002): 365–79.

54. Simopoulos, A. P., and N. Salem, "Omega-3 Fatty Acids in Eggs from Range-Fed Greek Chickens," *New England Journal of Medicine* 321, no. 20 (1989): 1412.

55. Ip, C., J. A. Scimeca, and H. J. Thompson, "Conjugated Linoleic Acid: A Powerful Anticarcinogen from Animal Fat Sources," *Cancer* 74, 3 supp. (1994): 1050–54.

56. Lavillonniere, F., V. Chajes, J-C. Martin, et al., "Dietary Purified cis-9, trans-11 Conjugated Linoleic Acid Isomer Has Anticarcinogenic Properties in Chemically Induced Mammary Tumors in Rats," *Nutrition and Cancer* 45, no. 2 (2003): 190–94.

57. Bougnoux, P., A. Barascu, M.-L. Jourdain, et al., "Acide Linoléique Conjugué et Cancer du Sein," *Oléagineux, Corps Gras, Lipides* 2005; 12(1): 56–60.

58. Dubnov, G., and E. M. Berry, "Omega-6/Omega-3 Fatty Acid Ratio: The Israeli Paradox," *World Review of Nutrition & Dietetics* 92 (2003): 81–91.

59. Weill, *Tous Gros Demain?*

60. van Kreijl, C., Knaap, A., Busch, M., et al. *"Ons eten gemeten. Gezonde voeding en veilig voedsel in Nederland."* Amsterdam NL: Public Health Department of the Netherlands; 2004. Report No.: RIVM report 27055509, available at Bohn, Stafleu, Van Loghum.

61. Nationaal Kompas Volksgezondheid. *"Verkeersongevallen. Omvang van het probleem. Verkeersongevallen naar leeftijd en geslacht, 2003–2007":* Public Health Department, Netherlands, 2004.

62. Chajes, V., et al., "Serum Trans-Monounsaturated Fatty Acids Are Associated with an Increased Risk of Breast Cancer in the E3N-EPIC Study," *American Journal of Epidemiology* (2008). DOI: 10.1093/aje/kwn069.

63. Hibbeln, J., W. Lands, and E. Lamoreaux, "Quantitative Changes in the Availability of Fats in the US Food Supply," 5th Congress of the International Society for Study of Fatty Acids and Lipids, May 7–11, 2002 Montreal, Canada, 2002, p. 10.

64. Bougnoux, P., et al., "Alpha-Linolenic Acid Content of Adipose Breast Tissue: A Host Determinant of the Risk of Early Metastasis in Breast Cancer," *British Journal of Cancer* 70, no. 2 (1994): 330–34.

65. Maillard, V., P. Bougnoux, P. Ferrari, et al., "N-3 and N-6 Fatty Acids in Breast Adipose Tissue and Relative Risk of Breast Cancer in a Case-Control Study in Tours, France," *International Journal of Cancer* 98, no. 1 (2002): 78–83.

66. Pollan, M., "Power Steer," *New York Times Magazine*, March 31, 2002.

67. Pollan, M., "Unhappy Meals," *New York Times Magazine*, January 28, 2007.

68. Pollan, M., *The Omnivore's Dilemma* (New York: Penguin Press, 2006).

69. Cunnane, S., and L. U. Thomson, *Flaxseed in Human Nutrition* (Champaign, IL: AOCS Press, 1995).

70. Weill, Schmitt, Chesneau, et al., "Effects of Introducing Linseed in Livestock Diet on Blood Fatty Acid Composition of Consumers of Animal Products."

71. Weill, *Tous Gros Demain?*

72. Ailhaud, Massiera, Weill, et al., "Temporal Changes in Dietary Fats."

73. World Cancer Research Fund, *Food, Nutrition and the Prevention of Cancer: A Global Perspective* (London: World Cancer Research Fund and American Institute for Research on Cancer, 2007).

74. Pollan, "Unhappy Meals."

75. Pollan, *The Omnivore's Dilemma.*

76. Ribeiro, C. A. O., Y. Vollaire, A. Sanchez-Chardi, et al., "Bioaccumulation and the Effects of Organochlorine Pesticides, PAH and Heavy Metals in the Eel (*Anguilla anguilla*) at the Camargue Nature Reserve, France," *Aquatic Toxicology* 74, no. 1 (2005): 53–69.

77. "Campagne Detox du WWF," World Wildlife Fund, 2005. (Accessed at www.panda.org/detox.)

78. Centers for Disease Control, *Third National Report on Human Exposure to Environmental Chemicals* (Atlanta: Centers for Disease Control and Prevention, 2005).

79. Davis, D. L., and B. H. Magee, "Cancer and Industrial Chemical Production," *Science* 206, no. 4425 (1979): 1356.

80. Ibid.

81. Davis, *The Secret History of the War on Cancer.*

82. Davis, D. L., *When Smoke Ran Like Water: Tales of Environmental Deception and the Battle Against Pollution* (New York: Basic Books, 2004).

83. Clapp R., G. Howe, and J. Lefevre, *Environmental and Occupational Causes of Cancer: Review of Recent Scientific Literature* (Lowell, MA: University of Massachusetts Lowell, 2005).

84. WWF-France, ed., *Planète Attitude—Santé* (Paris, France: Seuil, 2006).

85. Steingraber, *Living Downstream.*

86. Belpomme, D., "L'Appel de Paris," in *Guérir du Cancer ou s'en Protéger* (Paris, France: Fayard, 2005): 27–36.

87. Belpomme, D., P. Irigaray, A. Sasco, et al., "The Growing Incidence of Cancer: Role of Lifestyle and Screening Detection," *International Journal of Oncology* 30, no. 5 (2007): 1037–49.

88. Kortenkamp, A., *Breast Cancer and Exposure to Hormonally Active Chemicals: An Appraisal of the Scientific Evidence* (London: Chemical Health Monitor Alliance, 2008).

89. Relyea, R. "A Cocktail of Contaminants: How Mixtures of Pesticides at Low Concentrations Affect Aquatic Communities," *Decologia* 159 (2008): 373–76.

90. Irigaray, P., V. Ogier, S. Jacquenet, et al., "Benzo[a]pyrene Impairs Beta-Adrenergic Stimulation of Adipose Tissue Lipolysis and Causes Weight Gain in Mice: A Novel Molecular Mechanism of Toxicity for a Common Food Pollutant," *Federation of European Biochemical Societies Journal* 273, no. 7 (2006): 1362–72.

91. Davis, D. L., et al., "Medical Hypothesis: Xenoestrogens as Preventable Causes of Breast Cancer," *Environmental Health Perspectives* 101, no. 5 (1993): 372–74.

92. WWW-France, ed. *Planète Attitude—Santé.*

93. Environmental Working Group. *A Survey of Bisphenol A in U.S. Canned Foods* (2007). (Accessed March 23, 2009, at http://www.ewg.org/reports/bisphenola.)

94. LaPensee, E. W., et al., "Bisphenol A at Low Nanomolar Doses Confers Chemoresistance in Estrogen Receptor Alpha Positive and Negative Breast Cancer Cells," *Environmental Health Perspectives* (2008). doi: 10.1289/ehp.11788 (Accessed at http://dx.doi.org/.)

95. Carwile, J. L., et al., "Use of Polycarbonate Bottles and Urinary Bisphenol A Concentrations," *Environmental Health Perspectives* (2009).

96. Jin, H., et al., "High Dietary Inorganic Phosphate Increases Lung Tumorigenesis and Alters Akt Signaling," *American Journal of Respiratory and Critical Care Medicine* 179 (2009): 59–68.

97. Cho, E., et al., "Red Meat Intake and Risk of Breast Cancer Among Premenopausal Women," *Archives of Internal Medicine* 166, no. 20 (2006): 2253–59.

98. Norat, T., S. Bingham, P. Ferrari, et al., "Meat, Fish, and Colorectal Cancer Risk: The European Prospective Investigation into Cancer and Nutrition," *Journal of the National Cancer Institute* 97, no. 12 (2005): 906–16.

99. Eikelenboom, C., "Proof of Polychlorinated Biphenyls in Milk," *Zeitschrift fur Lebensmittel-Untersuchung und Forschung* 163, no. 4 (1977): 278.

100. Agence Française de Sécurité Sanitaire des Aliments, *Avis de l'agence française de sécurité sanitaire des aliments relatif à l'évaluation de l'exposition de la population française aux dioxines, furanes et PCB de type dioxine*, Agence Française de Sécurité Sanitaire des Aliments, 2005, Saisine no. 2005-SA-0372.

101. Kouba, M., "Quality of Organic Animal Products," *Lifestock Production Science* 80 (2003): 33–40.

102. Agence Française de Sécurité Sanitaire des Aliments, *Avis de l'agence française de de sécurité sanitaire . . .*

103. Kouba, "Quality of Organic Animal Products."

104. Observatoire des Résidus et Pesticides (2006). (Accessed at http://www.observatoire-pesticides.gouv.fr/index.php?pageid=381.)

105. Ibid.

106. Hayes, T., K. Haston, M. Tsui, et al., "Herbicides: Feminization of Male Frogs in the Wild," *Nature* 419, no. 6910 (2002): 895–96.

107. Hayes, T. B., A. Collins, M. Lee, et al., "Hermaphroditic, Demasculinized Frogs After Exposure to the Herbicide Atrazine at Low Ecologically Relevant Doses," *Proceedings of the National Academy of Sciences of the United States of America* 99, no. 8 (2002): 5476–80.

108. Batistatou, A., D. Stefanou, A. Goussia, et al., "Estrogen Receptor Beta (ERbeta) Is Expressed in Brain Astrocytic Tumors and Declines with Dedifferentiation of the Neoplasm," *Journal of Cancer Research & Clinical Oncology* 130, no. 7 (2004): 405–10.

109. Provost, D., A. Gruber, P. Lebailly, et al., "Brain Tumors and Exposure to Pesticides: A Case-Control Study in Southwestern France," *Occupational and Environmental Medicine* 2007.

110. Curl, C. L., R. A. Fenske, and K. Elgethun, "Organophosphorus Pesticide Exposure of Urban and Suburban Preschool Children with Organic and Conventional Diets," *Environmental Health Perspectives* 111, no. 3 (2003): 377–82.

111. Pesticide Action Network North America, "Chemical Trespass: Pesticides in Our Bodies and Corporate Accountability" (Pesticide Action Network of North America, 2004).

112. Aubert, C., *Présence de pesticides dans le lait maternel avec ou sans alimentation biologique.* In. Paris; 1986.

113. Lu, C., K. Toepel, R. Irish, et al., "Organic Diets Significantly Lower Children's Dietary Exposure to Organophosphorus Pesticides," *Environmental Health Perspectives* 114, no. 2 (2006): 260–63.

114. Doll, R., and R. Peto, "The Causes of Cancer: Quantitative Estimates of Avoidable Risks of Cancer in the United States Today," *Journal of the National Cancer Institute* 66, no. 6 (1981): 1191–1308.

115. Wynder, E. L., and E. A. Graham, "Tobacco Smoking as a Possible Etiological Factor in Bronchogienic Carcinoma," *JAMA* 143 (1950): 329–36.

116. Sasco, A. J., M. B. Secretan, and K. Straif, "Tobacco Smoking and Cancer: A Brief Review of Recent Epidemiological Evidence," *Lung Cancer* 45 Supp. 2 (2004): S3–9.

117. Bach, P. B., et al., "Variations in Lung Cancer Risk Among Smokers," *Journal of the National Cancer Institute* 95 (2003): 470–78.

118. Pimentel, D., *Techniques for Reducing Pesticide Use: Economic and Environmental Benefits* (Chichester, UK: John Wiley & Sons, 1997).

119. Cardis, Elizabeth, interview, *France Evening News,* June 15, 2008.

120. Hardell, L., M. Carlberg, and K. Mild, "Case-Control Study of the Association Between the Use of Cellular and Cordless Telephones and Malignant Brain Tumors Diagnosed During 2000–2003," *Environmental Research* 100 (2006): 232–41.

121. U.S. Department of Health and Human Services, *The Health Consequences of Smoking: A Report of the Surgeon General* (Atlanta, GA: U.S. Department of Health and Human Services, Centers for Disease Control and Prevention, National Center for Chronic Disease Prevention and Health Promotion Office on Smoking and Health, 2004).

122. Travis, L., et al., "Cancer Survivorship—Genetic Susceptibility and Second Primary Cancers: Research Strategies and Recommendations," *Journal of the National Cancer Institute* 98, no. 1 (2006): 15–25.

123. Dupont, G., "L'élevage Contribue Beaucoup au Réchauffement Climatique," *Le Monde,* December 5, 2006, sec. 9.

124. Bittman, M., "Rethinking the Meat-Guzzler," *New York Times,* January 27, 2008.

125. Environmental Working Group, "The Full List: 43 Fruits and Veggies," available at www.ewg.org, accessed 2006.

CHAPTER 7: LESSONS OF A RELAPSE

1. Baclesse, F., A. Ennuyer, and J. Cheguillaume, "May a Simple Tumorectomy Followed by Radiotherapy Be Performed in the Case of Mammary Tumor?" *Journal de Radiologie, d'Electrologie, et de Medecine Nucleaire* 41 (1960): 137–9.

2. Fisher, B., et al., "Twenty-Year Follow-up of a Randomized Trial Comparing Total Mastectomy, Lumpectomy, and Lumpectomy Plus Irradiation for the Treatment of Invasive Breast Cancer," *New England Journal of Medicine* 347, no. 16 (2002): 1233–41.

CHAPTER 8: THE ANTICANCER FOODS

1. Cao, Y., and R. Cao, "Angiogenesis Inhibited by Drinking Tea," *Nature* 398, no. 6726 (1999): 381.

2. Béliveau, R., and D. Gingras, *Les aliments contre le cancer* (Outremont, Canada: Trécarré, 2005).

3. Béliveau, R., and D. Gingras, *Foods That Fight Cancer: Preventing Cancer Through Diet* (New York: Random House, 2006).

4. Campbell, T. C., and T. M. Campbell, *Le Rapport Campbell: La plus vaste étude internationale à ce jour sur la nutrition par Colin Campbell, Thomas M Campbell, et Annie Ollivier* (Outremont, Canada: Editions Ariane, 2008).

5. Campbell, T. C., *The China Study* (Dallas, TX: BenBella Books, 2005).

6. Fidler, I. J., "Angiogenic Heterogeneity: Regulation of Neoplastic Angiogenesis by the Organ Microenvironment," *Journal of the National Cancer Institute* 93, no. 14 (2001): 1040–41.

7. Fidler, I. J., "Critical Factors in the Biology of Human Cancer Metastasis: Twenty-Eighth G. H. A. Clowes Memorial Award Lecture," *Cancer Research* 50, no. 19 (1990): 6130–38.

8. Paget, S., "The Distribution of Secondary Growths in Cancer of the Breast," *Lancet* 1 (1889): 571–3.

9. Coussens, L. M., Z. Werb, L. M. Coussens, et al., "Inflammation and Cancer," *Nature* 420, no. 6917 (2002): 860–67.

10. Jankun, J., S. H. Selman, R. Swiercz, et al., "Why Drinking Green Tea Could Prevent Cancer," *Nature* 387, no. 6633 (1997): 561.

11. Cao and Cao, "Angiogenesis Inhibited by Drinking Tea."

12. Demeule, M., B. Annabi, J. Michaud-Levesque, et al., "Dietary Prevention of Cancer: Anticancer and Antiangiogenic Properties of Green Tea Polyphenols," *Medicinal Chemistry Reviews-Online* 2 (2005): 49–58.

13. Ibid.

14. Zhou J.-R., L. Yu, Z. Mai, G. L. Blackburn, "Combined Inhibition of Estrogen-Dependent Human Breast Carcinoma by Soy and Tea Bioactive Components in Mice," *International Journal of Cancer*, 2004; 108(1): 8–14.

15. Zhou, J-R., L. Yu, Y. Zhong, et al., "Soy Phytochemicals and Tea Bioactive Components Synergistically Inhibit Androgen-Sensitive Human Prostate Tumors in Mice," *Journal of Nutrition* 133, no. 2 (2003): 516–21.

16. Inoue, M., et al., "Regular Consumption of Green Tea and the Risk of Breast Cancer Recurrence: Follow-up Study from the Hospital-Based Epidemiologic Research Program at Aichi Cancer Center (HERPACC), Japan," *Cancer Letters* 167, no. 2 (2001): 175–82.

17. Kurahashi, N., et al., "Green Tea Consumption and Prostate Cancer Risk in Japanese Men: A Prospective Study," *American Journal of Epidemiology* 167, no. 1 (2007): 71–77.

18. Knoops, K. T. B., et al., "Mediterranean Diet, Lifestyle Factors, and 10-Year Mortality in Elderly European Men and Women—The HALE Project," *JAMA* 292 (2004): 1433–39.

19. Oldways Trust Mediterranean Diet Foundation US, "Mediterranean Diet: The Scientific Evidence" (2009). (Accessed March 15, 2009, at http://www.oldwayspt .org/.)

20. Sofi, F., "Adherence to Mediterranean Diet and Health Status: Meta-Analysis," *British Medical Journal* (2008).

21. Owen, R. W., Haubner, R., Wurtele, G., Hull, E., Spiegelhalder, B., Bartsch, H., "Olives and Olive Oil in Cancer Prevention," *European Journal of Cancer Prevention* 13 (2004): 319–26.

22. Martin-Moreno, J. M., et al., "Dietary Fat, Olive Oil Intake and Breast Cancer Risk," *International Journal of Cancer* 58, no. 6 (1994): 774–80.

23. Stoneham, M., et al., "Olive Oil, Diet and Colorectal Cancer: An Ecological Study and a Hypothesis," *Journal of Epidemiology & Community Health* 54, no. 10 (2000): 756–60.

24. Lipworth, L., et al., "Olive Oil and Human Cancer: An Assessment of the Evidence," *Preventive Medicine* 26, no. 2 (1997): 181–90.

25. Menendez, J. A., et al., "Oleic Acid, the Main Monounsaturated Fatty Acid of Olive Oil, Suppresses Her-2/neu (erbB-2) Expression and Synergistically Enhances the Growth Inhibitory Effects of Trastuzumab (Herceptin) in Breast Cancer Cells with Her-2/neu Oncogene Amplification," *Annals of Oncology* 16, no. 3 (2005): 359–71.

26. Menendez, J. A., et al., "Analyzing Effects of Extra-Virgin Olive Oil Polyphenols on Breast Cancer–Associated Fatty Acid Synthase Protein Expression Using Reverse-Phase Protein Microarrays," *International Journal of Molecular Medicine* 22, no. 4 (2008): 433–39.

27. Wu, A. H., M. C. Pike, and D. O. Stram, "Meta-analysis: Dietary Fat Intake, Serum Estrogen Levels, and the Risk of Breast Cancer," *Journal of the National Cancer Institute* 91 (1999): 529–34.

28. Ravdin, P. M., K. A. Cronin, N. Howlader, et al., "The Decrease in Breast-Cancer Incidence in 2003 in the United States," *New England Journal of Medicine* 356, no. 16 (2007): 1670–74.

29. Agence Française de Sécurité Sanitaire des Aliments, *Sécurité et bénéfices des phyto-estrogènes apportés par l'alimentation*, Agence Française de Sécurité Sanitaire des Aliments, 2005, Saisine no. 2002–SA-231.

30. Aggarwal, B. B., H. Ichikawa, P. Garodia, et al., "From Traditional Ayurvedic Medicine to Modern Medicine: Identification of Therapeutic Targets for Suppression of Inflammation and Cancer," *Expert Opinion on Therapeutic Targets* 10, no. 1 (2006): 87–118.

31. Ferlay, J., F. Bray, P. Piesci, et al., eds., WHO International Agency for Research on Cancer (IARC), IARC Cancer Epidemiology Database, Globocan 2000, *Cancer Incidence, Mortality and Prevalence Worldwide* (Lyon, France: IARC Press, 2000).

32. Institute for Scientific Information, isihighlycited.com, 2005.

33. Shishodia, S., and B. B. Aggarwal, "Nuclear Factor-kappaB Activation: A Question of Life or Death," *Journal of Biochemistry & Molecular Biology* 35, no. 1 (2002): 28–40.

34. Mehta, K., P. Pantazis, T. McQueen, et al., "Antiproliferative Effect of Curcumin (Diferuloylmethane) Against Human Breast Tumor Cell Lines," *Anti-Cancer Drugs* 8, no. 5 (1997): 470–81.

35. Aggarwal, B. B., S. Shishodia, Y. Takada, et al., "Curcumin Suppresses the Paclitaxel-Induced Nuclear Factor-kappaB Pathway in Breast Cancer Cells and Inhibits Lung Metastasis of Human Breast Cancer in Nude Mice," *Clinical Cancer Research* 11, no. 20 (2005): 7490–98.

36. Carter, A., "Curry Compound Fights Cancer in the Clinic," *Journal of the National Cancer Institute* (2008). p. djn141.

37. Cheng, A. L., C. H. Hsu, J. K. Lin, et al., "Phase I Clinical Trial of Curcumin, a Chemopreventive Agent, in Patients with High-Risk or Pre-malignant Lesions," *Anticancer Research* 21, no. 4B (2001): 2895–900.

38. Shoba, G., D. Joy, T. Joseph, et al., "Influence of Piperine on the Pharmacokinetics of Curcumin in Animals and Human Volunteers," *Planta Medica* 64, no. 4 (1998): 353–56.

39. Gao, X., D. Deeb, H. Jiang, et al., "Curcumin Differentially Sensitizes Malignant Glioma Cells to TRAIL/Apo2L-Mediated Apoptosis Through Activation of Procaspases and Release of Cytochrome c from Mitochondria," *Journal of Experimental Therapeutics & Oncology* 5, no. 1 (2005): 39–48.

40. Ooi, V. E., and F. Liu, "Immunomodulation and Anti-Cancer Activity of Polysaccharide-Protein Complexes," *Current Medicinal Chemistry* 7, no. 7 (2000): 715–29.

41. Torisu, M., Y. Tayashi, T. Ishimitsu, et al., "Significant Prolongation of Disease-Free Period Gained by Oral Polysaccharide K (PSK) Administration After Curative Surgical Operation of Colorectal Cancer," *Cancer Immunology Immunotherapy* 31 (1999): 261–68.

42. Nakazato, H., A. Koike, S. Saji, et al., "Efficacy of Immunochemotherapy as Adjuvant Treatment After Curative Resection of Gastric Cancer," *Lancet* 343 (1994): 1122–26.

43. Hara, M., T. Hanaoka, M. Kobayashi, et al., "Cruciferous Vegetables, Mushrooms, and Gastrointestinal Cancer Risks in a Multicenter, Hospital-Based Case-Control Study in Japan," *Nutrition and Cancer* 46, no. 2 (2003): 138–47.

44. Torisu, Tayashi, Ishimitsu, et al., "Significant Prolongation of Disease-Free Period . . . "

45. Kikuchi, Y., I. Kizawa, K. Oomori, et al., "Effects of PSK on Interleukin-2 Production by Peripheral Lymphocytes of Patients with Advanced Ovarian Carcinoma During Chemotherapy," *Japanese Journal of Cancer Research* 79, no. 1 (1988): 125–30.

46. Tsujitani, S., Y. Kakeji, H. Orita, et al., "Postoperative Adjuvant Immunochemotherapy and Infiltration of Dendritic Cells for Patients with Advanced Gastric Cancer," *Anticancer Research* 12, no. 3 (1992): 645–48.

47. Kariya, Y., N. Inoue, T. Kihara, et al., "Activation of Human Natural Killer Cells by the Protein-Bound Polysaccharide PSK Independently of Interferon and Interleukin 2," *Immunology Letters* 31, no. 3 (1992): 241–45.

48. Mizutani, Y., and O. Yoshida, "Activation by the Protein-Bound Polysaccharide PSK (Krestin) of Cytotoxic Lymphocytes That Act on Fresh Autologous Tumor Cells and T24 Human Urinary Bladder Transitional Carcinoma Cell Line in Patients with Urinary Bladder Cancer," *Journal of Urology* 145, no. 5 (1991): 1082–87.

49. Torisu, Tayashi, Ishimitsu, et al., "Significant Prolongation of Disease-Free Period . . ."

50. Labrecque, L., S. Lamy, A. Chapus, et al., "Combined Inhibition of PDGF and VEGF Receptors by Ellagic Acid, a Dietary-Derived Phenolic Compound," *Carcinogenesis* 26, no. 4 (2005): 821–26.

51. Ibid.

52. Hanausek, M., Z. Walaszek, and T. J. Slaga, "Detoxifying Cancer Causing Agents to Prevent Cancer," *Integrative Cancer Therapies* 2, no. 2 (2003): 139–44.

53. Seeram, N., L. Adams, Y. Zhang, et al., "Blackberry, Black Raspberry, Blueberry, Cranberry, Red Raspberry, and Strawberry Extracts Inhibit Growth and Stimulate Apoptosis of Human Cancer Cells in Vitro," *Journal of Agricultural and Food Chemistry* 54 (2006): 9329–39.

54. Béliveau, R., and D. Gingras, *Les aliments contre le cancer*.

55. Stoner, G. D., et al., "Cancer Prevention with Freeze-Dried Berries and Berry Components," *Seminars in Cancer Biology* 17, no. 5 (2007): 403–10.

56. Stoner, G. D., "Commentary—Foodstuffs for Preventing Cancer: The Preclinical and Clinical Development of Berries," *Cancer Prevention Research* 187 (2009). DOI: doi: 10.1158/1940-6207.CAPR-08-0226.

57. Vizzotto, M., "Inhibition of Invasive Breast Cancer Cells by Selected Peach and Plum Phenolic Antioxidants" (PhD diss., Texas A&M University, August 2005).

58. Altman, L. K., "New Drug Fights Second Kind of Cancer," *New York Times*, May 14, 2001.

59. Folkman J., and R. Kalluri, "Cancer Without Disease," *Nature* 427, no. 6977 (2004): 787.

60. Plouzek, C. A., H. P. Ciolino, R. Clarke, et al., "Inhibition of P-glycoprotein Activity and Reversal of Multidrug Resistance in Vitro by Rosemary Extract," *European Journal of Cancer 35*, no. 10 (1999): 1541–45.

61. Lamy, S., et al., "The Dietary Flavonols Apigenin and Luteolin Inhibit PDGF-Dependent Vascular Smooth Muscle Cell Migration," *Cancer Research*, in submission.

62. Béliveau, R., and D. Gingras, *Cuisiner avec les aliments contre le cancer* (Outremont, Canada: Trécarré, 2006).

63. Yokoi, K., T. Sasaki, C. D. Bucana, et al., "Simultaneous Inhibition of EGFR, VEGFR, and Platelet-Derived Growth Factor Receptor Signaling Combined with Gemcitabine Produces Therapy of Human Pancreatic Carcinoma and Prolongs Survival in an Orthotopic Nude Mouse Model," *Cancer Research 65*, no. 22 (2005): 10371–80.

64. Ramesha, A., N. Rao, A. R. Rao, et al., "Chemoprevention of 7,12-Dimethylbenz-[a]anthracene-Induced Mammary Carcinogenesis in Rat by the Combined Actions of Selenium, Magnesium, Ascorbic Acid and Retinyl Acetate," *Japanese Journal of Cancer Research 81*, no. 12 (1990): 1239–46.

65. Ibid.

66. Canene-Adams, K., et al., "Combinations of Tomato and Broccoli Enhance Antitumor Activity in Dunning r3327-h Prostate Adenocarcinomas," *Cancer Research 67*, no. 2 (2007): 836–43.

67. Ramesha, et al., "Chemoprevention of 7,12-Dimethylbenz[a]anthracene-Induced Mammary Carcinogenesis . . . "

68. Chohan, M., G. Forster-Wilkins, and E. Opara, "Determination of the Antioxidant Capacity of Culinary Herbs Subjected to Various Cooking and Storage Processes Using the ABTS(*+) Radical Cation Assay," *Plant Foods for Human Nutrition 63*, no. 2 (June 2008): 47–52.

69. Lamy, S., et al., "The Dietary Flavonols . . . "

70. Campbell, *The China Study*.

71. Lanzmann-Petithory, D., *CANCERALCOOL: Consommation de boissons alcoolisées (vin, bière et alcools forts) et mortalité par différents types de cancers sur une cohorte de 100 000 sujets suivie depuis 25 ans.*, in *Premier Colloque Final—Programme National de Recherche en Alimentation et Nutrition Humaine (PNRA)*. (Paris: Agence Nationale de la Recherche et INRA, 2009).

72. Servan-Schreiber, D., R. Béliveau, and M. De Lorgeril, "Deux verres de vin rouge n'augmentent pas les risques de cancer," *Le Monde*, March 21, 2009.

73. De Lorgeril, M., and P. Salen, *Alcool, vin et santé* (Monaco: Alpen Editions, 2007).

74. Baglietto, L., et al., "Does Dietary Folate Intake Modify Effect of Alcohol Consumption on Breast Cancer Risk? Prospective Cohort Study," *BMJ 331*, no. 7520 (2005): 80.

75. Thorand, B., et al., "Intake of Fruits, Vegetables, Folic Acid and Related Nutrients and Risk of Breast Cancer in Postmenopausal Women," *Public Health Nutrition 1*, no. 3 (1998): 147–56.

76. Tjonneland, A., et al., "Folate Intake, Alcohol and Risk of Breast Cancer Among Postmenopausal Women in Denmark," European Journal of Clinical Nutrition, 60, no. 2 (2006): 280–86.

77. Chao, C., et al., Alcoholic Beverage Intake and Risk of Lung Cancer: The California Men's Health Study (2008).

78. Surh, Y.-J., "Cancer Chemoprevention with Dietary Phytochemicals," Nature Reviews Cancer 3, no. 10 (2003): 768–80.

79. Ibid.

80. DeVita, V. T., S. A. Rosenberg, and S. Hellman, eds., Cancer: Principles and Practice of Oncology, 7th ed. (Baltimore: Lippincott Williams & Wilkins, 2005).

81. American Cancer Society, "Nutrition for the Person with Cancer During Treatment: A Guide for Patients and Families," 2006.

82. Campbell, The China Sudy.

83. O'Keefe, J. J., and L. Cordain, "Cardiovascular Disease Resulting from a Diet and Lifestyle at Odds with Our Paleolithic Genome: How to Become a 21st-Century Hunter-Gatherer," Mayo Clinic Proceedings 79, no. 1 (2004): 101–8.

84. Cordain, L., S. Eaton, A. Sebastian, et al., "Origins and Evolution of the Western Diet: Health Implications for the 21st Century," American Journal of Clinical Nutrition 81, no. 2 (2005): 341–54.

85. Knoops, et al., "Mediterranean Diet . . . "

86. De Lorgeril, M., P. Salen, J. L. Martin, et al., "Mediterranean Diet, Traditional Risk Factors, and the Rate of Cardiovascular Complications After Myocardial Infarction: Final Report of the Lyon Diet Heart Study," Circulation 99, no. 6 (1999): 779–85.

87. Kris-Etherton, P., R. H. Eckel, B. V. Howard, et al., "AHA Science Advisory: Lyon Diet Heart Study. Benefits of a Mediterranean-Style, National Cholesterol Education Program/American Heart Association Step I Dietary Pattern on Cardiovascular Disease," Circulation 103, no. 13 (2001): 1823–25.

88. Renaud, S., M. de Lorgeril, J. Delaye, et al., "Cretan Mediterranean Diet for Prevention of Coronary Heart Disease," American Journal of Clinical Nutrition 61, no. 6, supp. (1995): 1360S–67S.

89. Pollan, M., "Unhappy Meals," New York Times Magazine, January 28, 2007.

90. World Cancer Research Fund, Food, Nutrition and the Prevention of Cancer: A Global Perspective (London: World Cancer Research Fund and American Institute for Research on Cancer, 2007).

91. Kikuzaki, H., and N. Nakatani, "Antioxidant Effects of Some Ginger Constituents," Journal of Food Science 58, no. 6 (1993): 1407–10.

92. Zhou, H.-Y., J.-K. Shen, J.-S. Hou, et al., "Experimental Study on Apoptosis Induced by Elemene in Glioma Cells," Aizheng 22, no. 9 (2003): 959–63.

93. Wang, G., "Element of Ginger Triggers Cell Death, Enhances Cisplatin—Abstract 2981," American Association for Cancer Research (2004).

94. Jaga, K., and H. Duvvi, "Risk Reduction for DDT Toxicity and Carcinogenesis Through Dietary Modification," Journal of the Royal Society of Health 121, no. 2 (2001): 107–13.

95. Cover, C. M., S. J. Hsieh, E. J. Cram, et al., "Indole-3-Carbinol and Tamoxifen Cooperate to Arrest the Cell Cycle of MCF-7 Human Breast Cancer Cells," *Cancer Research* 59, no. 6 (1999): 1244–51.

96. Gamet-Payrastre, L., P. Li, S. Lumeau, et al., "Sulforaphane, a Naturally Occurring Isothiocyanate, Induces Cell Cycle Arrest and Apoptosis in HT29 Human Colon Cancer Cells," *Cancer Research* 60, no. 5 (2000): 1426–33.

97. Singh, S. V., et al., "Sulforaphane Inhibits Prostate Carcinogenesis and Pulmonary Metastasis in TRAMP Mice in Association with Increased Cytotoxicity of Natural Killer Cells," *Cancer Research* 69 (2009): 2117–25.

98. Canane-Adams, et al., "Combinations of Tomato and Broccoli . . ."

99. Knoops, et al., "Mediterranean Diet . . ."

100. Ramesha, et al., "Chemoprevention of 7, 12-dimethylbenz[a]anthracene-Induced Mammary Carcinogenesis . . ."

101. Canane-Adams, et al., "Combinations of Tomato and Broccoli . . ."

102. Ballard-Barbash, R., and A. McTiernan, "Is the Whole Larger Than the Sum of the Parts? The Promise of Combining Physical Activity and Diet to Improve Cancer Outcomes," *Journal of Clinical Oncology* 25, no. 17 (2007): 2335–37.

103. Beljanski, M., and M. S. Beljanski, "Three Alkaloids as Selective Destroyers of Cancer Cells in Mice: Synergy with Classic Anticancer Drugs," *Oncology* 43, no. 3 (1986): 198–203.

104. Jacobs, D. R., et. al., "Food Synergy: An Operational Concept for Understanding Nutrition," *American Journal of Clinical Nutrirtion* 89, supp. (2009): 1S–6S.

105. Liu, R. H., "Potential Synergy of Phytochemicals in Cancer Prevention: Mechanism of Action," *Journal of Nutrition* 134, no. 12 supp., 3479S–3485S.

106. Pierce, J. P., et al., "Greater Survival After Breast Cancer in Physically Active Women with High Vegetable-Fruit Intake Regardless of Obesity," *Journal of Clinical Oncology* 25, no. 17 (2007): 2345–51.

107. Khaw, K.-T., et al., "Combined Impact of Health Behaviours and Mortality in Men and Women: The EPIC-Norfolk Prospective Population Study," *PLoS Medicine* 5, no. 1 (2008): e12.

108. Hsing, A. W., A. P. Chokkalingam, Y.-T. Gao, et al., "Allium Vegetable and Risk of Prostate Cancer: A Population-Based Study," *Journal of the National Cancer Institute* 94, no. 21 (2002): 1648–51; Thomson, M., and M. Ali, "Garlic [*Allium sativum*]: A Review of Its Potential Use as an Anti-Cancer Agent," *Current Cancer Drug Targets* 3, no. 15 (2003): 67–81.

109. Ingram, D., "Diet and Subsequent Survival in Women with Breast Cancer," *British Journal of Cancer* 69, no. 3 (1994): 592–95.

110. Chan, J. M., C. N. Holick, M. F. Leitzmann, et al., "Diet After Diagnosis and the Risk of Prostate Cancer Progression, Recurrence, and Death (United States)," *Cancer Causes & Control* 17, no. 2 (2006): 199–208.

111. Canene-Adams, et al., "Combinations of Tomato and Broccoli . . ."

112. Zhang, M., et al., "Dietary Intakes of Mushrooms and Green Tea Combine to Reduce the Risk of Breast Cancer in Chinese Women," *International Journal of Cancer* 15 (2009): 1404–8.

113. Maruyama, H., H. Tamauchi, M. Hashimoto, et al., "Antitumor Activity and Immune Response of Mekabu Fucoidan Extracted from Sporophyll of *Undaria pinnatifida*," *Vivo* 17, no. 3 (2003): 245–49.

114. Shimizu, J., "Proportion of Murine Cytotoxic T Cells Is Increased by High Molecular-Weight Fucoidan Extracted from Okinawa Mozuku (*Cladosiphon okamuranus*)," *Journal of Health Sciences* 51 (2005): 394–97.

115. Vizzotto, "Inhibition of Invasive Breast Cancer Cells . . ."

116. Taraphdar, A. K., M. Roy, and R. K. Bhattacharya, "Natural Products as Inducers of Apoptosis: Implication for Cancer Therapy and Prevention," *Current Science* 80 (2001): 1387–96.

117. Rooprai, H. K., A. Kandanearatchi, S. L. Maidment, et al., "Evaluation of the Effects of Swainsonine, Captopril, Tangeretin and Nobiletin on the Biological Behaviour of Brain Tumour Cells in Vitro," *Neuropathology & Applied Neurobiology* 27, no. 1 (2001): 29–39.

118. Pantuck, A. J., "Phase-II Study of Pomegranate Juice for Men with Prostate Cancer and Increasing PSA," American Urological Association Annual Meeting, San Antonio, TX, 2005.

119. Manna, S. K., A. Mukhopadhyay, B. B. Aggarwal, "Resveratrol Suppresses TNF-Induced Activation of Nuclear Transcription Factors NF-[kappa]B, Activator Protein-1, and Apoptosis: Potential Role of Reactive Oxygen Intermediates and Lipid Peroxidation," *Journal of Immunology* 164, no. 12 (2000): 6509–19.

120. Kaeberlein, M., T. McDonagh, B. Heltweg, et al., "Substrate-Specific Activation of Sirtuins by Resveratrol," *Journal of Biological Chemistry* 280, no. 17 (2005): 17038–45.

121. Lappe, J. M., K. Travers-Gustafson, K. M. Davies, "Vitamin D and Calcium Supplementation Reduces Cancer Risk: Results of a Randomized Trial," *American Journal of Clinical Nutrition* 85 (2007): 1586–91.

122. Woo, T. C. S., et al., "Pilot Study: Potential Role of Vitamin D (Cholecalciferol) in Patients with PSA Relapse After Definitive Therapy," *Nutrition & Cancer* 51, no. 1 (2005): 32–36.

123. Cannell, J. J. and B. W. Hollis, "Use of Vitamin D in Clinical Practice," *Alternative Medicine Review* 13 (2003).

124. Canadian Cancer Society, "La Société Canadienne du Cancer Annonce Ses Recommandations Concernant la Vitamine D," 2007. (Accessed June 10, 2007, at www.cancer.ca.)

125. Chan, Holick, Leitzman, et al., "Diet After Diagnosis and the Risk of Prostate Cancer Progression, Recurrence, and Death."

126. Gago-Dominguez, M., J. Yuan, C. Sun, et al., "Opposing Effects of Dietary n-3 and n-6 Fatty Acids on Mammary Carcinogenesis: The Singapore Chinese Health Study," *British Journal of Cancer* 89, no. 9 (2003): 1686–92.

127. Goodstine, S. L., T. Zheng, T. R. Holford, et al., "Dietary (n-3)/(n-6) Fatty Acid Ratio: Possible Relationship to Premenopausal but Not Postmenopausal Breast Cancer Risk in U.S. Women," *Journal of Nutrition* 133, no. 5 (2003): 1409–14.

128. Leitzmann, M., M. Stampfer, D. Michaud, et al., "Dietary Intake of n-3 and n-6 Fatty Acids and the Risk of Prostate Cancer," *American Journal of Clinical Nutrition* 80 (2004): 204–16.

129. Hedelin, M., "Association of Frequent Consumption of Fatty Fish with Prostate Cancer Risk Is Modified by COX-2 Polymorphism," *Internation Journal of Cancer* 120, no. 2 (2006): 398–405.

130. Norat, T., S. Bingham, P. Ferrari, et al., "Meat, Fish, and Colorectal Cancer Risk: The European Prospective Investigation into Cancer and Nutrition," *Journal of the National Cancer Institute* 97, no. 12 (2005): 906–16.

131. Terry, P., A. Wolk, H. Vainio, et al., "Fatty Fish Consumption Lowers the Risk of Endometrial Cancer: A Nationwide Case-Control Study in Sweden," *Cancer Epidemiology, Biomarkers & Prevention* 11, no. 1 (2002): 143–45.

132. Terry, P., P. Lichtenstein, M. Feychting, et al., "Fatty Fish Consumption and Risk of Prostate Cancer," *Lancet* 357, no. 9270 (2001): 1764–66.

133. Hooper, L. T., R. Thompson, R. Harrison, et al., "Risks and Benefits of Omega 3 Fats for Mortality, Cardiovascular Disease, and Cancer: Systematic Review," *British Medical Journal* 332 (2006): 752–60.

134. MacLean, C. H., S. J. Newberry, W. A. Mojica, et al., "Effects of Omega-3 Fatty Acids on Cancer Risk: A Systematic Review," *JAMA* 295, no. 4 (2006): 403–15.

135. Norat, Bingham, Ferrari, et al., "Meat, Fish, and Colorectal Cancer Risk."

136. George, S. L., et al., "Impact of Flaxseed Supplementation and Dietary Fat Restriction on Prostate Cancer Proliferation and Other Biomarkers: Results of a Phase II Randomized Controlled Trial (RCT) Using a Presurgical Model," *Journal of Clinical Oncology* 63S (2007).

137. Bougnoux, P., et al., "Alpha-Linolenic Acid Content of Adipose Breast Tissue: A Host Determinant of the Risk of Early Metastasis in Breast Cancer," *British Journal of Cancer* 70, no. 2 (1994): 330–34.

138. Wollowski, I., G. Rechkemmer, and B. L. Pool-Zobel, "Protective Role of Probiotics and Prebiotics in Colon Cancer," *American Journal of Clinical Nutrition* 73, no. 2 (2001): 451S–55.

139. Kim, H. S., et al., "Dietary Supplementation of Probiotic Bacillus Polyfermenticus, Bispan Strain, Modulates Natural Killer Cell and T Cell Subset Populations and Immunoglobulin G Levels in Human Subjects," *Journal of Medicinal Food* 9, no. 3 (2006): 321–27.

140. Rayman, M. P., "The Importance of Selenium to Human Health," *Lancet* 356, no. 9225 (2000): 233–41.

141. Kiremidjian-Schumacher, L., M. Roy, H. I. Wishe, "Supplementation with Selenium and Human Immune Cell Functions: II. Effect on Cytotoxic Lymphocytes and Natural Killer Cells," *Biological Trace Element Research* 41, no. 1–2 (1994): 115–27.

CHAPTER 9: THE ANTICANCER MIND

1. Dolbeault, S., "Quantité de survie versus qualité de vie: quel impact des interventions psychothérapeutiques en oncologie? Le point en 2008," *Revue de presse d'oncologie clinique* 17, no. 3 (2008).

2. Lerner, M., *Choices in Healing: Integrating the Best of Conventional and Complementary Approaches to Cancer* (Boston: MIT Press, 1994).

3. Simonton, C. O., S. Matthews-Simonton, and J. Creighton, *Guérir Envers et Contre Tout* (Paris: Desclée de Brouwer, 1990).

4. Baghurst, K. I., P. A. Baghurst, and S. J. Record, "Public Perceptions of the Role of Dietary and Other Environmental Factors in Cancer Causation or Prevention," *Journal of Epidemiology and Community Health* 46 (1992): 120–26.

5. Antoni, M. H., S. K. Lutgendorf, S. W. Cole, et al., "The Influence of Bio-Behavioural Factors on Tumour Biology: Pathways and Mechanisms," *Nature Reviews Cancer* 6, no. 3 (2006): 240–48.

6. Temoshok, L., "Biopsychosocial Studies on Cutaneous Malignant Melanoma: Psychosocial Factors Associated with Prognostic Indicators, Progression, Psychophysiology and Tumor-Host Response," *Social Science & Medicine* 20, no. 8 (1985): 833–40.

7. Temoshok, L., "Personality, Coping Style, Emotion and Cancer: Towards an Integrative Model," *Cancer Surveys* 6, no. 3 (1987): 545–67.

8. Simonton, et al., *Guérir Envers et Contre Tout.*

9. LeShan, L., *Cancer as Turning Point* (New York: Plume, 1990).

10. Gawler, I., *You Can Conquer Cancer—Prevention and Treatment* (South Yarra, Australia: Michelle Anderson, 2001).

11. Laplanche, J., and J. B. Pontalis, *Vocabulaire de la Psychanalyse* (Paris: Presses Universitaires de France, 1967).

12. Pace, T. T., T. Mletzko, O. Alagbe, et al., "Increased Stress-Induced Inflammatory Responses in Male Patients with Major Depression and Increased Early Life Stress," *American Journal of Psychiatry* 163, no. 9 (2006): 1630–33.

13. Palesh, O., et al., "Stress History and Breast Cancer Recurrence," *Journal of Psychosomatic Research* 63, no. 3 (2007): 233–39.

14. Visintainer, M. A., J. R. Volpicelli, and M. E. P. Seligman. "Tumor Rejection in Rats After Inescapable or Escapable Shock," *Science* 216 (1982): 437–39.

15. Ben-Eliyahu, S., et al., "Stress Increases Metastatic Spread of a Mammary Tumor in Rats: Evidence for Mediation by the Immune System," *Brain, Behavior, & Immunity* 5, no. 2 (1991): 193–205.

16. Sapolsky, R. M., and T. M. Donnelly, "Vulnerability to Stress-Induced Tumor Growth Increases with Age in Rats: Role of Glucocorticoids," *Endocrinology* 117, no. 2 (1985): 662–66.

17. Thaker, P. H., et al., "Chronic Stress Promotes Tumor Growth and Angiogenesis in a Mouse Model of Ovarian Carcinoma," *Nature Medicine* 12, no. 8 (2006): 939–44.

18. Visintainer, et al., "Tumor Rejection in Rats . . ."

19. Meares, A., "Regression of Osteogenic Sarcoma Metastases Associated with Intensive Meditation," *Medical Journal of Australia* 2, no. 9 (1978): 433.

20. Spiegel, D., and J. R. Bloom. "Group Therapy and Hypnosis Reduce Metastatic Breast Carcinoma Pain," *Psychosomatic Medicine* 45, no. 4 (1983): 333–39.

21. Spiegel, D., J. R. Bloom, and I. Yalom, "Group Support for Patients with Metastatic Cancer, a Randomized Outcome Study," *Archives of General Psychiatry* 38, no. 5 (1981): 527–33.

22. Spiegel, D., et al., "Effect of Psychosocial Treatment on Survival of Patients with Metastatic Breast Cancer," *Lancet* 2, no. 8673 (Nov. 18, 1989): 1209–10.

23. McCorkle, R., N. E. Strumpf, I. F. Nuamah, et al., "A Specialized Home Care Intervention Improves Survival Among Older Post-surgical Cancer Patients," *Journal of the American Geriatrics Society* 48, no. 12 (2000): 1707–13.

24. Kuchler, T., D. Henne-Bruns, S. Rappat, et al., "Impact of Psychotherapeutic Support on Gastrointestinal Cancer Patients Undergoing Surgery: Survival Results of a Trial," *Hepato-Gastroenterology* 46, no. 25 (1999): 322–35.

25. Richardson, J. L., D. R. Shelton, M. Krailo, et al., "The Effect of Compliance with Treatment on Survival Among Patients with Hematologic Malignancies," *Journal of Clinical Oncology* 8, no. 2 (1990): 356–64.

26. Fawzy, F. I., A. L. Canada, and N. W. Fawzy, "Malignant Melanoma: Effects of a Brief, Structured Psychiatric Intervention on Survival and Recurrence at 10-Year Follow-Up," *Archives of General Psychiatry* 60, no. 1 (2003): 100–103.

27. Linn, M. W., B. S. Linn, and R. Harris, "Effects of Counseling for Late Stage Cancer Patients," *Cancer* 49, no. 5 (1982): 1048–55.

28. Goodwin, P. J., M. Leszcz, M. Ennis, et al., "The Effect of Group Psychosocial Support on Survival in Metastatic Breast Cancer," *New England Journal of Medicine* 345, no. 24 (2001): 1719–26.

29. Edelman, S., J. Lemon, D. R. Bell, et al., "Effects of Group CBT on the Survival Time of Patients with Metastatic Breast Cancer," *Psycho-Oncology* 8, no. 6 (1999): 474–81.

30. Ilnyckyj, A., J. Farber, M. Chang, et al., "A Randomized Controlled Trial of Psychotherapeutic Intervention in Cancer Patients," *Annals of the Royal College of Physicians and Surgeons of Canada* 27 (1994): 93–96.

31. Cunningham, A. J., C. V. Edmonds, G. P. Jenkins, et al., "A Randomized Controlled Trial of the Effects of Group Psychological Therapy on Survival in Women with Metastatic Breast Cancer," *Psycho-Oncology* 7, no. 6 (1998): 508–17.

32. Kissane, D. W., A. Love, A. Hatton, et al., "Effect of Cognitive-Existential Group Therapy on Survival in Early-Stage Breast Cancer," *Journal of Clinical Oncology* 22, no. 21 (2004): 4255–60.

33. Spiegel, D., et al., "Effects of Supportive-Expressive Group Therapy on Survival of Patients with Metastatic Breast Cancer: A Randomized Prospective Trial," *Cancer* 110, no. 5 (2007): 1130–38.

34. Everson, S. A., et al., "Hopelessness and Risk of Mortality and Incidence of Myocardial Infarction and Cancer," *Psychosomatic Medicine* 58, no. 2 (1996): 113–121.

35. Chida, Y., et al., "Do Stress-Related Psychosocial Factors Contribute to Cancer Incidence and Survival?" *Nature Clinical Practice Oncology 5*, no. 8 (2008). Doi: 10.1038/ncponc1134.

36. Levy, S. M., R. B. Herberman, M. Lippman, et al., "Immunological and Psychosocial Predictors of Disease Recurrence in Patients with Early-Stage Breast Cancer," *Behavioral Medicine* 17, no. 2 (1991): 67–75.

37. Levy, S. M., R. B. Herberman, A. M. Maluish, et al., "Prognostic Risk Assessment in Primary Breast Cancer by Behavioral and Immunological Parameters," *Health Psychology* 4, no. 2 (1985): 99–113.

38. Levy, S., R. Herberman, M. Lippman, et al., "Correlation of Stress Factors with Sustained Depression of Natural Killer Cell Activity and Predicted Prognosis in Patients with Breast Cancer," *Journal of Clinical Oncology* 5, no. 3 (1987): 348–53.

39. Lutgendorf, S. K., A. K. Sood, B. Anderson, et al., "Social Support, Psychological Distress, and Natural Killer Cell Activity in Ovarian Cancer," *Journal of Clinical Oncology* 23, no. 28 (2005): 7105–13.

40. Servan-Schreiber, D., *Healing Without Freud or Prozac—Stress, Anxiety and Depression Without Drugs or Talk Therapy* (London: Pan MacMillan, 2004).

41. Servan-Schreiber, D., *The Instinct to Heal: Curing Depression, Anxiety and Stress Without Drugs and Without Talk Therapy* (New York: Rodale, 2004).

42. Kabat-Zinn, J., *Coming to Our Senses* (New York: Hyperion, 2005).

43. Rinpoche, S., *Le Livre Tibétain de la Vie et de la Mort* (Paris: Livre de Poche, 2005).

44. Dekker, J., E. Schouten, P. Klootwijk, et al., "Heart Rate Variability from Short-Term Electrocardiographic Recordings Predicts Mortality from All Causes in Middle-Aged and Elderly Men: The Zutphen Study," *American Journal of Epidemiology* 145, no. 10 (1997): 899–908.

45. Tsuji, H., F. Venditti, E. Manders, et al., "Reduced Heart Rate Variability and Mortality Risk in an Elderly Cohort: The Framingham Heart Study," *Circulation* 90, no. 2 (1994): 878–83.

46. Bernardi, L., P. Sleight, G. Bandinelli, et al., "Effect of Rosary Prayer and Yoga Mantras on Autonomic Cardiovascular Rhythms: Comparative Study," *British Medical Journal* 323 (2001): 1446–49.

47. Thayer, J. F., and E. Sternberg, "Beyond Heart Rate Variability: Vagal Regulation of Allostatic Systems," *Annals of the New York Academy of Sciences* 1008 (2006): 361–72.

48. Umetani, K., D. Singer, R. McCraty, et al., "Twenty-four Hour Time Domain Heart Rate Variability and Heart Rate: Relations to Age and Gender over Nine Decades," *Journal of the American College of Cardiology* 31, no. 3 (1999): 593–601.

49. Dekker, Schouten, Klootwijk, et al., "Heart Rate Variability from Short-Term Electrocardiographic Recordings . . ."

50. Bernardi, Sleight, Bandinelli, et al., "Effect of Rosary Prayer and Yoga Mantras on Autonomic Cardiovascular Rhythms."

51. Lutz, A., L. Greischar, N. Rawlings, et al., "Long-term Meditators Self-Induce High-Amplitude Gamma Synchrony During Mental Practice," *Proceedings of the National Academy of Sciences USA* 101 (2004): 16369–73.

52. Davidson, R. J., J. Kabat-Zinn, J. Schumacher, et al., "Alterations in Brain and Immune Function Produced by Mindfulness Meditation," *Psychosomatic Medicine* 65, no. 4 (2003): 564–70.

53. Rosenkranz, M. A., D. C. Jackson, K. M. Dalton, et al., "Affective Style and in Vivo Immune Response: Neurobehavioral Mechanisms," *Proceedings of the National Academy of Sciences* 100 (2003): 11148–52.

54. Gruzelier, J., A. Burgess, T. Baldewig, et al., "Prospective Associations Between Lateralized Brain Function and Immunte Status in HIV Infection: Analysis of EEG, Cognition and Mood over 30 Months," *International Journal of Psychophysiology* 23 (1996): 215–24.

55. Kiecolt-Glaser, J. K., R. Glaser, D. Williger, et al., "Psychosocial Enhancement of Immunocompetence in a Geriatric Population," *Health Psychology* 4, no. 1 (1985): 25–41.

56. Creswell, J. D., Myers, H. F., Cole, S. W., Irwin, M. R., "Mindfulness Meditation Training Effects on CD4+T Lymphocytes in HIV-1 Infected Adults: A Small Randomized Controlled Trial," *Brain Behav Immun* (2008).

57. Gawler, *You Can Conquer Cancer.*

58. Lillberg, K., P. K. Verkasalo, J. Kaprio, et al., "Stressful Life Events and Risk of Breast Cancer in 10,808 Women: A Cohort Study," *American Journal of Epidemiology* 157 (2003): 415–23.

59. Price, M. A., C. C. Tennant, P. N. Butow, et al., "The Role of Psychosocial Factors in the Development of Breast Carcinoma: Part II: Life Event Stressors, Social Support, Defense Style, and Emotional Control and Their Interactions," *Cancer* 91, no. 4 (2001): 686–97.

60. Bartrop, R. W., E. Luckhurst, L. Lazarus, et al., "Depressed Lymphocyte Function After Bereavement," *Lancet* 1, no. 8016 (1977): 834–36.

61. Ironson, G., C. Wynings, N. Schneiderman, et al., "Posttraumatic Stress Symptoms, Intrusive Thoughts, Loss, and Immune Function After Hurricane Andrew," *Psychosomatic Medicine* 59, no. 2 (1997): 128–41.

62. Irwin, M., M. Daniels, S. C. Risch, et al., "Plasma Cortisol and Natural Killer Cell Activity During Bereavement," *Biological Psychiatry* 24, no. 2 (1988): 173–78.

63. Weisberg, R. B., S. E. Bruce, J. T. Machan, et al., "Nonpsychiatric Illness Among Primary Care Patients with Trauma Histories and Posttraumatic Stress Disorder," *Psychiatric Services* 53, no. 7 (2002): 848–54.

64. Dong, M., W. H. Giles, V. J. Felitti, et al., "Insights into Causal Pathways for Ischemic Heart Disease: Adverse Childhood Experiences Study," *Circulation* 110, no. 13 (2004): 1761–66.

65. Dew, M., R. Kormos, L. Roth, et al., "Early Post-Transplant Medical Compliance and Mental Health Predict Physical Morbidity and Mortality 1–3 Years After Heart Transplantation," *Journal of Heart and Lung Transplantation* 18 (1999): 549–62.

66. Felitti, V., R. Anda, D. Nordenberg, et al., "Relationship of Childhood Abuse and Household Dysfunction to Many of the Leading Causes of Dealth in Adults," *American Journal of Preventive Medicine* 14 (1998): 245–58.

67. American Psychiatric Association, *Guidelines for the Psychiatric Treatment of Acute Stress Disorder and Posttraumatic Stress Disorder* (Washington: American Psychiatric Association, 2004).

68. Bradley, R., J. Greene, E. Russ, et al., "A Multidimensional Meta-Analysis of Psychotherapy for PTSD," *American Journal of Psychiatry* 162 (2005): 214–27.

69. Bisson, J. I., A. Ehlers, R. Matthews, et al., "Psychological Treatments for Chronic Post-Traumatic Stress Disorder: Systematic Review and Meta-Analysis," *British Journal of Psychiatry* 190 (2007): 97–104.

70. Antoni, Lutgendorf, Cole, et al., "The Influence of Bio-Behavioral Factors on Tumour Biology."

71. Reiche, E. M. V., S. O. V. Nunes, and H. K. Morimoto, "Stress, Depression, the Immune System, and Cancer," *Lancet Oncology* 5, no. 10 (2004): 617–25.

72. Petrie, K., R. Booth, J. Pennebaker, et al., "Disclosure of Trauma and Immune Response to Hepatitis B Vaccination Program," *Journal of Consulting & Clinical Psychology* 63 (1995): 787–92.

73. Zaslow, J., *The Girls from Ames: A Story of Women and Friendship* (New York: Penguin Group, 2009).

74. Parker-Pope, T., "What Are Friends For? A Longer Life," *New York Times*, April 21, 2009.

75. Kroenke, C. H., et al., "Social Networks, Social Support, and Survival After Breast Cancer Diagnosis," *Journal of Clinical Oncology* 24, no. 7 (2006): 1105–11.

76. Orth-Gomer, K., A. Rosengren, and L. Wilhelmsen, "Lack of Social Support and Incidence of Coronary Heart Disease in Middle-Aged Swedish Men," *Psychosomatic Medicine* 55, no. 1 (1993): 37–43.

77. Lerner, *Choices in Healing.*

78. Solomon, S., E. T. Gerrity, and A. M. Muff, "Efficacy of Treatments for Posttraumatic Stress Disorder," *JAMA* 268 (1992): 633–38.

79. Brady, K., T. Pearlstein, G. Asnis, et al., "Efficacy and Safety of Sertraline Treatment of Posttraumatic Stress Disorder," *JAMA* 283 (2000): 1837–44.

80. Davidson, J. R. T., B. O. Rothbaum, B. Van Der Kolk, et al., "Multicenter, Double-Blind Comparison of Sertraline and Placebo in the Treatment of Posttraumatic Stress Disorder," *Archives of General Psychiatry* 58 (2001): 485–92.

81. Asnis, G. M., S. R. Kohn, M. Henderson, et al., "SSRIs Versus Non-SSRIs in Post-Traumatic Stress Disorder: An Update with Recommendations," *Drugs* 64, no. 4 (2004): 383–404.

82. van Etten, M.L. and S. Taylor, "Comparative Efficacy of Treatments for Post-Traumatic Stress Disorder: A Meta-Analysis," *Clinical Psychology & Psychotherapy* 5 (1998): 126–144.

83. Maxfield, L., and L. A. Hyer, "The Relationship Between Efficacy and Method-

ology in Studies Investigating EMDR Treatment of PTSD," *Journal of Clinical Psychology* 58 (2002): 23–41.

84. Sack, M., W. Lempa, and F. Lamprecht, "Study Quality and Effect Sizes—a Meta-Analysis of EMDR Treatment for Posttraumatic Stress Disorder," *Psychotherapie, Psychosomatik, Medizinische Psychologie* 51, no. 9–10 (2001): 350–355.

85. Expertise Collective INSERM, et al., *Psychothérapie: Trois approches évaluées,* eds., INSERM Unité d'Evaluation et d'Expertise Collective, et al., Paris: 2004, Institut National de la Santé et de la Recherche Médicale France, 2004.

86. Shapiro, F., *Eye-Movement Desensitization and Reprocessing: Basic Principles, Protocols and Procedures* (New York: Guilford, 2001).

87. Kübler-Ross, E., *On Death and Dying* (New York: Touchstone, 1969).

88. Bisson, J. and M. Andrew, "Psychological Treatment of Post-Traumatic Stress Disorder (PTSD) (Review)," *Cochrane Database of Systematic Reviews,* no. 3 (2007): CD004046.

89. Shapiro, F., *Manuel d'EMDR (Intégration neuro-émotionnelle par les mouvements oculaires)—principes, protocoles, procédures* (Paris: Dunod, 2007).

90. Stickgold, R., "EMDR: A Putative Neurobiological Mechanism," *Journal of Clinical Psychology* 58 (2002): 61–75.

91. Anderson, B. L., et al., "Psychological, Behavioral, and Immune Changes After a Psychological Intervention: A Clinical Trial," *Journal of Clinical Oncology* 22, no. 17 (2004): 3570–80.

92. Anderson, B. L., et al., "Distress Reduction from a Psychological Intervention Contributes to Improved Health for Cancer Patients," *Brain, Behavior, & Immunity* 21, no. 7 (2007): 953–61.

93. Thornton, L. M., et al., "Individual Trajectories in Stress Covary with Immunity During Recovery from Cancer Diagnosis and Treatments," *Brain, Behavior, & Immunity* 21, no. 2 (2007): 185–94.

CHAPTER 10: DEFUSING FEAR

1. Peck, M. S., *Further Along the Road Less Travelled: Going to Omaha—The Issue of Death and Meaning* (New York: Simon and Schuster Audio, 2004).

2. Nuland, S. B., *Mourir: Reflexions sur le Dernier Chapitre de la Vie* (Paris: Interéditions, 1994).

3. Johanson, G. A., *Physician's Handbook of Symptom Relief in Terminal Care* (Sonoma County, CA: Home Hospice of Sonoma County, 1994).

4. Frankl, V. E., *Découvrir un sens à sa vie* (Montréal, QC: Editions de l'Homme, 2005).

5. Ring, K., *Heading Toward Omega: In Search of the Meaning of the Near-Death Experience* (New York: Morrow, 1985).

6. Van Lommel, P., R. van Wees, V. Meyers, et al., "Near-Death Experience in Survivors of Cardiac Arrest: A Prospective Study in the Netherlands," *Lancet* 358, no. 9298 (2001): 2039–45.

7. Rinpoche, S., *The Tibetan Book of Living and Dying* (San Francisco: Harper-Collins, 1992).

8. Spiegel, D., "A 43-Year-Old Woman Coping with Cancer," *JAMA* 282, no. 4 (1999): 371–78.

9. House, J. S., K. R. Landis, and D. Umberson, "Social Relationships and Health," *Science* 241 (1988): 540–45.

10. House, J. S., C. Robbins, and H. L. Metzner, "The Association of Social Relationships and Activities with Mortality: Prospective Evidence from the Tecumseh Community Health Study," *American Journal of Epidemiology* 116, no. 1 (1982): 123–40.

11. Berkman, L. F., and S. L. Syme, "Social Networks, Host Resistance, and Mortality: A Nine-Year Follow-Up Study of Alameda County Residents," *American Journal of Epidemiology* 109, no. 2 (1979): 186–204.

12. Berkman, L. F., L. Leo-Summers, and R. I. Horwitz, "Emotional Support and Survival After Myocardial Infarction: A Prospective, Population-Based Study of the Elderly," *Annals of Internal Medicine* 117, no. 12 (1992): 1003–9.

13. Hoffman, J., "Doctors' Delicate Balance in Keeping Hope Alive," *New York Times*, December 24, 2005.

CHAPTER 11: THE ANTICANCER BODY

1. Field, T., S. M. Schanberg, F. Scafidi, et al., "Tactile/Kinesthetic Stimulation Effects on Preterm Neonates," *Pediatrics* 77 (1986): 654–58.

2. Schanberg, S., "Genetic Basis for Touch Effects," in *Touch in Early Development*, ed. T. Field (Hillsdale, NJ: Erlbaum, 1994), 67–80.

3. Hernandez-Reif, M., T. Field, G. Ironson, et al., "Natural Killer Cells and Lymphocytes Increase in Women with Breast Cancer Following Massage Therapy," *International Journal of Neuroscience* 115, no. 4 (2005): 495–510.

4. Hernandez-Reif, M., G. Ironson, T. Field, et al., "Breast Cancer Patients Have Improved Immune and Neuroendocrine Functions Following Massage Therapy," *Journal of Psychosomatic Research* 57, no. 1 (2004): 45–52.

5. Field, T. M., "Massage Therapy Effects," *American Psychologist* 53 (1998): 1270–81.

6. Tehard, B., C. M. Friedenreich, J.-M. Oppert, et al., "Effect of Physical Activity on Women at Increased Risk of Breast Cancer: Results from the E3N Cohort Study," *Cancer Epidemiology, Biomarkers & Prevention* 15, no. 1 (2006): 57–64.

7. Meyerhardt, J. A., E. L. Giovannucci, M. D. Holmes, et al., "Physical Activity and Survival After Colorectal Cancer Diagnosis," *Journal of Clinical Oncology* 24, no. 22 (2006): 3527–34.

8. Meyerhardt, J. A., D. Heseltine, D. Niedzwiecki, et al., "Impact of Physical Activity on Cancer Recurrence and Survival in Patients with Stage III Colon Cancer: Findings from CALGB 89803," *Journal of Clinical Oncology* 24, no. 22 (2006): 3535–41.

9. Holmes, M. D., W. Y. Chen, D. Feskanich, et al., "Physical Activity and Survival After Breast Cancer Diagnosis," *JAMA* 293, no. 20 (2005): 2479–86.

10. Giovannucci, E., Y. L. Liu, M. F. Leitzmann, et al., "A Prospective Study of Physical Activity and Incident and Fatal Prostate Cancer," *Archives of Internal Medicine* 165 (2005): 1005–10.

11. Ornish, D., G. Weidner, W. R. Fair, et al., "Intensive Lifestyle Changes May Affect the Progression of Prostate Cancer," *Journal of Urology* 174, no. 3 (2005): 1065–69.

12. Patel, A. V., C. Rodriguez, E. J. Jacobs, et al., "Recreational Physical Activity and Risk of Prostate Cancer in a Large Cohort of U.S. Men," *Cancer Epidemiology, Biomarkers & Prevention* 14, no. 1 (2005): 275–79.

13. Nilsen, T. I. L., "Recreational Physical Activity and Risk of Prostate Cancer: A Prospective Population-Based Study in Norway (the HUNT Study)," *International Journal of Cancer*, 2006.

14. Bardia, A., L. C. Hartmann, C. M. Vachon, et al., "Recreational Physical Activity and Risk of Postmenopausal Breast Cancer Based on Hormone Receptor Status," *Archives of Internal Medicine* 166, no. 22 (2006): 2478–83.

15. Barnard, R. J., J. H. Gonzalez, M. E. Liva, et al., "Effects of a Low-Fat, High-Fiber Diet and Exercise Program on Breast Cancer Risk Factors in Vivo and Tumor Cell Growth and Apoptosis in Vitro," *Nutrition and Cancer* 55, no. 1 (2006): 28–34.

16. Irwin, M. L., "Randomized Controlled Trials of Physical Activity and Breast Cancer Prevention," *Exercise & Sport Sciences Reviews* 34, no. 4 (2006): 182–93.

17. Abrahamson, P. E., M. D. Gammon, M. J. Lund, et al., "Recreational Physical Activity and Survival Among Young Women with Breast Cancer," *Cancer* 107, no. 8 (2006): 1777–85.

18. Adams, S. A., C. E. Matthews, J. R. Hebert, et al., "Association of Physical Activity with Hormone Receptor Status: The Shanghai Breast Cancer Study," *Cancer Epidemiology, Biomarkers & Prevention* 15, no. 6 (2006): 1170–78.

19. Mutrie, N., A. M. Campbell, F. Whyte, et al., "Benefits of Supervised Group Exercise Programme for Women Being Treated for Early Stage Breast Cancer: Pragmatic Randomised Controlled Trial," *British Medical Journal* 334, no. 7592 (2007): 517.

20. Friedenreich, C. M., "Overview of the Association Between Physical Activity, Obesity and Cancer," *Eurocancer* (Paris: John Libbey Eurotex, 2005).

21. Friedenreich, C. M., and M. R. Orenstein, "Physical Activity and Cancer Prevention: Etiologic Evidence and Biological Mechanisms," *Journal of Nutrition* 132, no. 11, supp. (2002): 3456S–64S.

22. Barnard, Gonzalez, Liva, et al., "Effects of a Low-Fat, High-Fiber Diet and Exercise Program . . ."

23. Leung, P-S., W. J. Aronson, T. H. Ngo, et al., "Exercise Alters the IGF Axis in Vivo and Increases p53 Protein in Prostate Tumor Cells in Vitro," *Journal of Applied Physiology* 96, no. 2 (2004): 450–54.

24. Barnard, R. J., T. H. Ngo, P-S. Leung, et al., "A Low-Fat Diet and/or Strenuous Exercise Alters the IGF Axis in Vivo and Reduces Prostate Tumor Cell Growth in Vitro," *Prostate* 56, no. 3 (2003): 201–6.

25. Colbert, L. H., M. Visser, E. M. Simonsick, et al., "Physical Activity, Exercise, and Inflammatory Markers in Older Adults: Findings from the Health, Aging and Body Composition Study," *Journal of the American Geriatrics Society* 52, no. 7 (2004): 1098–104.

26. LaPerriere, A., M. H. Antoni, N. Schneiderman, et al., "Exercise Intervention Attenuates Emotional Distress and Natural Killer Cell Decrements Following Notification of Positive Serologic Status of HIV-1," *Biofeedback and Self-Regulation* 15 (1990): 229–42.

27. LaPerriere, A., A. Fletcher, M. Antoni, et al., *International Journal of Sports Medicine*, 12 supp., no. 1 (1991): S53–57.

28. Sood, A., and T. J. Moynihan, "Cancer-Related Fatigue: An Update," *Current Oncology Reports* 7, no. 4 (2005): 277–82.

29. National Cancer Institute, "Herceptin Combined with Chemotherapy Improves Disease-Free Survival for Patients with Early-Stage Breast Cancer," 2005 (accessed at http://www.cancer.gov/newscenter/pressreleases/HerceptinCombination2005).

30. Bardia, Hartmann, Vachon, et al., "Recreational Physical Activity and Risk of Postmenopausal Breast Cancer Based on Hormone Receptor Status."

31. Adams, Matthews, Hebert, et al., "Association of Physical Activity with Hormone Receptor Status."

32. Meyerhardt, J. A., E. L. Giovannucci, M. D. Holmes, et al., "Physical Activity and Survival After Colorectal Cancer Diagnosis," *Journal of Clinical Oncology* 24, no. 22 (2006): 3527–34.

33. Meyerhardt, J. A., D. Heseltine, D. Niedzwiecki, et al., "Impact of Physical Activity on Cancer Recurrence and Survival in Patients with Stage III Colon Cancer: Findings from CALGB 89803," *Journal of Clinical Oncology* 24, no. 22 (2006): 3535–41.

34. Holmes, M. D., W. Y. Chen, D. Feskanich, et al., "Physical Activity and Survival After Breast Cancer Diagnosis," *JAMA* 293, no. 20 (2005): 2479–86.

35. Giovannucci, E., Y. L. Liu, M. F. Leitzmann, et al., "A Prospective Study of Physical Activity and Incident and Fatal Prostate Cancer," *Archives of Internal Medicine* 165 (2005): 1005–10.

36. Ornish, D., G. Weidner, W. R. Fair, et al., "Intensive Lifestyle Changes May Affect the Progression of Prostate Cancer," *Journal of Urology* 174, no. 3 (2005): 1065–69.

37. Patel, A. V., C. Rodriguez, E. J. Jacobs, et al., "Recreational Physical Activity and Risk of Prostate Cancer in a Large Cohort of U.S. Men," *Cancer Epidemiology, Biomarkers & Prevention* 14, no. 1 (2005): 275–79.

38. Nilsen, T. I. L., "Recreational Physical Activity and Risk of Prostate Cancer: A Prospective Population-Based Study in Norway (the HUNT Study)," *International Journal of Cancer* 2006.

39. Bardia, A., L. C. Hartmann, C. M. Vachon, et al., "Recreational Physical Activity and Risk of Postmenopausal Breast Cancer Based on Hormone Receptor Status," *Archives of Internal Medicine* 166, no. 22 (2006): 2478–83.

40. Barnard, R. J., J. H. Gonzalez, M. E. Liva, et al., "Effects of a Low-Fat, High-Fiber Diet and Exercise Program on Breast Cancer Risk Factors in Vivo and Tumor Cell Growth and Apoptosis in Vitro," *Nutrition and Cancer* 55, no. 1 (2006): 28–34.

41. Irwin, M. L., "Randomized Controlled Trials of Physical Activity and Breast Cancer Prevention," *Exercise & Sport Sciences Reviews* 34, no. 4 (2006): 182–93.

42. Abrahamson, P. E., M. D. Gammon, M.J. Lund, et al., "Recreational Physical Activity and Survival Among Young Women with Breast Cancer," *Cancer* 107, no. 8 (2006): 1777–85.

43. Adams, S. A., C. E. Matthews, J. R. Hebert, et al., "Association of Physical Activity with Hormone Receptor Status: The Shanghai Breast Cancer Study," *Cancer Epidemiology, Biomarkers & Prevention* 15, no. 6 (2006): 1170–78.

44. Mutrie, Campbell, Whyte, et al., "Benefits of Supervised Group Exercise Programme . . ."

45. Friedenreich, "Overview of the Association Between Physical Activity, Obesity and Cancer."

46. Beck, A., *Cognitive Therapy and the Emotional Disorders* (New York: International Universities Press, 1976).

47. National Institute for Clinical Excellence, *Depression: The Management of Depression in Primary and Secondary Care, NICE Guideline, Second draft consultation* (London, 2003).

48. Csikszentmihalyi, M., *Flow: The Psychology of Optimal Experience* (New York: Harper Perennial, 1991).

49. Kawano, R., "The Effect of Exercise on Body Awareness and Mood," *Dissertation Abstracts International: Section B—The Sciences and Engineering*, vol. 59 (7–8), January 1999: 3387.

50. Woolery, A., H. Myers, B. Sternlieb, et al., "A Yoga Intervention for Young Adults with Elevated Symptoms of Depression," *Alternative Therapies in Health & Medicine* 10, no. 2 (2004): 60–63.

51. Netz, Y., and R. Lidor, "Mood Alterations in Mindful Versus Aerobic Exercise Modes," *Journal of Psychology* 137, no. 5 (2003): 405–19.

52. Sandlund, E., and T. Norlander, "The Effects of Tai Chi Chuan Relaxation and Exercise on Stress Responses and Well-Being: An Overview of Research," *International Journal of Stress Management* 7 (2000): 139–49.

53. Li, F., P. Harmer, E. McAuley, et al., "An Evaluation of the Effects of Tai Chi Exercise on Physical Function Among Older Persons: A Randomized Contolled Trial," *Annals of Behavioral Medicine* 23, no. 2 (2001): 139–46.

54. Jin, P., "Changes in Heart Rate, Noradrenaline, Cortisol and Mood During Tai Chi," *Journal of Psychosomatic Research* 33, no. 2 (1989): 197–206.

55. Fletcher, G. F., G. J. Balady, E. A. Amsterdam, et al., "Exercise Standards for Testing and Training: A Statement for Healthcare Professionals from the American Heart Association," *Circulation* 104, no. 14 (2001): 1694–740.

CHAPTER 12: LEARNING TO CHANGE

1. Groopman, J., "Dr. Fair's Tumor," *New Yorker*, October 26, 1998, 78.

2. "The War on Cancer Townsend Letter for Doctors and Patients," April 2002. (Accessed May 29, 2007, at http://findarticles.com/p/articles/mi_m0ISW/is_2002_April/ai_84211149/pg_1.)

3. Groopman, "Dr. Fair's Tumor."

4. Cunningham, A. J., C. V. Edmonds, C. Phillips, et al., "A Prospective, Longitudinal Study of the Relationship of Psychological Work to Duration of Survival in Patients with Metastatic Cancer," *Psycho-Oncology* 9, no. 4 (2000): 323–39.

5. Cunningham, A. J., and K. Watson, "How Psychological Therapy May Prolong Survival in Cancer Patients: New Evidence and a Simple Theory," *Integrative Cancer Therapies* 3, no. 3 (2004) 214–29.

6. Cunningham, Edmunds, Phillips, et al., "A Prospective, Longitudinal Study . . ."

7. Cunningham and Watson, "How Psychological Therapy May Prolong Survival . . ."

8. Aristotle, *Nicomachean Ethics* (New York: Penguin Classics, 2003).

9. Jung, C. G., ed., *The Development of Personality (The Collected Works of C. G. Jung)*, vol. 17 (Princeton: Princeton University Press, 1981).

10. Maslow, A., *The Further Reaches of Human Nature* (New York: Viking, 1971).

11. Walsh, R., *Essential Spirituality: The Seven Central Practices to Awaken Heart and Mind* (New York: John Wiley & Sons, 1999).

CHAPTER 13: CONCLUSION

1. Hambrecht, R., C. Walther, S. Mobius-Winkler, et al., "Percutaneous Coronary Angioplasty Compared with Exercise Training in Patients with Stable Coronary Artery Disease: A Randomized Trial," *Circulation* 109, no. 11 (2004): 1371–78.

2. Folkman, J., and R. Kalluri, "Cancer Without Disease," *Nature* 427, no. 6977 (2004): 787.

3. Faggiano, F., T. Partanen, M. Kogevinas, et al., "Socioeconomic Differences in Cancer Incidence and Mortality," *International Agency for Research on Cancer Scientific Publications* 138 (1997): 65–176.

4. Davis, D. L., *The Secret History of the War on Cancer* (New York: Basic Books, 2007).

5. Campbell, T. C., *The China Study* (Dallas, TX: BenBella Books, 2005).

6. Marshall, B., "The *Campylobacter pylori* Story," *Scandinavian Journal of Gastroenterology* 146 (supp.): 58–66.

7. Ornish, D., G. Weidner, W. R. Fair, et al., "Intensive Lifestyle Changes May Affect the Progression of Prostate Cancer," *Journal of Urology* 174, no. 3(2005): 1065–69; discussion 1069–70.

8. Andersen, B. L., et al., "Psychologic Intervention Improves Survival for Breast Cancer Patients: A Randomized Clinical Trial," *Cancer* 113 (2008): 3450–58.

9. Ballard-Barbash, R. and A. McTiernan, "Is the Whole Larger Than the Sum of the Parts? The Promise of Combining Physical Activity and Diet to Improve Cancer Outcomes," *Journal of Clinical Oncology* 25, no. 17 (2007): 2335–2337.

10. Pierce, J. P., et al., "Greater Survival After Breast Cancer in Physically Active Women with High Vegetable-Fruit Intake Regardless of Obesity," *Journal of Clinical Oncology* 25, no. 17 (2007): 2345–51.

11. World Cancer Research Fund, *Food, Nutrition and the Prevention of Cancer: A Global Perspective* (London: World Cancer Research Fund and American Institute for Research on Cancer, 2007), xxiii.

Index